TOWARD HEALTHCARE RESOURCE STEWARDSHIP

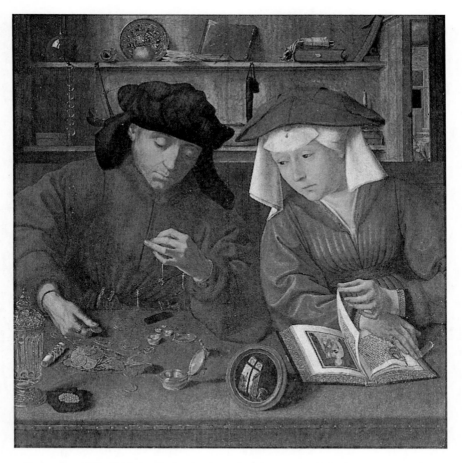

"The Money Changer and His Wife," painting by Quentin Massys, 1514; in the Louvre, Paris.

HEALTH CARE ISSUES, COSTS AND ACCESS

Additional books in this series can be found on Nova's website
under the Series tab.

Additional E-books in this series can be found on Nova's website
under the E-book tab.

HEALTH CARE IN TRANSITION

Additional books in this series can be found on Nova's website
under the Series tab.

Additional E-books in this series can be found on Nova's website
under the E-book tab.

TOWARD HEALTHCARE RESOURCE STEWARDSHIP

JOE SAM ROBINSON
M. SAMI WALID
AND
AARON C.M. BARTH
EDITORS

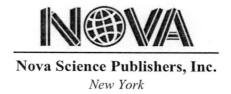

Nova Science Publishers, Inc.
New York

Library of Congress Cataloging-in-Publication Data

Toward healthcare resource stewardship / editors, Joe Sam Robinson and M. Sami Walid.
    p. ; cm.
 Includes bibliographical references and index.
 ISBN 978-1-62100-182-9 (hardcover)
 I. Robinson, Joe Sam. II. Walid, M. Sami.
 [DNLM: 1. Delivery of Health Care--economics. 2. Health Policy. 3. Hospital Costs. W 84.1]
 LC classification not assigned
 362.1'0425--dc23
                    2011031641

Published by Nova Science Publishers, Inc. † New York

CONTENTS

Preface   ix

Chapter 1   Healthcare Insights from the Front Line: "System Efficiency Not
                 Government-Regulated Rationing"   1
                 Joe Sam Robinson, M. Sami Walid
                 and Aaron C. M. Barth

Chapter 2   The Economics of Regional Trauma Centers -
                 The Georgia Model   11
                 Greg Bishop, Dennis W. Ashley
                 and Joe Sam Robinson Jr.

Chapter 3   Economic Viability of Stroke Centers -
                 The Georgia Model   29
                 Aaron C. M. Barth, M. Sami Walid,
                 Michael J. Conforti and Margaret C. Boltja

Chapter 4   Strategies to Improve Cost-Efficiency of Stroke Care:
                 Bolstering and Linking Stroke and Trauma Care
                 Networks - The Georgia Model   35
                 Joe Sam Robinson and M. Sami Walid

Chapter 5   Strategies to Improve Cost-Efficiency of Stroke Care:
                 Stroke Units and Telestroke   49
                 Minal Jain, Anunaya Jain and Babak S. Jahromi

Chapter 6   Strategies to Improve Cost-Efficiency of Stroke Care:
                 Integrating Automated Prompts into Standard
                 Physical Assessments to Reduce Aspiration
                 Risk in Dysphagic Stroke Patients   75
                 Brandi S. Rambo, Kimberly F. Mancin,
                 Aaron C. M. Barth, M. Sami Walid,
                 Patricia Bertram-Arnett, Laura Yarbrough,
                 Sheri Leslein, Margaret Boltja
                 and Delanor D. Doyle

Chapter 7   Hospitalist and Perioperative Care   **81**
                M. Sami Walid and Joe Sam Robinson Jr.

Chapter 8   The Effect of Comorbidities on Length of Stay
                and Hospital Charges of Spine Surgery Patients   **87**
                M. Sami Walid and Tracey Blalock

Chapter 9   The Impact of Preoperative Screening on Spine Surgery Cost   **93**
                Mohammed Ajjan, Aaron C. M. Barth, M. Sami Walid,
                Vicki L. Conlon, Kimberly F. Mancin
                and Joe Sam Robinson Jr.

Chapter 10   The Impact of Surgical Material on Hospital Cost:
                Economic Analysis of Allograft vs. Autograft
                for Elective One- and Two-level Anterior
                Cervical Decompression and Fusion Surgery   **97**
                Aaron C. M. Barth, Robert A. Lummus, M. Sami Walid,
                Kostas N. Fountas, Aleksandar Tomic,
                Joe Sam Robinson III and Joe Sam Robinson Jr.

Chapter 11   Prevalence and Economic Impact of Postoperative Anemia
                following Lumbar Spine Fusion   **111**
                M. Sami Walid and Nadezhda Zaytseva

Chapter 12   A New Concept of Inpatient Care: Acuity-Adaptable Patient Room
                Decreases Length of Stay and Cost - Results of a Pilot Study   **115**
                Nena Bonuel, Alma deGracia and Sandra Cesario

Chapter 13   Obesity – The American Epidemic: The Impact of Obesity
                on Hospital Cost in Obstetrics and Gynecology: A Review   **139**
                Courtney L. Barnes, Mistie P. Mills and Mira Aubuchon

Chapter 14   Perspectives on Psychiatric Comorbidities of Late
                Life and Their Cost Implications for Medical Care   **155**
                Lee A. Hyer, Ciera V. Scott and Catherine A. Yeager

Chapter 15   Hospital Costs and the Emergency Department   **181**
                Ulf Martin Schilling

Chapter 16   Long –Term Economic Analysis of Outpatient Follow-up   **203**
                Fernando Alfageme Roldan
                and Almudena Bermejo Hernando

Chapter 17   A Reemerging Bacteria: Cost Analysis of Care
                and Treatment of Tuberculosis (TB) in Childhood   **217**
                Reka Bodnar, Laszlo Kadar and Agnes Meszaros

Chapter 18   Physician-Hospital Relations: Current Realities
                and Partnership Possibilities   **231**
                Aaron C. M. Barth and Louis Goolsby

Chapter 19	Bureaucracy and Cost-Inefficiency in the Healthcare System *Richard L. Heaton and M. Sami Walid*	**241**
Chapter 20	An Economic Analysis of the Physician Workforce Shortage *Don K. Nakayama*	**249**
Chapter 21	Cost Awareness in Clinical Research: Lack of Cost Inclusion in the Clinical Methodology in Spine Fusion Literature *M. Sami Walid, Joe Sam Robinson III* *and Joe Sam Robinson Jr.*	**257**
Chapter 22	Physicians as Guardians of Healthcare Resources *M. Sami Walid, Aaron C. M. Barth,* *Edward R. M. Robinson and Joe Sam Robinson Jr.*	**273**

About the Editors **279**

Index **281**

PREFACE

As the 21st Century continues, the United States (U.S.) as well as both developed and undeveloped countries around the World grapple with escalating healthcare costs. Diffuse reasons exist for such increases. Importantly the number of healthcare consumers is on the march worldwide. Stimulated by improved nutrition and a more readily available uncontaminated water supply, better vaccination rates, better pre and post natal care, the world's population is expected to exceed the extraordinary figure of 9 billion by the year 2050. While most of such an increase tilts the demographic curve toward younger age groups, older age cohorts, unavoidably afflicted with the degenerative diseases inherent in our species, are also on the increase. These older age cohorts are particularly noticeable in developed countries where useful scientific progress has evolved substantial and extensive healthcare technologies. Access to such expensive technologies, often inefficiently provided, has both been widely sought and become available to needful healthcare consumers. Though undeniably adding substantial value in the broadest sense of the word, moderating these escalating healthcare expenses has been a widely sought goal.

Varying countries have developed different technologies in efforts to minimize such costs. Though the United States excels in technological innovation in an environment where healthcare expenses appear to be the most burdensome, efforts at cost restraints may be described as less than successful. In the resulting national debate over improving healthcare efficiency of particular consequence has been the often marginalized and neglected viewpoint of the practicing physician. Several reasons exist for this. Firstly, the Stark Law considerations and government regulations tend to separate physicians from hospital and other care organizations. Secondly, physicians have no real background in economic issues and often from a relatively early age amerced themselves in scientific intricacies of their profession leaving economic issues to accountants. Thirdly, because of unreasonable patient expectation unrestrained expenditure of healthcare resources has often been a reflexive physician practice. Such unfortunate factors have often left the many useful opinions of healthcare providers outside regular public discourse.

Additionally, substantial political and culture ambiances mandate against any standardized universal cost restraints in the United States. Our country, with its carefully demarcated system of checks and balances, and restraint of centralized power, is a federation, not a unitary state. In such a national system, a unified managerial structure for managing healthcare costs does not exist. Moreover by well-established tradition, individuals accept responsibility for their personal welfare, jealously guarding against the perceived threat of arbitrary and capricious state intrusion into their daily lives. Lastly the country's pervasive legal system closely protected by its proponents, has aggressively sought and succeeded imposing powerful Tort Law limitations on easy healthcare cost reductions.

For a long time the prosperity of the United States along with its' triumph in the political conflicts of the 20th century and resulting role of the dollar as a worldwide reserve currency, has masked the problems associated with healthcare expense; however, it has become apparent to all participants in the American healthcare system that a significant change is needed. Many different suggestions have been undertaken to reform American healthcare; different models have been floated; different geographical entities have experimented in different ways of diminishing costs while maintaining quality. After years of controversy and concern, the U.S. plan for healthcare reform inspired by President Barack Obama was recently signed into law (though at this time the plan appears quite complicated and will undoubtedly require substantial changes as it makes its way into actuality). What the final picture will be is quite cloudy.

In this volume, many different authors have offered prescient insights upon various ways to diminish healthcare expenses. Their ideas are eclectic and arise from variegated circumstances. One could hope this could serve as a useful addition to national debate and encourage others to put forth their opinion. In general, as the causes for the complexities of healthcare in the United States are multifactorial, solutions necessarily will have to comport with the complicated political and social structures of the United States. Many different experiments will be necessary to successfully solve the difficulties this issue causes. In any event, we hope some of the suggestions offered in this book find applications in practice and not remain merely stated words in a book.

The editors
06/02/2011

In: Toward Healthcare Resource Stewardship
Editors: J. S.Robinson, M. S.Walid et al.

ISBN: 978-1-62100-182-9
© 2012 Nova Science Publishers, Inc.

Chapter 1

HEALTHCARE INSIGHTS FROM THE FRONT LINE: "SYSTEM EFFICIENCY NOT GOVERNMENT-REGULATED RATIONING"

Joe Sam Robinson,[1,2,3] *M. Sami Walid*[3]* *and Aaron C. M. Barth*[3]

[1]Georgia Neurosurgical Institute, Macon, GA, US
[2]Mercer University School of Medicine, Macon, GA, US
3Medical Center of Central Georgia, Macon, GA, US

I. INTRODUCTION: IMPORTANCE OF HEALTHCARE IN AMERICA

While Americans of earlier generations haphazardly sought healthcare - often living their whole lives without entering the confines of the hospital or consulting with a physician; today, every American is embraced by a system unimaginable to our forefathers. Paradoxically, at the same time that profound healthcare advances have expensively promoted some possibility of earthly bliss, the spiritual underpinnings that consoled earlier generations are declining. Fewer repose hope for the next world. Yet the need for something better than a Hobbsian life - short, nasty and brutish is part of our deepest nature.

Much of these displaced internal longings and hopes have been transferred to what one may call a great new secular church- the American healthcare system. Its priests wear white coats, its divine service occur in diagnostic machines, its miracles performed in brightly lit operation rooms, and its great hospitals are cathedrals, while not promising everlasting life. The secular church does seem to promote life without pain (thanks to a superior anesthetic agent). It can afford life without work (if the system approves healthcare related disability payments). Plastic surgeon can defeat old age and disfigurements, cripples are healed, the blind are made to see and nearly every boundary of reproductive difficulty is breached. Now, like the biblical Sarah, elderly women conceive children. When death is encountered, physicians are at hand to make sure that the grim reaper is met in pleasant narcotic haze. If

* Corresponding Author: M. Sami Walid, 840 Pine Street, Suite 880, Medical Center of Central Georgia, Macon, GA 331201. Email: mswalid@yahoo.com.

any of these results are less than satisfactory, the parishioner/ patient may consult a trial lawyer who often obtains considerable financial compensation. And just as in traditional religion, paradise is equally available to the rich and the poor. Americans expect a system that supports superior and equal healthcare in which a sick child from a poor family receives comparable care to one from wealthier circumstances. Importantly in an increasingly diverse, even fragmented nation, the great new American secular healthcare church provides its service to every soul like a great universal religion increasing the sense of community and national identity.

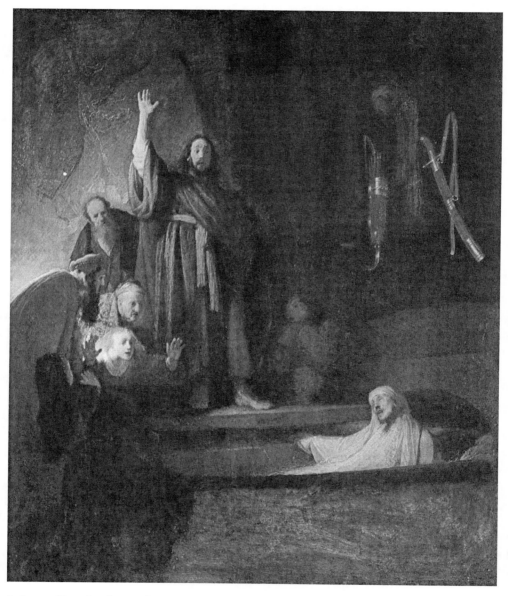

Man's Innate Yearning for Healing (Rembrandt's "The Raising of Lazareth" c. 1630).

Politicians of every stripe should take care that Americans continue to possess the possibility of physical temporal salvation in this great national healing secular church. When spiritual and quasi spiritual national values are injured, the responsible political establishments are invariably bruised by such an encounter. While politicians may argue in many ways healthcare salvation needs to be earned by personal responsibility and financial restraint, the centrality of this institution to the American culture should never be underestimated - of this in our electoral cycles politicians need to be intensely aware.

II. COMPLEXITIES OF THE MODERN U.S. HEALTHCARE SYSTEM

A System with Great Merit

For many points of view, despite the dismissive appraisal of often politically motivated detractors, the American healthcare system is arguably the best in the World. Markers of healthcare progress, medical education and post-graduate training leads the world. Students from every nation aspire to study at an American institute. Biomedical research is unexcelled in the United States where 91 Nobel Prize doctors and scientists in physiology and medicine received the privileged prize [1]. The National Institute of Health Budget for Drug and Biological Product Development is $27 billion dollars, approximately four times greater than the European expenditure [2]. In comparison with other systems, the United States healthcare arrangements are far more impressive and convenient on many fronts. Access to appropriate pharmaceutical regimens and hospital and specialty service is generally quick and flexible. Moreover in other public health arenas such as diminution among healthy tobacco users, the United States outpaces the rest of the world.

Difficulties in a Good System

Expense: Unfortunately the United States Healthcare System is expensive, with overall costs doubling between 1993 and 200 [3]. In 2004, spending topped $1.9 billion dollars [3]. The cost of developing new drugs has also expanded in the past decade, with some estimates exceeding $800 billion dollars despite federal funding cuts [2].

Projected National Health Expenditures by Source of Funds (Billions)

	2006	2015	% Change
Medicare	$ 420	$ 792	88.6%
Medicaid(Fed)	$ 184	$ 384	108.7%
Medicaid(State)	$ 136	$ 285	109.6%
Private Health Ins.	$ 745	$ 1,397	87.5%
Out of Pocket Pymt	$ 246	$ 421	71.1%
Total	$ 2,163	$ 4,031	86.4%

Source: HealthAffairs.org; 25 No. 2 (2006).

With increasing life expectancy and escalation in medical technology and utilization, national healthcare expenditures are expected to grow at an average rate of 7.2% a year. As a result, the share of gross national product devoted to healthcare rose to 16% of the national Gross National Product (GNP) and in 2004 is expected to climb to 20% by 2015 [3]. Such an increase in expenditure to any reasonable observer in not sustainable.

Access: There are also substantial limits to healthcare access for an estimated 43 million people are without health insurance and 120 million without dental coverage including illegal immigrants [4]. Concern over healthcare insurance makes the economy more brittle as it prevents job migration. Moreover because of increasing population growth and expansion of government entitlement programs, Medicaid in many states has erected access barriers to their client population. Fortunately there is a failsafe method which guarantees healthcare coverage. Anyone who visits a hospital emergency room finds access to the system for serious diseases. Regrettably however if someone is insured but has no substantial financial resource, an extensive hospitalization is often a prelude to bankruptcy.

Extraordinary Complexities of the U.S. Healthcare System

Many Key Players: Even small healthcare institutions are complex places. The American Healthcare System is like a giant ocean liner; its complicated relationships and interactions make quick maneuvers difficult, even dangerous, Intervention needs to be measured and restrained by the law of unintended consequences. The system is composed of varying stakeholders with often competing interests and ambitions. Notoriously independent and self-directed physicians control frontline healthcare decisions and thus ultimately economic expenses. The hospital system is a mixed bag of for-profit and non-profit institutions that many times are hostages to local politics, each with a confused oversight arrangement. These institutions are stretched to the breaking point. The hospital administrators who control much of the day-to-day function of healthcare industry likewise have their own sense of place in the establishment. Mid-level care providers (nurses) are progressively attempting to enlarge the boundaries of their practice skills. These interests often collide with other parts of the healthcare establishment. Millions of workers in these institutions who do the day-to-day work are often subject to arbitrary union authority and work rules.

Complex Issues: Moreover, the healthcare payment structure may be best described as chaotic and irrational. Over all of this, a host of complicated government regulations and legal precedence stretch back for years, while the variance in jurisdiction and circumstance confuse well meaning decisions. Embedded in these matrices are the patients who understandably demand the best possible care and treatment, and are quick to point out any deviation from their perceptions of merit often enhanced by internet information. Finally, those confused system must cope with enormous changes as demographic, technological innovation, and provider shortages confuse stability.

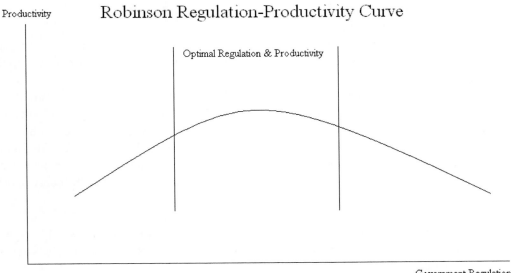

III. POLITICS AND HEALTHCARE

Responding to their constituents' interests and their own philosophy of the direction of the country, politicians make changing the American healthcare apparatus central in their electoral campaign. In general, politicians make little reference to individual responsibility for healthy lifestyle or minimizing healthcare expenditure. They expand entitlements and offer favorite classes' special attention. Barrier entrances to healthcare are substantially diminished.

This increase in healthcare demands will be paid for by increasing taxes on wealthy American, on drug companies, and on employing varying devices to restrain and recycle insurance company profits. Provider income will decrease while centralized management will rocket upward. Healthcare will become far more doctrinal. Imposed inefficiencies will be discovered by use of electronic records and centralized financial coercion instituted. The details of much of this are not clearly stated and certainly no mention of increasing national productivity in regards to the nation's healthcare system.

Solutions that rely on external pressures to bring change to the healthcare delivery system will likely result in greater inefficiency and problems. Increased taxes and regulation will result in government centralization that hinders those immediately involved in healthcare delivery to affect change.

Negative Bi-Products of Healthcare Overhaul Proposals

(1) No financial penalty or any other penalty for patients undertaking bad habits and abusing the system;

(2) The idea that patient information or patient awareness of different treatment options and outcomes can serve to more appropriately direct patients has substantial limits as

patients endure a time of emotional distress when healthcare crises occur and moreover even the sophisticated can be defeated;

(3) Increasing regulation of drug companies and insurance companies is a sure way to cause these institutions to retract and become less efficient and minimize their capital investment;

(4) Efforts to control a complicated healthcare system by external regulations are bound to encounter substantial difficulties, resentment and create a dispirited workforce;

(5) Because of demographic growth and shortfalls in the healthcare system, politicians would be forced to propose rationing healthcare. As such rationing became more commonly appreciated, the country's allegiance to its quasi religious healthcare institutions would be disturbed. These difficulties are bound to cause voter resentment which can be profound.

If regulations are so onerous, it places immense burden on caregivers and will likely lead to worse outcomes. The following Robinson curve (akin to Laver curve) provides a gross visual demonstration of detrimental excessive taxation and regulation.

Opportunity for Politicians to Promote System Efficiencies

There is great value in empowering clinicians involved in delivery of healthcare to work with current systems and structures to expand efficiency efforts and thereby curtail unsustainable national expenditure.

Better healthcare policy could be obtained by empowering clinicians to increase efficiency rather than enforcing government rationing. We provide 10 of our suggestions for how individuals involved in the front-lines of healthcare delivery can contribute to the national goals of decreasing healthcare expenditure:

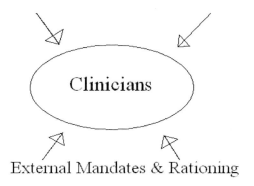
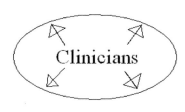

External Mandates & Rationing   Internal System Efficiency

Ten Ways to Enable System Efficiencies

1. Paradigm Shift-View Healthcare as Investment.
   - Investing into healthcare results in positive return in investment to government.
   - Important to shift mindset of healthcare as "investment" that results in more lives saved, increasingly productive citizens, greater economic development, higher tax revenues.
2. Provide coverage for Indigent Care.

- Recommend that healthcare costs for illegal immigrant are paid for by Federal Government.
- Financial burden to care for indigent patients is placed on caregivers who then "cost-shift" by charging higher to private insurance.

3. Address Healthcare Bureaucracy.
   - Bureaucracy within fragmented healthcare system leads to inefficiencies.
4. Encourage collaboration
   - Clinical collaboration leads to improved healthcare delivery.
   - Encourage collaborative cost-savings projects.
5. Facilitate better understanding of healthcare costs.
   - Determining true healthcare costs is difficult both at micro and macro levels.
6. Promote Economic Outcome Analysis
   - Outcome analysis in biomedical literature has generally failed to make appropriate economic inquiries.
   - Physicians often utilize these resources to track new ideas, but are not provided with cost numbers. Physicians need incentive to pay attention to healthcare expenditure.
7. Curb Professional Clinician Shorfalls
   - Inconsistent connection between social needs and supply of specific clinicians (e.g. need more MDs, Pas, RNs).
   - Nursing Instructor shortfall driving RN Shortfall. Public salaries not competitive - supply and demand not allowed to interact.
8. Address Unfunded Mandates
   - Unfunded government mandates forced on healthcare system
   - Financial risk to taking care of society's needs.
9. Reform Balanced Budget Act
   - Currently limits the number of clinical residents in the south.
   - Mechanism needed where physician gaps can be filled on national scale.
10. Promote Individual Patient Responsibility
    - e.g. Swiss Model-patient's insurance payments impacted by results to annual check-up, lifestyle and behavior, etc.

Preservation and Expansion of Doctor-Patient Relationship

Proposals for more regulation will extend the reach and power of our government institution, leading it to become ever more intrusive and threaten to disturb a fundamental American cultural icon - balance of powers, and checks and balances. In this, if one believes the healthcare system is a quasi of secular religion, the takeover of this institution by centralized government mirrors in many ways the medieval monarch's seizure of the universal church on the way to absolute monarchy [5]. The modern health care shortfalls can be compared with the corruption of church in the Middle Ages. The priests became corrupted when the King named himself as the head of the church of England because they began trying to please him instead of seeking the pleasure of God. In the same way, we believe that physicians are being corrupted or will be further corrupted as the government becomes the modern "king" of healthcare, which for many people is what they look to for hope and salvation, instead of to God.

If the doctor-patient relationship can be strengthened to its previous pattern this will act as a brogue against an undesirable concentration of power. The physician could serve as the protector of the patient's rights and his champion and struggling against any system that arbitrarily injured his patient. Unfortunately, these notions have been under assault from varying government legal establishments focused mainly on issues involving restraint of trade. The priestly role of physicians has been degraded. They cannot currently even offer charity to their patients in form of dropping physician copayments.

As a point on this, payment for good outcome would be supported in a doctor-patient relationship. It would remove the suspicion that a patient might have if a physician was merely attempting to line his pockets with excessive treatment. One however should be careful that the patient's risk:benefit ratio is not jeopardized by formulas that discourage treatment of patients with high chance of a bad outcome and thus no compensation.

What should be done? More medical society role and regulations of physicians should be undertaken. Ethical instruction and residency in medical school and post-graduate training are excellent ideas. The doctor-patient relationship can also be maximized by an altered tort reform system which reassures the physician that his best efforts will not lead him to the court room.

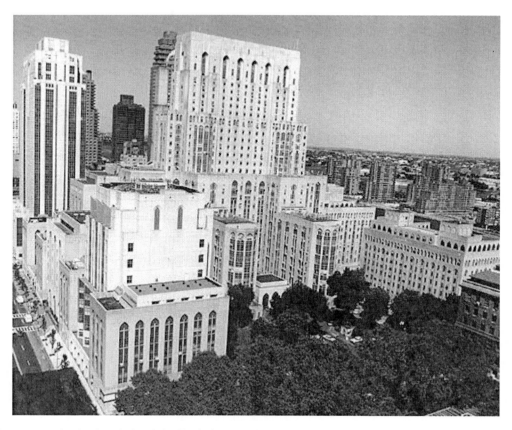

The New York City hospital, originally designed to look like a cathedral, now rises high to offer the hope of healing.

What Is Different about Our Point of View?

A variable cornucopia of suggestions for improving the US Healthcare system have emanated from many quarters. These voices have provided useful sage advice, statistics, and much well earned erudition.

Surprisingly, most suggestions have arisen from either academic economists or business professors who predicated upon a by-the-book logic of cost containment. Our approach, as clinicians serving patients on a daily basis, is meant as a frontline battlefield report back to general headquarters. Our Plea is to let the participants of the healthcare battlefield have some responsibility and possibly some benefit for increasing healthcare efficiency. Externally directed regulation did not work for the Soviet Union and it will not work in this country.

REFERENCES

[1]   The Nobel Prize in Medicine. JAMA 2008;299:114.

[2]   McClellan MB. Speech before first international colloquium on generic medicine. Washington, DC: US food and drug administration, 2003.

[3]   National health expenditure projections 2006-2016. http://www.cms.hhs.gov/ NationalHealthExpendData/03_NationalHealthAccountsProjected.asp

[4]   Hutchinson B. Medical tourism growing worldwide. University of Delaware. http://www.udel.edu/PR/UDaily/2005/mar/tourism072505.html

[5]   King Henry VIII. http://www.greatsite.com/timeline-english-bible-history/king-henry.html

In: Toward Healthcare Resource Stewardship
Editors: J. S.Robinson, M. S.Walid et al.

ISBN: 978-1-62100-182-9
© 2012 Nova Science Publishers, Inc.

Chapter 2

THE ECONOMICS OF REGIONAL TRAUMA CENTERS - THE GEORGIA MODEL

Greg Bishop,[1] Dennis W. Ashley[2,3,4] and Joe Sam Robinson Jr.[2,3,4,5]*

[1]Bishop+Associates, Irvine, CA
[2]Georgia Trauma Commission, Atlanta, GA, US
[3]Medical Center of Central Georgia, Macon, Georgia, US
[4]Mercer University School of Medicine, Macon, Georgia, US
[5]Georgia Neurosurgical Institute, Macon, Georgia, US

This chapter provides an overview of the economic factors impacting regional trauma centers, with the Georgia Trauma Commission's work in assessing Georgia's trauma centers for 2006-2008 (with funding arriving in 2008) used as a case study.

BACKGROUND

The U.S. military learned lessons during the Vietnam War that led to dramatic changes in the care of the seriously injured in America in the 1970's and 80's. Upon returning home, medical personnel pointed out that a soldier wounded in the jungles of Southeast Asia had a better chance of survival than those injured in auto crashes in communities across this nation.[1]

In those two decades, the first trauma centers were developed, trauma center standards were established by the American College of Surgeons, training programs were created, and regional trauma systems developed in a number of States.[2] Trauma centers proliferated in the 80's, driven by a passionate group of physicians, nurses and emergency personnel committed to saving the lives of the injured. At the end of the eighties, development stalled and trauma centers started closing due to economic challenges.[3, 4]

---

* Corresponding Author: Dennis W. Ashley, 840 Pine Street, Suite 710, Macon, GA 31201.
  Email: ashley.dennis@mccg.org.

Today, while many still struggle economically, about 600 [5] of the nation's hospitals serve as regional trauma centers. They dedicate extensive staff, physician and facility resources at all times so that seriously injured patients have the best possible chance of survival and productivity. [6]

THE REGIONAL TRAUMA CENTER

When a regional trauma center opens, paramedics transport injury victims past local hospitals to its waiting trauma team, composed of a trauma surgeon, emergency physician, trauma nurses and personnel from radiology, blood bank and other departments. Fifteen surgical and medical specialties from neurosurgery to OB/GYN are on standby, and nursing teams are ready in the operating room and critical care unit. [6]

The difference between the severity and type of injuries treated by an emergency department versus a regional trauma center is indicated in this table.

Paramedics use formal triage criteria [7] to determine whether injury victims will be transported to the closest hospital or to one of the 10% of the nation's hospitals that serves as a regional trauma center.

Across the U.S. regional trauma centers are categorized as Level I or II, depending upon their level of resources. Some are specialized pediatric trauma centers. Level I trauma centers conduct education and research and are typically based in teaching hospitals, and Level II trauma centers are usually based in community hospitals. There are also Level III and IV trauma centers that are typically based in smaller rural hospitals where they treat lower severity injury patients and stabilize and transfer the more seriously injured to a regional trauma center. [6]

Typical Patient Injuries Treated	
Emergency Room	Trauma Center
Broken Leg	Multiple Fractures
Back Sprain	Paralysis
Broken Rib	Punctured Lung
Laceration	Stab Wound
Concussion	Brain Injury

Trauma Medical Staff Specialties	
Trauma Surgery	Emergency Medicine
Anesthesiology	Neurosurgery
Orthopedic Surgery	Ophthalmology
Plastic Surgery	Micro Surgery
Hand Surgery	Cardiac Surgery
Thoracic Surgery	Critical Care
Oral Surgery	Radiology
Pediatric Surgery	Ob/Gyn Surgery

Regional trauma centers are the cornerstone of state trauma systems, which also incorporate emergency medical services (paramedics, air medical transport, etc.), referral hospitals (rehabilitation, burn centers), and other hospitals in a systematic approach to optimizing care for the seriously injured at all stages of treatment. [8, 9]

GEORGIA'S TRAUMA CENTERS: A CASE STUDY

Georgia experienced a crisis in trauma care in the mid 2000's due to closures of trauma centers in a state with an inadequate supply to begin with.[10] The most critical issues were the declining number of physicians available to participate in trauma care, a substantial proportion of uninsured trauma victims, the lack of a system to direct patients to the most appropriate hospital, and an antiquated emergency medical services (EMS) system that is fragmented and under resourced. [11,12] These issues are common in states across the nation, and particularly in the South and Southwest where there are high proportions of uninsured and large rural areas. [13]

Georgia's trauma surgeons, nurses and other system stakeholders worked for years to get the state to act, and developed strong alliances with EMS, Georgia's hospital and medical associations, and the Chamber of Commerce. The State Legislature acted to create the Georgia Trauma Care Network Commission and allocated $58.9 million to stabilize and expand Georgia's trauma system. [14] The Commission met in December 2007 for the first time and set about assessing Georgia trauma center's financial performance. The assessment was conducted on information provided by trauma centers on 2006 patients meeting Georgia trauma registry criteria. [15]

FUNDING FOR REGIONAL TRAUMA CENTERS

In June 2008, the Commission approved the 2008-2009 $59 million trauma system-funding plan, which included funding of $17,888,539 for Level I and II trauma center readiness costs and another $17,888,539 for trauma center uninsured patient care costs (for a total of $35,777,078). The four Level I and nine Level II trauma centers were responsible for passing on 25% of this funding to their medical staff who participated in trauma care. [16, 17]

Additional assessments of Level I and II trauma center financial performance were conducted for 2007 and 2008, the period in which initial state funding arrived at the trauma centers. This case study summarizes the results of all three years as a basis for exploring the economic factors that impact acute trauma care.

A COMPREHENSIVE TRAUMA SYSTEM

While this case study focuses on the financial viability of regional trauma centers, an essential issue addressed in Goal #2 below, a comprehensive trauma system is necessary for trauma patients to be treated and transported from the scene, stabilized and transferred by

Level III/IV trauma centers and local hospitals to higher level trauma centers, and for those who need it, transfer to rehabilitation and burn care.

In 2008, the GTCNC assessed Georgia's trauma system and found it to be rich in opportunities. This is reflected in the broad range of goals in the GTCNC strategic plan, which expands the concept of a comprehensive trauma system. It includes economically beneficial partnerships with Georgia organizations responsible for emergency communications, telemedicine, all EMS, pediatric emergencies, disaster/ terror preparedness, injury prevention, other types of medical emergencies, and all local/regional emergency care systems. [9]

Primary Goals

1. Obtain Permanent Funding
2. Maintain/Expand Georgia Trauma Centers
3. Strengthen Emergency Medical Services
4. Develop Trauma Communication System
5. Build Trauma System Infrastructure
6. Establish Exceptional Accountability

Secondary Goals

1. Pilot/Build Trauma Telemedicine System
2. Enhance Pediatric Trauma Subsystem
3. Strengthen Trauma Physician Support
4. Address Rehab, Burn and Interstate Transfers
5. Assist Initiatives to Reduce Traumatic Injury
6. Integrate with Disaster/Terror Preparedness
7. Expand System to All Emergency Care Needs
8. Develop Trauma System Regionalization
9. Develop Policy/Stakeholder Structure

Progress has also been broad and includes:

*   All 2007 trauma centers have maintained their status, four hospitals have become trauma centers, two have upgraded, and others are in process.
*   A cutting edge performance-based payment program to improve quality and reduce costs with financial incentives has been established.
*   A state-of-the-art system to assure all injured are quickly moved to the appropriate level of care is developing, using Sweden's trauma communication system software.
*   EMS is stronger throughout Georgia for all emergencies due to new ambulances, pediatric training, and a robust stakeholder structure within the GTCNC.

The components of the GTCNC Strategic Plan above impact many of the economic factors of trauma care, and they provide a broader basis for exploring these factors in this case study.

GEORGIA REGIONAL TRAUMA CENTER 2006-2008 FINANCIAL PERFORMANCE

This component summarizes the results of 2008 in comparison to 2006 and 2007.

Trauma Center Volume and Severity

The table below indicates the breakdown of admitted patients treated in 2008 in Georgia trauma centers by injury severity score (ISS) and comparative 2006-7 data.

Georgia Admitted Trauma Center Patients

Injury Severity	2008	%	2007	%	2006	%
ISS 0-8 Minor	4,057	37%	3,425	31%	4,132	36%
ISS 9-14 Moderate	4,133	38%	3,972	36%	3,816	34%
ISS 15-24 Major	1,800	16%	2,158	20%	2,016	18%
ISS >24 Severe	993	9%	1,410	13%	1,354	12%
Totals	10,983	100%	10,965	100%	11,318	100%

In 2008 the average patient volume was 1,564 for Georgia's Level I trauma centers, and 521 for Level II trauma centers. The total number of admitted patients with an ISS above 15 (major/severe injuries) was 2,733, or 25% of the total, in comparison to 3,568 (33%) in 2007 and 3,370 (30%) in 2006.

For 2008, information on non-admitted patients meeting state trauma registry criteria was also provided by Georgia trauma centers and is summarized in the table below.

Georgia Admitted Trauma Center Patients 2008

Type Non Admit	All Trauma Centers	Treatment Cost	Average Cost
Dead On Arrival	22	$44,570	$2,026
ED Deaths	233	$1,140,866	$4,896
OR Deaths	51	$555,755	$10,897
ED Transfers Out	320	$2,159,483	$6,748
Transfers In and ED Discharge	403	$745,271	$1,849
Totals	1,027	$4,916,568	$4,787

The total of 1,027 patients adds 9.3% to overall volume, and the cost of $4.9 million adds 2.1% to $237.9 million in patient treatment costs (see below).

Trauma Center Patient Treatment Costs by Payer Class

The table below indicates fully allocated treatment costs, composed of both direct and indirect costs, for admitted trauma patient under each payer class:

Trauma Center Treatment Costs by Payer Class

Payer Class	CY 2008 Costs	Payer Mix	CY 2007 Costs	CY 2006 Costs
Private Insurance	97,185,231	41%	$84,758,174	$86,991,732
Other	23,214,860	10%	$11,103,058	$14,604,157
Medicare	28,140,570	12%	$22,452,714	$25,707,732
Medicaid	46,747,856	20%	$41,491,140	$37,181,827
Uninsured	42,578,211	18%	$59,529,585	$56,199,126
Total	$237,866,728	100%	$219,334,671	$220,684,574

Georgia's 39% trauma center proportion of privately insured patients in relation to the 51% national norm [13] is low and is offset by a higher proportion of uninsured/underinsured patients. Total costs in 2008 were 8.5% higher than in 2007, with about the same number of patients. The application of the "other" category was inconsistent over previous years in that some poorly insured patients were included in 2008 that resulted in a corresponding decrease in uninsured patient costs. There is no evidence that actual uninsured patient costs decreased in 2008.

Trauma Center Readiness Costs

Trauma centers incur substantial costs over and above patient treatment costs that are not normally allocated to trauma patient care by hospital cost allocation formulas. These extraordinary "readiness costs" would be eliminated if the trauma center were to close.

The GTCNC's Trauma Care Economic Subcommittee developed a new methodology to assess such costs, based upon previous trauma center readiness cost surveys in Georgia and Florida [18], and using the American College of Surgeon's standards for trauma centers. [6] Summarized results of the survey are as follows:

Trauma Center Readiness Costs

Readiness Cost Category	LI Total	LI Average	LII Total	LII Average	Georgia Totals
Administrative	2,431,530	607,883	3,339,644	371,072	5,771,174
Medical Staff	18,003,208	4,500,802	12,836,008	1,426,223	30,839,216
In House OR	1,744,231	436,058	2,284,553	253,839	4,028,784
Education/Outreach	222,518	55,630	1,437,046	159,672	1,659,564
Totals	$22,401,487	$5,600,372	$19,897,251	1,992,890	$42,298,738

The 2008 results total $42.3 million, compared to $46.3 million in CY 2007, and $44.0 million in CY 2006.

2008 Revenue and Total Costs and Payer Class

The table below incorporates total trauma center costs (including readiness costs) allocated by payer, revenue produced by each payer source, the cost recovery rate (CRR) or revenue divided by costs, and the percentage of overall loss contributed by each payer class.

2008 Trauma Center Total Costs Revenue by Payer Class

Payer Class	Total Costs	Revenue	Surplus /Loss	CRR %	Overall Contri.
Private Ins.	$114,467,230	$128,194,547	$13,727,317	112.0%	4.9%
Other	$27,343,051	$16,873,772	($10,469,279)	61.0%	-3.8%
Medicare	$33,144,677	$28,111,038	($5,033,639)	84.0%	-1.9%
Medicaid	$55,060,811	$36,752,712	($18,308,099)	66.0%	-6.7%
Uninsured	$50,149,697	$3,079,352	($47,070,345)	6.1%	-16.8%
Total	$280,165,466	$213,011,421	($67,154,045)	76.0%	-24.0%

Readiness costs were allocated proportionally to treatment costs and together total $280.2 million. Patient revenue was $213 million, leaving a loss (before state funding is considered) of $67.7 million.

Georgia 2008 Trauma Center Financial Performance

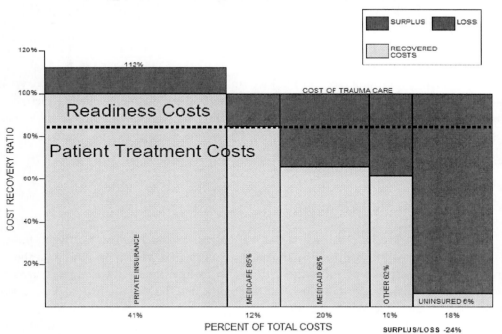

The green area reflects a surplus generated by a payer class; the red area represents a loss, and the yellow area represents recovered costs. Readiness and patient treatment costs are also indicated. Of the loss on trauma care in Georgia (red), 17% is generated by uninsured patients, and Other, Medicaid and Medicare patients generate another 12% in losses. [19]

2008 Georgia Trauma Center Reimbursement Profile

The reimbursement profile below depicts the above table in graphic form. The width of each column reflects the proportion of full costs incurred by patients in each payer class, and the height of each column reflects the proportion of total costs covered by each payer class. [19]

Total 2006-2008 Financial Performance of Georgia's Regional Trauma Centers

The table below presents the overall financial performance of Georgia's trauma centers in 2008 in comparison to 2007 and 2006.

Georgia Trauma Centers	CY 2008	CY 2007	CY 2006
Patient Care Revenue	$213,011,421	$201,052,174	$193,999,255
Direct Patient Treatment Costs	$159,370,708	$146,954,230	$147,858,665
Indirect Patient Treatment Costs	$78,496,020	$72,380,441	$72,825,909
Trauma Patient Treatment Costs	$237,866,728	$219,334,671	$220,684,574
Readiness Costs	$42,298,738	$46,284,440	$44,063,224
Total Trauma Patient Costs	$280,165,466	$265,619,111	$264,747,798
Loss on Trauma Care	($67,154,045)	-$64,566,937	-$70,748,543
State Funding	$47,041,166		
Remaining Loss	($20,112,979	-$64,566,937	-$70,748,543

In CY 2008, with revenue of $213 million, total costs of $280.2 million, and a payer mix with 59% of patients either uninsured or underinsured, Georgia trauma centers experienced a combined financial loss on trauma care of $67.2 million. In 2008, $47 million in state funding was provided, which reduced this loss from a 2006-2008 average of $68.2 million to $20.1 million.

Trauma Medical Staff Costs

In addition to the $237.9 million in hospital costs for trauma patient treatment, there are also substantial costs for treatment by trauma specialists such as trauma surgery, orthopedic surgery, neurosurgery and plastic surgery. This also includes hospital based physicians such as emergency medicine, anesthesiology and radiology, and other specialists such as urology, ophthalmology and infectious disease.

Based on previous assessments, trauma center physician costs are estimated at 30-35% of patient treatment costs incurred by trauma hospitals. [21] If 33%, this would add $78.5 million in trauma patient treatment costs for physician care.

Total Acute Trauma Care Costs

Total trauma center costs, or those incurred in the acute care phase of trauma patient care, are estimated as follows:

Trauma Center Treatment Costs	$ 237,866,728
Trauma Center Readiness Costs	$ 42,298,738
Trauma Center Physician Costs	$ 78,496,020
Total Acute Trauma Center Costs	$ 358,661,486

This does not include costs for care of the seriously injured who do not reach trauma centers, pre-hospital care, rehabilitation and burn care, and out-of-state treatment.

THE ECONOMIC FACTORS OF ACUTE TRAUMA CARE

For decades, trauma centers have reported problems with high costs, low payment and unstable physician support. They have learned to overcome these challenges and, trauma systems continue to slowly but inexorably expand. Georgia presents an excellent example and case study for understanding the variety of economic factors, many unique, that impact the acute phase of care for the injured.

THE VALUE OF TRAUMA CARE

The intrinsic value of trauma care is reflected in polls demonstrating high favorability to government support of trauma care (a 2008 poll in Georgia indicated 78% support for paying $10 per year for trauma care [22]), and rankings of health services by cost/benefit that placed trauma care at the top [23] (since it heals injured young people who go on to a long, productive life). This intrinsic value is a key reason why the public and their legislators make it a priority, and trauma systems inexorably expand to meet needs.

REGIONALIZATION OF COMPLEX HEALTH CARE SERVICES

Before trauma centers, each hospital did its best to treat the seriously injured under emergent circumstances, but the low numbers of such patients did not support the resources necessary to effectively care for them. When a trauma system is established, serious injury victims from throughout a region are transported past local hospitals to the regional trauma center, a designated hospital offering specially trained, immediately available staff and the necessary equipment and facilities. [24]

In essence, trauma centers are able to offer high-quality medical care because of the proficiency of the surgeons and trauma specific resources supported by high patient volumes (i.e., economies of scale) [25]. This concept of regionalization of complex health care services, the efficacy of which was first demonstrated with cardiac surgery, provides the economic foundation for regional trauma systems and centers. [26]

TRAUMA CENTER READINESS COSTS

Trauma patient treatment costs are relatively well defined by standardized hospital cost-accounting systems. The costs required by trauma center regulations to maintain essential infrastructure and capacity to provide emergent services on a 24/7 basis are not. These are non-patient care costs the hospital would not have to pay if it were not a trauma center. They are referred to as trauma center readiness costs [18], and were definitively defined by the GTCNC in the course of their assessments. [27] They can include:

- Medical staff payments for trauma call
- 24 hour operating room staffing
- Added staff for lab/diagnostic services
- Injury prevention activities
- Training of nurses and physicians
- Program administrative infrastructure
- Performance improvement programs
- Trauma specific equipment

In Georgia, these costs amounted to $42.3 million, or 15% of total trauma center costs.

ADVERSE SELECTION AND DISPROPORTIONATE SHARE

Young adults (particularly young men) and the poor have an increased propensity for injury; these groups make up a high proportion of the patients in trauma centers. They are also less likely to have commercial insurance coverage or be eligible for public assistance programs; as a result, trauma centers attract a *disproportionate share* of patients unable to pay for their care.

Trauma systems also seek the sickest and thus the most expensive patients in a classic example of *adverse selection*. This means higher costs over which to spread the same revenue on uninsured, Medicaid, Medicare and insured patients paid on a case or day rate. The combination of adverse selection and disproportionate share act as multipliers to produce high levels of uncompensated care. [19, 28]

COST SHIFTING

Charging insured patients more to cover the uncompensated costs of treating un/under insured patients is cost shifting, which has become a fundamental trauma center financing mechanism. This profile of the financial performance of Georgia's trauma centers shows a surplus of 12% on privately insured patients and losses on all others, a classic example of cost shifting. It is more prevalent in states with high levels of uninsured like Georgia.[13]

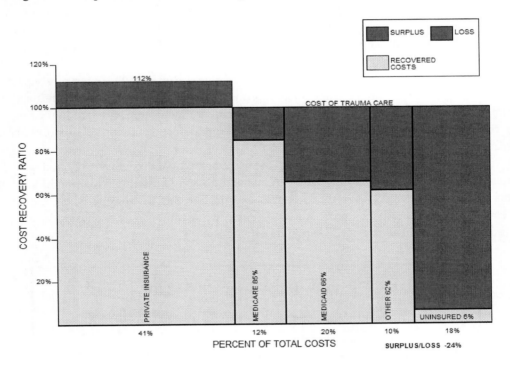

OUT-OF-NETWORK AND REPATRIATION

With the development of managed care, payers use their leverage to direct patients to contracted, low-cost providers. With trauma care, EMS triage policy and paramedics determine patient destination, leaving health plans with little control. Health plans consider trauma patients out-of-network and "out-of-control." This is what enables extensive cost-shifting. [29, 30]

Managed care organizations with a high market share have responded by leveraging the high amount of non-trauma business they do with trauma hospitals to force down their costs for trauma care. Those with a low market share pay a much higher rate for trauma care. Another response is repatriation, in which health plans seek to bring patients back into network by arranging their post-stabilization transfer from trauma centers to lower cost, contracted facilities.

INCREASING SHORTAGES AND COSTS FOR TRAUMA MEDICAL STAFF

Up to 200 physicians in 16 specialties are needed to support a regional trauma center. For most, trauma care is a small and often problematic part of their practice. It is a responsibility they have taken over from their brethren at other hospitals in the region, and most find it incompatible with their private practice and would like to limit the "opportunity cost" to their lifestyle from trauma call. In essence, their *costs* participating in trauma care have increased, and like any other producer, they raised their prices. [13]

Trauma hospitals are now paying substantial and increasing amounts of call pay or other forms of compensation, but are finding it increasingly problematic to have all trauma specialties staffed at all times. This is in addition to increased difficulty in recruiting surgeons to many areas of the country. [31]

Professional fee billing on trauma care is unique because of the unusual sources of payment (e.g., auto insurance), the disproportionate share of uninsured patients, surgery billing codes that do not reflect the demands of emergent trauma care and very limited means for cost-shifting. Also problematic is obtaining adequate documentation to support charges under emergent circumstances. [13]

The shortage of surgeons developing in many areas of the country [32] bodes ill for trauma care at multiple levels because the remaining ones are busier, making trauma call that much more disruptive. Perhaps the U.S. will end up like Eastern Europe where their very effective trauma centers are staffed only with emergency physician/surgeons, anesthesiologist/critical care specialists and radiologists.

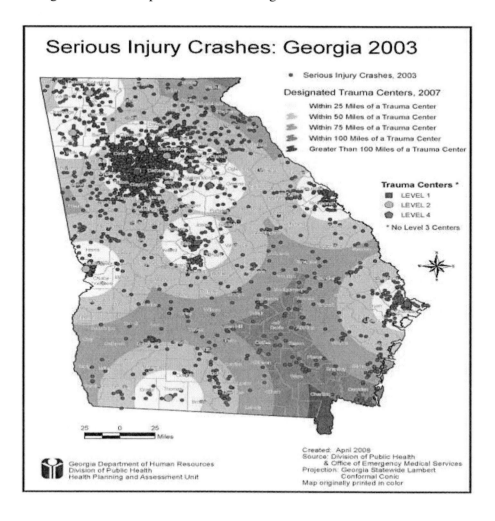

SCARCE RURAL TRAUMA CARE RESOURCES

Rural, lowly populated regions have limited public health structures, small numbers of medical care providers, volunteer emergency medical systems, and long travel distances. Despite these limitations, rural ambulance services and hospitals play a critical role in trauma care. [13]

Georgia presents an excellent example. The map on the right indicates the location of serious injury crashes and adult Level I and II trauma centers, and the areas within 25, 50, 75 and 100 miles of each. The result is that there are large portions of very rural southern Georgia that are beyond 50 miles of a trauma center. [33] The time it will take to stabilize and transport the seriously injured from these areas (medium and dark blue) to a trauma center will exceed the "golden hour", the point at which their prospects for survival start declining rapidly.

COMMUNICATION ENABLES EFFICIENT USE OF SCARCE RESOURCES

A key economic factor driving plans for the Georgia Trauma System is the efficient use of scarce resources. Strategies include the following [9]:

Trauma Communication Center - Functioning like an air traffic control system, it will route inbound ambulances and helicopters with injured patients to the closest hospital staffed and equipped to meet the patient's needs. It would also help rural doctors transfer critical patients to a trauma center or tertiary care hospital, and can be expanded to other medical emergencies like strokes and heart attacks if the experts in these fields wish to utilize the trauma infrastructure.

Trauma Telemedicine System – The Commission has partnered with Georgia Tele-Health to link regional trauma centers with rural providers using telemedicine to enable real time observation of the patient's emergency care course to enable offsite evaluations by specialists, guide resuscitation measures, and assess radiology and lab test results.

Statewide GPS EMS Vehicle Locater System

This will enable all dispatch and transports by ambulances in Georgia to be managed based upon the vehicle's location. This is critical in high severity trauma cases where time is of the essence, as well as other time critical medical emergencies.

All communication components are being integrated to add new capability to Georgia disaster/terror response organizations.

PERFORMANCE: AN ECONOMIC ISSUE

Getting the most out of health care dollars is now imperative. Performance based payment (PBP) is an evolving concept in health care that is gaining traction as a means of improving quality and reducing costs by financially incentivizing providers to do so. Its application in trauma care is very limited, although it has strong potential in terms of quality and costs, particularly in states that fund trauma centers.

Georgia has taken on PBP as an opportunity to squeeze the best value out of Georgia's resources by developing a cutting edge program with financial incentives that is fostering the needed participation in trauma system development, cost effectiveness, injured patients' access to trauma care, meeting trauma center standards, and most importantly, patient outcomes. [34]

A New Public Service for Georgia

When trauma systems start breaking down, the overburdened emergency care sector of the overall health care system starts breaking down as well. When a trauma center is full and cannot handle the next seriously injured patient, such patients go to other hospitals and physicians, who are then impacted like dominos and react to avoid such cases. Surgeons opt out of call panels for all patients, and paramedics are left to search for another hospital willing to accept the injured patient.

The converse can be true too. When a state builds a trauma system, it can strengthen its overall emergency care system. The surgeons available for trauma care are also available for other surgical emergency cases. Within a trauma hospital, a strong trauma service takes a major load off the overburdened ER. Ambulance GPS systems benefit all emergency patients. The regional infrastructure built to coordinate trauma patient triage, transport and transfer can also help consolidate fragmented county EMS programs into efficient regional EMS agencies. This is what is happening in Georgia.

A Public Good

Trauma systems, like fire and police departments, are defined as a public good in economic terms; i.e., the absence of purchase decisions, immediate access to all, and extensive stand-by resources. In response to closures of trauma centers, many states with relatively high proportions of uninsured patients, developed various means to fund trauma centers, including surcharges on vehicle registrations. Georgia has recognized the importance of trauma centers with funding, and due to the high proportion (51%) of motor vehicle crash victims among its trauma patients [35], the funding source of choice is the vehicle registration fee, with a surcharge on speeding violations playing an important role in funding (and injury prevention due to excessive speeding).

Partnering to Make the most of Public Resources

One of the central characteristics of the Georgia Trauma Commission's strategic plan is partnerships with other organizations to maximize the use of Georgia's resources. This includes partnering with public and private organizations whose role involves:

- Terror And Disaster Preparedness
- EMS/Hospital Communications

- Telemedicine
- State EMS And Health Department
- Injury Prevention
- Emergency Medical Services
- Local Hospitals
- Trauma Centers
- Surgeons/Medical Specialists
- Pediatric Resources
- Interstate Trauma Providers
- Specialized Tertiary Care
- Highway Patrol
- Other

There is also an opportunity for having a strong trauma system serve as a new pillar of support for the larger emergency health care sector throughout the state. Evolving problems with facility capacity and physician supply and participation in emergency care go well beyond trauma care and will require this new regional support structure for trauma care to be broadened to address other "time sensitive" health care issues such as stroke, heart attack and other conditions requiring emergency surgery.

Partnering with Stakeholders

There are many stakeholders for Georgia's trauma system, and each has something to gain as well as contribute to the system. Pediatric trauma providers are an excellent example of leveraging the trauma system. Georgia enjoys an exceptionally strong array of pediatric trauma centers that are well located to care for seriously injured children under age 15. They account for 12% of trauma center patients and require a parallel system to adults due to their specialized needs.

The pediatric stakeholders have worked to make this component an exceptional part of the trauma system– including 911, pediatric trained and equipped EMS, local hospitals with pediatric training and equipment, telemedicine consults, the trauma communication system, air transport, and the pediatric trauma centers. This system can also serve children who are not injured but need emergent tertiary care (e.g., emergency surgery).

Partnering with the Ultimate Stakeholders – Georgians

Fire and police services are strong, established public goods with strong constituencies, broad public support, and exceptional means of communicating their message. When they do something good, their communities are well aware of it.

As a public good, trauma and EMS sectors are highly fragmented, and just bringing the stakeholders together is a major accomplishment. Moving further to build coalitions with related interests, conduct advocacy to build public support, and build connections with local legislators – all critical steps for building a new public service - is uncommon, but this is what trauma system stakeholders in Georgia did to get the necessary resources described in this case study.

A referendum was placed on the ballot in November amid the anti-tax fervor of the 2010 elections to add a $10 tag fee onto motor vehicle registration to generate funding for trauma. One of the lessons learned was that the Commission's highest priority - rural regions – voted against it because they believed the resources would favor urban hospitals. Obviously, more education and communication will be needed in these areas.

There will be more opportunities for funding, and once this critical public service effectively communicates with its ultimate stakeholders, its sustainability will be assured. Rome was not built overnight and police and fire public services took many decades to evolve into the strong positions they enjoy today. Trauma and emergency care public services will also take time to fully develop, and Georgia is well on its way. Unfortunately, once the resources were in hand, the Georgia Trauma Commission became fully engrossed in building an exceptional trauma system for Georgians, but did not communicate with their ultimate stakeholders what they were doing.

REFERENCES

[1]   West JG, Trunkey D, et al: Trauma Systems: Current status – future challenges. *JAMA* 259:3597, 1988.

[2]   American College of Surgeons, Committee on Trauma: Resources for Optimal Care of the Injured Patient, 1999.

[3]   United States General Accounting office: Trauma Care, Lifesaving System Threatened by Un-reimbursed Cost and Other Factors: A Report to the Chairman of the Subcommittee on Health for Families and the Uninsured, Committee on Finance, U.S. Senate. Washington D.C., No. HRD 91-57, May 1991.

[4]   The American Association for the Surgery of Trauma: Trauma Center Economic Study – Report on comprehensive survey of nation's trauma centers. December 1994.

[5]   Coalition for Trauma Care: Number of U.S. Trauma Centers by Level, 2004.

[6]   American College of Surgeons, Committee on Trauma: Resources for Optimal Care of the Injured Patient 2006.

[7]   Sasser, SM, Hunt RC, Sulivent, EE, et al: Guidelines for Field Triage of Injured Patients – Recommendations of the National Expert Panel on Field Triage. Figure 1. Field triage decision scheme – United States, 2006.

[8]   U. S. Department of Health and Human Services, Health Resources and Services Administration. Model Trauma System Planning and Evaluation. February 2006.

[9]   Georgia Trauma Care Network Commission: Our Emerging Vision – A new Public Service for Georgia. February 2009.

[10]   Personal communication with Pat O'Neal, Director, Office of EMS/Trauma, Georgia Department of Community Health, 2008.

[11]   Bishop + Associates: Ideas from and for Georgia's Trauma System. January 2009.

[12]   American College of Surgeons Trauma System Consultation Program, Georgia Site Visit, January 5, 2009.

[13]   National Foundation for Trauma Care: U.S. Trauma Center Economic Status, 2003.

[14] Georgia State Legislature, Senate Bill 60: Establish Georgia Trauma Commission, May 11, 2007.

[15] Georgia Trauma Care Network Commission, 2006 Georgia Trauma Center Economic Analysis, March 2008.

[16] Georgia Trauma Care Network Commission, Minutes, June 8 2008.

[17] Ashley DW. The quest for sustainable trauma funding: The Georgia Story. Bulletin of the American College of Surgeons, October 2010.

[18] Taheri PA, Butz DA et al. The cost of trauma center readiness. *Am J Surg.* 2004 Jan; 187(1):7-13.

[19] Eastman AB, Rice CL, Bishop GS, et al: An analysis of the critical problem of trauma center reimbursement. *J. Trauma* 31:920, 1991.

[20] Trauma Center Association of America, Member communications, 2010.

[21] Bishop+Associates, Information from trauma centers operating comprehensive trauma medical staff billing programs, 1999.

[22] Healthcare Georgia Foundation. Trauma care in Georgia: Georgians are willing to pay for a statewide system. *HealthVoices.* 2008;23(2).

[23] Oregon Medicaid Program, Oregon Health Plan 1992.

[24] Trunkey DD, Lewis FR: Current Therapy of Trauma 4th Edition. The Economics of Trauma Care. Eastman AB, Bishop GS: 27, 1999.

[25] Birkmeyer, JD, Siewers AE, Finlayson, EV et al: Hospital Volume and Surgical Mortality in the United States; NEJM, 2002; 293:112-1137.

[26] Nathens, AB, Jurkovich, GJ, Maier, RV, Grossman, DC et al: Relationship Between Trauma Center Volume and Outcomes; *JAMA*, 2001; 285: 1164-1171.

[27] Georgia Trauma Care Network Commission, Trauma Center Readiness Costs, Webinar, December 16, 2009.

[28] Eastman AB, Bishop GS et al: The Economic Status of Trauma Centers on the Eve of Health Care Reform. *J. Trauma*, volume 36, number, 1994.

[29] Bishop+Associates, Managed Trauma Care Project, 1998.

[30] Campbell AR and Villinghoff E: Trauma centers in a managed care environment, 1 Trauma 39:246-251, 1995.

[31] Rachel Fields, Sullican Cotter and Associates: 5 Factors Affecting Physician On-Call Pay, March 22, 2011.

[32] American College of Surgeons. Sheldon, George. The Looming Challenge for Small Medical Practices: The Future Physician Shortage and How Health Care Reforms Can Address the Problem. July 8, 2009.

[33] Division of Public Health and Office of Emergency Medical Services. Serious Injury Crashes: Georgia 2003. April 2008.

[34] Georgia Trauma Care Network Commission, Performance Based Payment For Georgia Trauma, March 1, 2010.

[35] Georgia Department of Human Resources, Division of Public Health, Office of Emergency Medical Services/Trauma Operations Research and Analysis Section. Trauma in Georgia: Analysis of 2003 Trauma System Data. December 17, 2004. p. 30.

In: Toward Healthcare Resource Stewardship
Editors: J. S.Robinson, M. S.Walid et al.

ISBN: 978-1-62100-182-9
© 2012 Nova Science Publishers, Inc.

Chapter 3

ECONOMIC VIABILITY OF STROKE CENTERS - THE GEORGIA MODEL

Aaron C. M. Barth,[1] M. Sami Walid,[1]*
Michael J. Conforti[1] and Margaret C. Boltja[1,2]
[1]The Medical Center of Central Georgia, Macon, GA, US
[2]Neurology Associates, Macon, GA, US

ABSTRACT

Introduction: Hospitals serving regions with unfavorable payor mixes face a tension between providing optimal care and remaining financially viable. To demonstrate this fact we present our stroke center data with objective analysis of profit-loss ratios.

Materials and Methods: The hospital charges of stroke treated at the Georgia NeuroCenter between 2006 and 2008 were retrospectively analyzed. These included 535 hemorrhagic stroke patients, 1151 ischemic stroke patients, 2071 transient ischemic attack (TIA) patients. Approximately 82% of TIA patients were treated in an outpatient setting.

Results: DRGs 61-63 (Acute ischemic stroke with tPA) and DRGs 25-27 (Endovascular Intracranial Procedures) yield positive margins while DRGs 64-69 (Intracranial Hemorrhage, nonspecific CVA, transient ischemia) yield negative margins.

Conclusion: Hospitals with stroke centers struggle to balance the desire to provide optimal stroke care with the need to remain financially stable.

INTRODUCTION

The detrimental impact of stroke in the United States (U.S.) cannot be overstated. Approximately, 500,000 people suffer their first stroke annually and additional 250,000 suffer recurrent strokes [1,2]. Despite having one of the lowest mortality rates in the world, stroke is

---

* Corresponding Author: Aaron C.M. Barth, MBA. The Medical Center of Central Georgia, 777 Hemlock Street, Macon, GA 31201, USA. Email: aaron.barth@gmail.com.

the third most common cause of death in the U.S. behind heart disease and cancer [1-3]. Approximately 167,000 stroke-related deaths (33.4% of incidence) occur each year [2]. Stroke incidence, prevalence and death rates are highest in the southeastern states known as "The Stroke Belt." This is attributed to the high prevalence of minority races and people of lower socio-economic statuses [2, 4]. Blacks, American Indians/Alaska Natives, Asians/Pacific Islanders, and Hispanics die from stroke at younger ages than Whites [2-8], a phenomenon consistent with James Neel's 'thrifty genotype' hypothesis [6, 7] and the demographic transition paradigm.[8] The importance role of economics in stroke prevalence is highlighted through international comparison, with a ten-fold difference in burden of disease seen between the least affected and most affected countries and the national per capita income being the strongest predictor [1].

Stroke patients generally receive more consistent care with better outcome at nationally certified stroke centers. Thrombolysis is the key life-saving therapy for acute ischemic stroke patients. Recent Medicare reimbursement for providing this type of therapeutic treatment is sufficient. However, this is not the case for other types of stroke. Hospitals serving regions with unfavorable payor mixes face a tension between providing optimal care and remaining financially viable. To demonstrate this fact we present our stroke center data with objective analysis of profit-loss ratios.

MATERIALS AND METHODS

The hospital charges of stroke treated at the Georgia NeuroCenter between 2006 and 2008 were retrospectively analyzed. These included 535 hemorrhagic stroke patients, 1151 ischemic stroke patients, 2071 transient ischemic attack (TIA) patients. Approximately 82% of TIA patients were treated in an outpatient setting (Tables 1-3).

Table 1 shows the number of patients belonging to the hemorrhagic stroke category with the total and average values of hospital length of stay and cost associated with their treatment.

Table 2 shows the number of patients belonging to the ischemic stroke category with the total and average values of hospital length of stay and cost associated with their treatment.

Table 3 shows the number of patients belonging to the TIA category with the total and average values of hospital length of stay and cost associated with their treatment.

Hospital costs for stroke related DRGs were analyzed and compared to actual reimbursements based on our actual payor mix.

RESULTS

DRGs 61-63 (Acute ischemic stroke with tPA) and DRGs 25-27 (Endovascular Intracranial Procedures) yield positive margins. In most cases, reimbursement for DRGs 64-69 (Intracranial Hemorrhage, nonspecific CVA, transient ischemia) fails to cover the costs of providing the core measures required of national stroke centers. In other words, reimbursement for interventional DRGs results in profit while other stroke-related DRGs fail to cover the costs of providing core stroke measures (Figure 1)

Table 1.

Fiscal Year	Cases	Avg. Los	Total Cost	Total Cost/Case	Contribution Margin	Contribution Margin/Case	Profit Loss	Profit Loss/Case	Expired Cases
FY06	220	7.05	$3,577,300	$16,260	$1,921,621	$8,735	$115,083	$523	44
FY07	252	7.10	$4,352,921	$17,273	$2,179,881	$8,650	$81,564	$324	54
FY08 (Oct-Jun)	264	10.09	$7,350,470	$27,843	$3,770,208	$14,281	$337,481	$1,278	40
Hemorrhagic Total	736	8.16	$15,280,691	$20,762	$7,871,709	$10,695	$534,129	$726	138

Table 2.

Fiscal Year	Cases	Avg. Los	Total Cost	Total Cost/Case	Contribution Margin	Contribution Margin/Case	Profit Loss	Profit Loss/Case	Expired Cases
FY06	648	3.50	$4,100,225	$6,328	$1,458,802	$2,251	($806,862)	($1,245)	21
FY07	783	3.09	$4,522,708	$5,776	$1,779,491	$2,273	($641,268)	($819)	18
FY08 (Oct-Jun)	492	3.38	$3,305,300	$6,718	$1,189,149	$2,417	($559,923)	($1,138)	22
Ischemic Total	1923	3.30	$11,928,232	$6,203	$4,427,442	$2,302	($2,008,052)	($1,044)	61

Table 3.

Fiscal Year	Cases	Avg. Los	Total Cost	Total Cost/Case	Contribution Margin	Contribution Margin/Case	Profit Loss	Profit Loss/Case	Expired Cases
FY06	794	0.43	$1,008,078	$1,270	$355,880	$448	($231,668)	($292)	0
FY07	629	0.65	$1,114,495	$1,772	$514,117	$817	($136,678)	($217)	0
FY08 (Oct-Jun)	465	0.76	$1,027,175	$2,209	$304,019	$654	($285,715)	($614)	1
TIA Total	1888	0.58	$3,149,748	$1,668	$1,174,016	$622	($654,061)	($346)	1

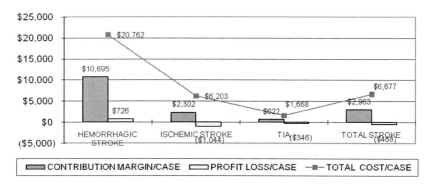

Figure 1. MCCG Stroke Financial Data - FY06-08 (Oct-Jun).

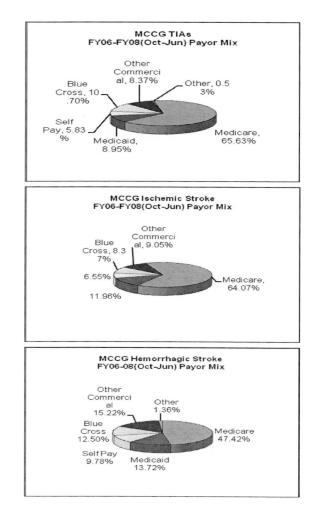

Figure 2. MCCG Stroke Data by Payor - FY06-08 (Oct-Jun).

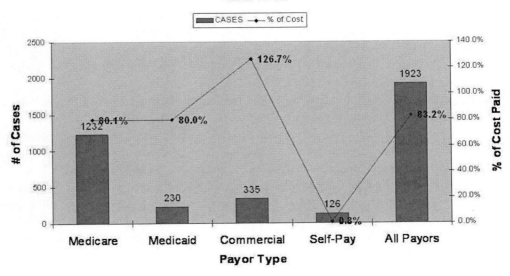

Figure 3. MCCG ischemic Stroke Data by Payor - FY06-08 (Oct-Jun).

Reimbursement for interventional diagnosis-related groups (DRGs) come close to break-even or result in profit depending on payor type (Figure 2). Studying the percentages of patients with the 4 major payment sources, slight variations in the percentages of indigent, Medicaid, Medicare, or private payors result in variations as to whether a hospital is able to break even in providing optimal stroke care. Approximately 80% of ischemic stroke costs are covered by Medicare and Medicaid whose beneficiaries make 76% of patients (Figure 3).

DISCUSSION

Nationwide, direct and indirect costs related to stroke are increasing steadily. In 2007 these costs reached $63 billion from $53 billion in 2004 [2, 9] The direct and indirect costs of stroke are formidable. Direct costs include ambulance services, expensive surgery, hospital stays, intensive rehabilitation, outpatient clinic visits, and drug therapy. Indirect costs to both patients and caregivers in form of lost wages, nursing home resources and other social coping costs are also substantial. The per capita cost of stroke is estimated at around $20,000 [9] The mean lifetime cost from an ischemic stroke is estimated at around $140,000 per patient [2]. Disability compensation and losses of earnings are the biggest cost contributor.

Tertiary care institutions with stroke centers must balance the desire to provide optimal stroke care with the need to simultaneously remain financially viable. This task proves more difficult when serving a higher percentage of patients with low funding sources. Developing telemedicine and stroke care networks, educating community members regarding the importance of rapid treatment, and encouraging payors to correctly align incentives for hospitals are vital tasks in promoting the provision of leading stroke care.

REFERENCES

[1]   Johnston SC, Mendis S, Mathers CD. Global variation in stroke burden and mortality: estimates from monitoring, surveillance, and modelling. *Lancet* 2009; DOI:10.1016/S1474-4422(09)70025-0.

[2]   Sarti C, Rastenyte D, Cepaitis Z, et al. International Trends in Mortality From Stroke, 1968 to 1994. *Stroke* 2000; 31 (7): 1588-601.

[3]   King H, Aubert RE, Herman WH. Global burden of diabetes, 1995-2025: prevalence, numerical estimates, and projections. *Diabetes Care* 1998; 21 (9): 1414-31.

[4]   Danaei G, Lawes CM, Van der Hoorn S, et al. Global and regional mortality from ischaemic heart disease and stroke attributable to higher-than-optimum blood glucose concentration: comparative risk assessment. *Lancet* 2006; 368 (9548): 1651-9.

[5]   Tassone EC, Waller LA, Casper ML. Small-Area Racial Disparity in Stroke Mortality: An Application of Bayesian Spatial Hierarchical Modeling. *Epidemiology* 2009: Epub ahead of print.

[6]   Chakravarthy MV, Booth FW. Eating, exercise, and "thrifty" genotypes: connecting the dots toward an evolutionary understanding of modern chronic diseases. *J. Appl. Physiol.* 2004; 96 (1): 3-10.

[7]   Neel JV. Diabetes mellitus a "thrifty" genotype rendered detrimental by "progress"? *Am. J. Hum. Genet.* 1962; 14: 353-62.

[8]   Yusuf S, Reddy S, Ounpuu S, et al. Global burden of cardiovascular diseases: part I: general considerations, the epidemiologic transition, risk factors, and impact of urbanization. *Circulation* 2001; 104: 2746-53.

[9]   NSA. National Stroke Association website: Recovery and rehabilitation Englewood CO National Stroke Association. Available from: http://www.stroke.org/site/PageServer?pagename=REHABT

In: Toward Healthcare Resource Stewardship
Editors: J. S.Robinson, M. S.Walid et al.

ISBN: 978-1-62100-182-9
© 2012 Nova Science Publishers, Inc.

Chapter 4

STRATEGIES TO IMPROVE COST-EFFICIENCY OF STROKE CARE: BOLSTERING AND LINKING STROKE AND TRAUMA CARE NETWORKS - THE GEORGIA MODEL

*Joe Sam Robinson[1,2,3] and M. Sami Walid[2]**

[1]Georgia Neurosurgical Institute, Macon, Georgia, US
[2]Medical Center of Central Georgia, Macon, Georgia, US
[3]Mercer University School of Medicine, Macon, Georgia, US

ABSTRACT

Access to trauma and stroke care in the United States is reasonably influenced by the profitability of those institutions that render care. Institutions existing in areas where geographic and demographic composition diminishes hospital profitability often are unable to offer these services. Hospitals facing these circumstances may choose not to offer these expensive services to their catchment area. This dysfunction causes significant discrepancies in patient mortality and morbidity related to trauma and stroke among different neighboring areas. Consequently, productive citizens are substracted from the National Labor Force and substantial governmental money is spent on treating the sequelae of trauma and stroke. The Gross National Product is thereby diminished. Rectification of this dysfunction can be solved by the establishment of a centralized system which will uniformly serve trauma and stroke patients as well as other citizens with compelling medical emergencies. An opportunity exists to better coordinate stroke care via bolstering the stroke system and combining it with the existing trauma care network. With limited resources available it is importance to make use of existent structures and find creative and cost-effective means for providing high quality stroke and trauma care.

---

* Corresponding Author: M. Sami Walid, PhD. 840 Pine Street, Suite 880, Medical Center of Central Georgia, Macon, GA 331201. Email: mswalid@yahoo.com.

INTRODUCTION

Stroke is the third most common cause of death after heart disease and cancer with significant differences across the states and within each state from one county to another [1, 2]. The age-adjusted mortality rate among adults over 35 years of age is on a range from 89 per 100,000 in New York State to 169 per 100,000 in South Carolina (1991-1998 data) [3]. Stroke is also a major cause of disability, with enormous physical and psychological impacts. The majority of strokes are ischemic, with a minority of hemorrhagic strokes and a residual amount being indistinguishable. Patients who suffer from strokes fare differently; 15% expire, 40% suffer from moderate to severe impairments that will require special rehabilitative care, 25% recover with minor impairments, 10% will require care in a long term facility, and 10% recover almost completely [4]. Acute-care costs incurred in the first two years following a stroke account for 45.0%, long-term ambulatory care account for 35.0%, and nursing home costs account for 17.5% of the aggregate lifetime cost of stroke [5]. Stroke care requires substantial health-care expenditures. The mean lifetime cost for an ischemic stroke is estimated at around $140,000 per patient [2]. The overall per capita cost of stroke is estimated at around $20,000, but per case cost estimates are highest among African Americans ($25,782), followed by Hispanics ($17,201), and non-Hispanic whites ($15,597) [6]. The direct costs of stroke come from ambulance services, expensive surgery, hospital stays, intensive rehabilitation, outpatient clinic visits, and drug therapy. Indirect costs to patients in terms of lost wages are also substantial. Nationwide, direct and indirect costs related to stroke were estimated around $69 billion in 2009, up from $53 billion in 2004 [7].

Stroke incidence, prevalence and death rates are highest in the southeastern states of the USA, nicknamed "The Stroke Belt." Our state, Georgia, is in the center of that belt. Georgia is home to a wide spectrum of socio-economic classes with clearly delineated areas of greater or lesser rates of poverty. The detrimental burden of stroke may be more pronounced among people of lower socio-economic statuses and especially among some minorities who carry higher risks of suffering from strokes with diabetes and hypertension being the main culprits and accounting for 10-15% of the disparity in the region and 30-40% of the disparity among blacks in the region [6, 8-10]. The total cost of stroke from 2005 to 2050 was projected to be $1.52 trillion (2005 US$) for non-Hispanic whites, $313 billion for Hispanics, and $379 billion for African Americans with disability compensation and loss of earnings being the highest cost contributor in each race-ethnic group [6].

Parallel to stroke problems, trauma contribute to a substantial number of deaths and disabilities annually. It is the leading cause of death for those under the age of 45 and the fourth leading cause of death for all Americans [11]. It is estimated by the Centers for Disease Control and Prevention (CDC) that 1.4 million sustain a traumatic brain injury each year in the United States; among these, 50,000 (3.6%) die, 235,000 (16.8%) are hospitalized and 1.1 million (78.6%) are treated and released from an emergency department [12]. In the early 1990s, the Trauma Care Systems Planning and Development Act of 1990 (P.L. 101-590) provided the ground for many states to develop publicly administered trauma systems leading to better outcomes and greater savings [13-15].

HYPOTHESIS

Recent studies have shown the important role of per capita income as a determinant of stroke and trauma mortality rate and disability-adjusted life-years loss [16-19]. In the State of Georgia, persistently high stroke and trauma mortality rates have become a clinical concern despite the invaluable servies provided by stroke and trauma centers accross the state [15]. Economic disparities among regions seem to impact the distribution of stroke and trauma care services which consequently affects mortality rates. In this paper we study the relationship between mortality rates for stroke and trauma patients and the distribution of stroke and trauma systems across the 10 Emergency Medical Services (EMS) regions of Georgia. We will also discuss the possible solutions for existing networks and ways to enhance their efficacy.

METHODS

As of June 2009, the State of Georgia had twenty-three stroke centers certified by the Joint Commission as "Primary Stroke Centers." These centers provide treatment according to nationally recognized measures and standards of care. It is reasonable that proximity to certified stroke centers is vital in dealing with ischemic stroke. Eligibility for rtPA therapy or the services of a neuro-interventionalist depends on quick triage. Delays in presentation to emergency rooms (ERs) have been reported as the primary reason behind missing the therapeutic 3-hour window for administering rtPA [20]. The same golden window applies to trauma patients, especially traumatic brain injury cases. Georgia has fifteen Level I and II Trauma Centers accross the state. A review of the geographic location of stroke and trauma centers reveals that the majority lie in EMS regions corresponding to large metropolitan areas of the state, primarily Atlanta, with at least two centers located in other major cities including Augusta, Columbus, Macon, Rome, and Savannah. The southernmost counties lying far from any certified stroke care services seem to be underserved compared to other Emergency Medical Service (EMS) regions (Figure 1). Ultimately, the goal of EMS services in situations of stroke and trauma is to provide timely transfer of patients to the next point of definitive care, the stroke or trauma center.

In our study the relationship between mortality rates for stroke and trauma patients and the distribution of stroke and trauma systems was investigated. We studied the following stroke-related variables: stroke morbidity rate, stroke mortality rate, the number of Stroke Centers per EMS regions, and the number of EMS vehicles in each region. In a parallel way we studied the following trauma-related variables: the number of Level I and II Trauma Centers, the number of EMS vehicles per region and the rate of traumatic death in each EMS region (Table 1). We used SPSS v16 to run analysis of covariance controlling for confounding variables.

Table 1. Trauma and stroke data in the State of Georgia per EMS regions

	EMS1	EMS2	EMS3	EMS4	EMS5	EMS6	EMS7	EMS8	EMS9	EMS10
Population (Thousand)	951	530	338	707	637	434	284	661	845	405
Population Density Per Square Mile	173	151	1441	184	74	82	82	69	67	135
Licenced Ambulance Services	31	21	68	28	26	17	17	35	34	13
Vehicles	176	108	673	129	143	77	63	157	158	58
Vehicles Per 100 Square Mile	3.2	3.1	29	3.4	1.7	1.5	1.5	1.5	1.3	1.8
Stroke Centers	3	0	11	0	1	2	2	0	2	1
Stroke Morbidity	180	201	192	243	249	223	241	224	219	222
Stroke Mortality	48	51	43	53	60	54	63	62	56	46
Stroke Incidence	1604	1093	5059	1583	1610	963	845	1332	1746	836
Stroke Deaths	410	262	1054	324	353	226	226	366	432	173
100 X Stroke Deaths/Incidence	26	24	21	20	22	23	27	27	25	21
Trauma Centers	2	0	6	0	1	1	1	1	1	2
Trauma Centers Levels I & II	2	0	5	0	1	1	1	1	1	0
Traumatic Deaths 2006	68	72	54	64	76	99	75	69	78	71
MVA 2000-2004	136742	83055	765811	115172	104272	81527	49735	88051	136684	67624
Fatalities from MVA	932	605	1995	640	806	454	235	880	979	461
Probability Of Dying From A Car Accident Per 1000	6.8	7.3	2.6	5.6	7.7	5.6	4.7	10.0	7.2	6.8
Neurosurgeons	7	4	65	1	8	22	3	8	13	6
Neurosurgeons Per 100000	1	1	2	0	1	5	1	1	2	1
Orthopedic Surgeons	48	36	283	34	43	63	31	62	66	15
Orthopedic Surgeons Per 100000	5	7	8	5	7	15	11	9	8	4
Trauma Surgeons	0	0	9	1	1	2	1	0	3	0
Trauma Surgeons Per 100000	0	0	0	0	0	0	0	0	0	0
Neurologists	10	9	159	18	12	41	5	14	25	9
Neurologists Per 100000	1	2	5	3	2	9	2	2	3	2

Probability Of Dying From A Car Accident Per 1000 = Fatalities from MVA / MVA 2000-2004.

RESULTS

A comparison of stroke resources between the EMS regions reveals a distorted pattern where most resources are concentrated in the large metropolitan area corresponding to EMS #3 region. We also see that the mortality rate from stroke per 100,000 population is lowest in this region. All other regions suffer from a higher mortality rate. Even EMS#1 region with a stroke morbidity rate that is lower than EMS#3 region has a higher mortality rate than EMS#3. This points to the strong relationship between tertiary care provided by specialized stroke centers and stroke outcome (Figure 2). Statistically, the number of stroke centers is a signifcant determinant of stroke mortality after controlling for the number of EMS vehicles per 100,000 population ($p<0.05$). The model accounts for 88% of the variance.

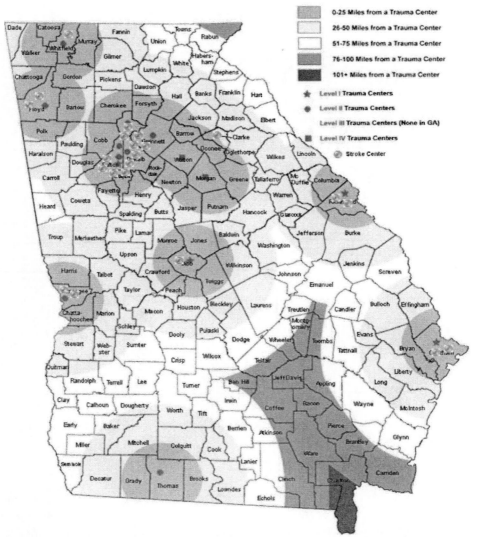

The original map was obtained from Georgia Office of Emergency Medical Servies/Trauma.

Figure 1. Distribution of stroke and trauma centers across the State of Georgia.

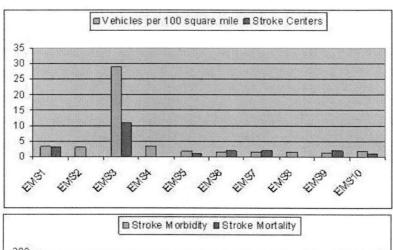

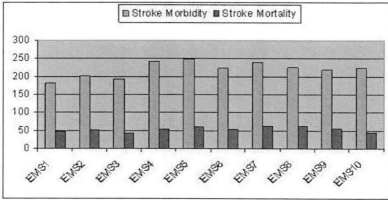

Dependent Variable:Stroke Mortality

Source	Type III Sum of Squares	df	Mean Square	F	Sig.
Corrected Model	393.837ª	5	78.767	15.323	.010
Intercept	42.011	1	42.011	8.172	.046
Vehiclesper100000	190.771	1	190.771	37.110	.004
StrokeCenters	196.539	4	49.135	9.558	.025
Error	20.563	4	5.141		
Total	29144.000	10			
Corrected Total	414.400	9			

a. R Squared = .950 (Adjusted R Squared = .888)

Data from the Division of Public Health, Office of Health Information and Policy, Georgia Department of Community Health.

Figure 2. Stroke morbidity, mortality and treatment resources in the State of Georgia per EMS regions.

Looking at the situation of the trauma network we find that EMS# 3 (Atlanta) region has the highest resources in terms of trauma centers and EMS vehicles per 100,000 population and lowest mortality rate from traumatic death (Figure 3). Statistically, the number of level I and II Trauma centers is close to statistical significance if we control for the number of vehicles per population. This speaks to a similar trend in the trauma system as well.

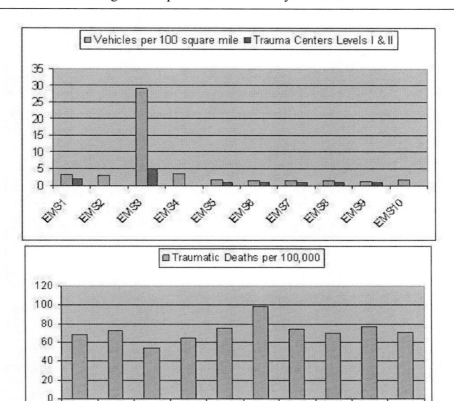

Dependent Variable:Traumatic Deaths					
Source	Type III Sum of Squares	df	Mean Square	F	Sig.
Corrected Model	853.001ª	4	213.250	3.100	.123
Intercept	1427.674	1	1427.674	20.756	.006
Vehiclesper100000	207.872	1	207.872	3.022	.143
TraumaCentersLevelsIII	837.810	3	279.270	4.060	.083
Error	343.915	5	68.783		
Total	53730.420	10			
Corrected Total	1196.916	9			

a. R Squared = .713 (Adjusted R Squared = .483)

Data from the Division of Public Health, Office of Health Information and Policy, Georgia Department of Community Health.

Figure 3. Incidence of traumatic death and trauma treatment resources in the State of Georgia per EMS regions.

The regions with the highest poverty rates in Georgia, as indicated by the US census Bureau, seem to inversely correlate with the availability of stroke and trauma centers. If we compare EMS#3 and EMS#8 regions we see wide divergence in trauma and stroke resources and outcomes (Figure 4).

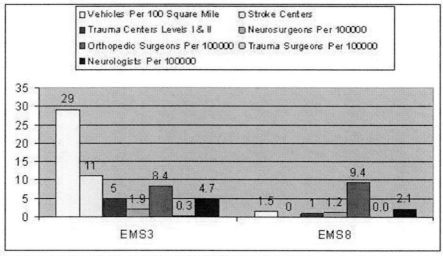

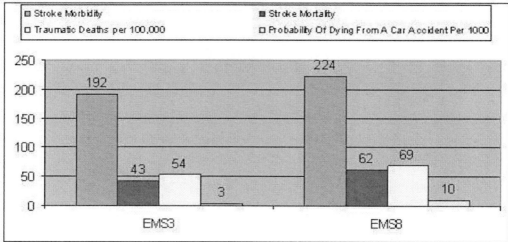

Data from the Division of Public Health, Office of Health Information and Policy, Georgia Department
of Community Health.

Figure 4. Comparison of trauma and stroke resources and outcome between EMS#3 (Atlanta) region
and EMS#8 (Southwest Georgia) region.

It appears that issues of population density seem to play a pivotal role among the reasons
why tertiary care centers have not spread throughout Georgia. We will discuss why we need
to work hard to address the stroke and trauma needs of the state as a whole as opposed to
merely in the urban centers where tertiary care centers are preferably located.

DISCUSSION

The findings above demonstrate the necessity to improve stroke and trauma situation.
This will require local and federal payors and private healthcare providers to spend more
effort on three fronts: addressing risk factors of stroke and methods of prevention, improving

the efficacy of treatment and intervention protocols, and promoting better rehabilitation for these patients in order to speed up their return to society. From an acute standpoint, effective treatment depends on an efficient emergency transportation system. Ideally, these transporters would transfer patients with suspected stroke diagnosis to centers that specialize in stroke care and trauma patients to hospitals where specialized trauma units are available that can provide the best care for these patients. Certified stroke centers rapidly assess patients and provide complete diagnostic testing within 45 minutes of arrival to the hospital with acute stroke symptoms. A significant advancement in the management of acute ischemic stroke has been the advent of thrombolytic therapy. Recombinant tissue plasminogen activator (rtPA) is administered within three hours of symptom onset, with recent studies suggesting that the window be extended to 4.5 hours [21-23]. Advances in neuro-interventional technology have allowed for more window extension in some instances of ischemic stroke with the use of thrombectomy devices [24, 25], although possession of these technologies are not indispensable requirements for establishing a primary stroke center. Overall, stroke centers are generally equipped with state-of-the-art technology and staffed with highly trained clinicians, including neurologists and neurosurgeons, which enable these centers to provide high-quality treatment for stroke patients. The the American Heart Association (AHA) and the American Stroke Association (ASA) have recently introduced a hospital-based quality improvement initiative to improve the care of patients with cardiac diseases and stroke and support the AHA mission to reduce death and disability from these diseases [26] .

Hospitals in regions with higher rates of poverty may be discouraged from establishing stroke centers because of the foreseen financial loss associated with it. The investments that are required of hospitals to establish a stroke center are usually formidable. As previously described, certified stroke centers must possess the essential staff and technology to meet national guidelines for stroke care. Reimbursement arrangements force caregivers to consider the profit and loss of investing in a stroke center, especially with the current financial pressures that create disincentives for acute stroke treatment. In light of the unfavorable reimbursement rates, hospitals must often look to other sources of funding or rely on treatment of higher volumes of non-government patients in order to achieve balance leverage. In regions with higher poverty rates, patients rely more heavily on government healthcare funding. This reality may inhibit hospitals that treat these patients from earning sufficient reimbursement required to sustain their operations. A 2006 Duke University study revealed that in 2005, US hospitals lost an average of $2,100-$3,700 for treating Medicare patients with strokes [27]. In this study, Medicare patients represented 72% of the patients. Analysis of 2006-2008 data from the Medical Center of Central Georgia in Macon reveals similar results: only 80.1% of the hospital's total costs have been paid by the government for Medicare ischemic stroke patients, who represent 64% of the total number of patients.

Hospital system viability depends on the ability of providers to cope with the cost of rendered care, and these providers cannot do so without sufficient reimbursement. A question worthy of further investigation is whether there is a trapping cycle whereby populations in poorer regions unable to provide enough reimbursement to justify building new stroke centers experience worse healthcare outcomes which result in greater economic privation further encouraging self-neglect and health deterioration. Eventually, society as a whole end up carrying the expenses associated with bad health outcomes and long-term care cost.

There is a real need to find ways to establish stroke centers more broadly throughout Georgia to provide high-quality stroke care. A bolstered stroke system and coordination with the already established trauma care network may be a plausible solution. An effective pre-hospital acute stroke triage, advanced hospital notification by the EMS, the creation of an acute stroke team in each hospital, reducing delays in performing computed tomography imaging and delivering thrombolysis treatment right in the emergency department (ED) are measures that have been suggested as possible solutions to increase stroke care efficiency [28-32]. Emergency physicians are trained to receive and assess patients with possible stroke and can integrally be involved in the delivery of thrombolysis to patients with acute ischemic stroke through communication and collaboration with local neurologists and radiologists [31]. The concept of "telemedicine" is another option that may be a less expensive alternative to building new stroke centers. It involves using emergency departments with remote visual and phonic guidance from distant neurologists to treat incoming stroke patients [33-35]. With such guidance, appropriate treatment therapies could then be administered in the rural setting or a determination could be made to immediately transfer the patient to a stroke center.

State legislators have taken initial steps to promote this type of networking through the Coverdell-Murphy Act (GA Senate Bill 549) which passed in 2008 [36]. This bill seeks to establish standards and practices regarding stroke care centers and aims to create a systematized network of certified stroke centers. Ultimately, with better funding the hope is that all citizens of Georgia would have access to either a nearby primary stroke center or a local treatment center that can connect efficiently with a primary stroke center. This would be important for improving the coordination of care and timely treatment for stroke patients. The key point in this period of economic travail is to efficiently use pre-existing networks without a great deal of additional cost.

Similarities between the trauma and stroke systems abound. Trauma victims experience the best chances of recovery if they can be treated in the "golden hour" after injury and stroke victims similarly face an urgency to receive care within the "golden window" in order to have the best possible clinical outcomes [37]. Both types of patients require access to care centers that have invested in appropriate readiness costs, can provide emergency transportation, have rapid triage capabilities and centralized resource allocation. A coordinated stroke network would appear to naturally fit with the trauma network already existent in the state. It has already been argued that a coordinated trauma network would result in tremendous economic savings for the State of Georgia [15]. The trauma system investment and development experience in Georgia can be used as a paradigm to help structure an efficient state-wide stroke network.

Developing a coordinated statewide stroke network alongside the pre-established trauma network might offer great benefits to citizens and savings to the healthcare system. Collaboration between the centers that serve as part of both the trauma and stroke networks could also yield positive potential returns for infrastructure investment and benefit of the state. If such systems were successful, the citizens of Georgia might see a positive long-term decrease in stroke and trauma mortality rates, particularly in the areas without immediate access to specialized centers. As a palliative strategy in the absence of a comprehensive stroke policy that addresses disparities in health and healthcare, supporting primary care medicine may serve the stroke cause by early recognition of stroke symptoms and promoting stroke awareness in the population [38, 39].

CONCLUSION

Stroke and trauma care are two healthcare challenges for the State of Georgia and the U.S. healthcare systems. Legitimate concerns face Georgia healthcare providers as they seek to provide adequate stroke care to their citizens. Many of the State's poorest regions are located farthest from certified stroke centers and suffer from the highest stroke mortality rates. Addressing these disparities requires focused and creative efforts on the part of both healthcare providers and policymakers. With limited resources available it is of paramount importance to make use of existent structures and find creative and cost-effective means for providing care. While stroke prevention is an imperative State responsibility, linking the State's stroke and trauma centers via a centralized coordinated network may be a key step in diminishing the deleterious effects of stroke and trauma incidence.

It is vital to consider the health impact of strengthening the stroke and trauma network along with the expense. The long-term economic benefits of effectively treating stroke victims and restoring them to productivity are understandable. By returning people to normal life they subsequently make substantial societal contributions and provide the state with a worthwhile return on its initial investment. More economic analysis studies are needed to determine the potential positive returns from investment in stroke research [40]. Further investment is warranted not only to find new ways for treating stroke, but also to expand the capacity of the healthcare system to ensure equitable access to population groups that need it most. The positive correlation between population health, healthcare resources, and productivity should always be the basis for healthcare decisions, not only related to stroke, but for all health-related issues.

A final word, a National and State-wide coordinated stroke-trauma policy would be advantageous. Such policies would have the potential to affect stroke and trauma outcome across the states and populations. The Heart Disease and Stroke Prevention Policy Project introduced lately by the Centers for Disease Control and Prevention (CDC) is a good example [41]. More economic statistics are needed to allow full assessment of stroke-related healthcare costs. The long term financial benefit of additional expenditures on stroke centers can be difficult to comprehend when healthcare decision makers contemplate cost-benefit ratios. Consequently, a direct analysis of stroke economics will help understand the potential benefits that might result from improvements in the stroke care systems.

REFERENCES

[1]   Rosamond, W., et al., Heart disease and stroke statistics--2007 update: a report from the American Heart Association Statistics Committee and Stroke Statistics Subcommittee. *Circulation*, 2007. 115(5): p. e69-171.

[2]   Prevalence of stroke--United States, 2005. *MMWR Morb. Mortal. Wkly Rep*, 2007. 56(19): p. 469-74.

[3]   Casper, M.L., et al., Atlas of Stroke Mortality: Racial, Ethnic, and Geographic Disparities in the United States. 2003, Department of Health and Human Services, Centers for Disease Control and Prevention.: Atlanta, GA.

[4]   Stroke Rehabilitation Information. 06/22/07 08/17/09]; Available from:

http://www.ninds.nih.gov/disorders/stroke/stroke_rehabilitation.htm.

[5]   Taylor, T.N., et al., Lifetime cost of stroke in the United States. *Stroke*, 1996. 27(9): p. 1459-66.

[6]   Brown, D.L., et al., Projected costs of ischemic stroke in the United States. *Neurology*, 2006. 67(8): p. 1390-5.

[7]   Lloyd-Jones, D., et al., Heart disease and stroke statistics--2009 update: a report from the American Heart Association Statistics Committee and Stroke Statistics Subcommittee. *Circulation*, 2009. 119(3): p. 480-6.

[8]   Racial/ethnic and socioeconomic disparities in multiple risk factors for heart disease and stroke--United States, 2003. *MMWR Morb. Mortal. Wkly Rep*, 2005. 54(5): p. 113-7.

[9]   Tassone, E.C., L.A. Waller, and M.L. Casper, Small-area racial disparity in stroke mortality: an application of bayesian spatial hierarchical modeling. *Epidemiology*, 2009. 20(2): p. 234-41.

[10]   Longstreth, W.T., Jr., The REasons for Geographic And Racial Differences in Stroke (REGARDS) Study and the National Institute of Neurological Disorders and Stroke (NINDS). *Stroke*, 2006. 37(5): p. 1147.

[11]   Goldfarb, M.G., G.J. Bazzoli, and R.M. Coffey, Trauma systems and the costs of trauma care. *Health Serv. Res*, 1996. 31(1): p. 71-95.

[12]   Langlois, J.A., W. Rutland-Brown, and K.E. Thomas, Traumatic brain injury in the United States: emergency department visits, hospitalizations, and deaths. 2004, Centers for Disease Control and Prevention, National Center for Injury Prevention and Control: Atlanta, GA.

[13]   Hulka, F., et al., Influence of a statewide trauma system on pediatric hospitalization and outcome. *J. Trauma*, 1997. 42(3): p. 514-9.

[14]   Miller, T.R. and D.T. Levy, The effect of regional trauma care systems on costs. *Arch. Surg*, 1995. 130(2): p. 188-93.

[15]   Robinson, J.S., Jr., et al., Economic impact model for the development of a statewide trauma system in Georgia. *J. Med. Assoc. Ga*, 2007. 96(3): p. 10-3.

[16]   Johnston, S.C., S. Mendis, and C.D. Mathers, Global variation in stroke burden and mortality: estimates from monitoring, surveillance, and modelling. *Lancet Neurol*, 2009. 8(4): p. 345-54.

[17]   Feigin, V.L., et al., Worldwide stroke incidence and early case fatality reported in 56 population-based studies: a systematic review. *Lancet Neurol*, 2009. 8(4): p. 355-69.

[18]   van Beeck, E.F., et al., Determinants of traffic accident mortality in The Netherlands: a geographical analysis. *Int. J. Epidemiol*, 1991. 20(3): p. 698-706.

[19]   Shafi, S., et al., Effect of trauma systems on motor vehicle occupant mortality: A comparison between states with and without a formal system. *J. Trauma*, 2006. 61(6): p. 1374-8; discussion 1378-9.

[20]   Barber, P.A., et al., Why are stroke patients excluded from TPA therapy? An analysis of patient eligibility. *Neurology*, 2001. 56(8): p. 1015-20.

[21]   Hill, M.D., ACP Journal Club. Alteplase given 3 to 4.5 hours after stroke reduced disability and improved global outcome. *Ann. Intern. Med*, 2009. 150(2): p. JC1-13.

[22]   Uyttenboogaart, M., et al., [Treatment of acute ischemic stroke with intravenous thrombolysis: extension of the time window should not delay initiation of treatment]. *Ned. Tijdschr. Geneeskd*, 2008. 152(49): p. 2653-5.

[23] Hacke, W., et al., Thrombolysis with alteplase 3 to 4.5 hours after acute ischemic stroke. *N. Engl. J. Med*, 2008. 359(13): p. 1317-29.

[24] Gobin, Y.P., et al., MERCI 1: a phase 1 study of Mechanical Embolus Removal in Cerebral Ischemia. *Stroke*, 2004. 35(12): p. 2848-54.

[25] Bose, A., et al., The Penumbra System: a mechanical device for the treatment of acute stroke due to thromboembolism. *AJNR Am. J. Neuroradiol*, 2008. 29(7): p. 1409-13.

[26] Smaha, L.A., The American Heart Association get with the guidelines program. *American Heart Journal*, 2004. 148(5): p. S46-48.

[27] Marotta, C., et al., Impact of length of stay and costs on the ability of hospitals to adopt new technology for the treatment of acute ischemic stroke patients, in International Stroke Conference. 2006: Kissimmee, FL.

[28] Quain, D.A., et al., Improving access to acute stroke therapies: a controlled trial of organised pre-hospital and emergency care. *Med. J. Aust*, 2008. 189(8): p. 429-33.

[29] Nazir, F.S., I. Petre, and H.M. Dewey, Introduction of an acute stroke team: an effective approach to hasten assessment and management of stroke in the emergency department. *J. Clin. Neurosci*, 2009. 16(1): p. 21-5.

[30] Abdullah, A.R., et al., Advance hospital notification by EMS in acute stroke is associated with shorter door-to-computed tomography time and increased likelihood of administration of tissue-plasminogen activator. *Prehosp. Emerg. Care*, 2008. 12(4): p. 426-31.

[31] Kendall, J., Thrombolysis for acute ischaemic stroke: a new challenge for emergency medicine. *Emerg. Med. J*, 2008. 25(8): p. 471-5.

[32] Mehdiratta, M., et al., Reducing the delay in thrombolysis: is it necessary to await the results of renal function tests before computed tomography perfusion and angiography in patients with code stroke? *J. Stroke Cerebrovasc. Dis*, 2008. 17(5): p. 273-5.

[33] Hess, D.C., et al., REACH: clinical feasibility of a rural telestroke network. *Stroke*, 2005. 36(9): p. 2018-20.

[34] Vaishnav, A.G., L.C. Pettigrew, and S. Ryan, Telephonic guidance of systemic thrombolysis in acute ischemic stroke: safety outcome in rural hospitals. *Clin. Neurol. Neurosurg*, 2008. 110(5): p. 451-4.

[35] Semplicini, A., et al., Intravenous thrombolysis in the emergency department for the treatment of acute ischaemic stroke. *Emerg. Med. J*, 2008. 25(7): p. 403-6.

[36] Coverdell-Murphy Act, in Official Code of Georgia Annotated.

[37] Blow, O., et al., The golden hour and the silver day: detection and correction of occult hypoperfusion within 24 hours improves outcome from major trauma. *J. Trauma*, 1999. 47(5): p. 964-9.

[38] Shi, L., et al., Primary care, income inequality, and stroke mortality in the United States: a longitudinal analysis, 1985-1995. *Stroke*, 2003. 34(8): p. 1958-64.

[39] York, K.A., Rural case management for stroke: the development of a community-based screening and education program. *Lippincotts Case Manag*, 2003. 8(3): p. 98-114; quiz 115-6.

[40] Johnston, S.C., The 2008 William M. Feinberg lecture: prioritizing stroke research. *Stroke*, 2008. 39(12): p. 3431-6.

[41] Ford Lattimore B, O.N.S., Besculides M., Tools for developing, implementing, and evaluating state policy. *Prev. Chronic. Dis*, 2008. 5(2): p. A58.

In: Toward Healthcare Resource Stewardship
Editors: J. S.Robinson, M. S.Walid et al.

ISBN: 978-1-62100-182-9
© 2012 Nova Science Publishers, Inc.

Chapter 5

STRATEGIES TO IMPROVE COST-EFFICIENCY OF STROKE CARE: STROKE UNITS AND TELESTROKE

Minal Jain, Anunaya Jain and Babak S. Jahromi*

Department of Neurosurgery,
University of Rochester Medical Center, Rochester, NY, US

ABSTRACT

Background: New treatments, protocols and technologies have been emerging for effective management of stroke. Establishment of a Stroke Unit (SU) has been one of the oldest concepts that has undergone constant change over time while consistently improving outcomes in stroke patients. On the other hand, Telestroke, a relatively new concept has also proven its mettle in expediting diagnosis and decision making for inaccessible stroke patients. This chapter presents a brief literature review comparing outcome and costs of care in SU versus conventional care (CC). As a secondary aim we also analyze which SU subtype is the most cost effective. We also present a business case for cost effectiveness of Telestroke.

Methods: A Pubmed search was performed with the search term "stroke unit" to access all English language studies published from 01/01/1996 to 01/01/2011. Of these, articles reporting length of stay and/or cost and outcomes were included for the review. Articles wherein research was conducted before 01/01/1996; articles reporting only on rehabilitation units and all review articles were excluded. Costs of care were documented from the studies themselves or by using length of stay as a surrogate. Logistic regressions from literature were used to convert all non-QALY (quality-adjusted life year) outcome measures to QALYs. All cost were reported in 2010 US \$. Incremental Cost Effectiveness ratios (ICER) were calculated for care at SU versus CC. Cost/QALY and weighted average of the cost effectiveness ratios were calculated for different types of stroke units [acute only SU, acute + rehabilitation SU (acute + rehab SU), acute + rehabilitation + early supported discharge (acute + Rehab + ESD SU) and SU with

---

* Corresponding Author: Jain Minal, 601, Elmwood Ave. Box 670, University of Rochester Medical Center, Rochester, NY 14642. Email: minal_jain@urmc.rochester.edu.

continuous monitoring]. Ratios less than $50,000/QALY were considered cost effective and ratios greater than $100,000 /QALY were considered non-cost effective.

We also searched Pubmed for all studies on "Telestroke" networks conducted across the developed world in English language. For simplicity we have presented an overall perspective of this technology from the perspective of the healthcare system. Further, we did a meta-analysis comparing the cost savings offered by a Telestroke networks to traditional care models for treating acute ischemic stroke patients. We also simulated revenue generation and compared them to reported costs of initiation of Telestroke networks to conduct a break-even probability analysis. A sensitivity analysis was also done to comment on the robustness of this model to changing variable costs of Telestroke mediated care.

Results: Review of Stroke Units - A total of 5537 articles in Pubmed were studied, of which 19 studies met the inclusion criteria. 7 studies had comparison reported between SU and CC. Length of stay for patients managed at SU ranged from 9.2-32.3 days versus 8-35.3 days for CC units and average incremental QALY between them were 0.09. The average incremental cost/QALY was $41,204.37. The average cost/QALY for different types of SU were $19,428.64 for acute only SU, $44,228.81 for acute +rehab SU, $29,145.93 for acute +rehab+ESD SU and $20,460.56 for SU with continuous monitoring. In comparison to an acute only SU, SU with continuous monitoring and acute+rehab+ESD SU were cost effective alternatives. (ICER SU with continuous monitoring – $25,120.89, ICER acute+rehab+ESD - $24,574.59).

Review of Telestroke – A total of 15 Telestroke networks were analyzed. Of almost 24,000 consultations nearly 10.8% had received IV thrombolytic therapy, which translated into cost savings of $90,000 per 100 consultations. The average duration of consultation reported by these networks was 28.25 minutes (SD 18.86 minutes) generating an average revenue of $48.7 per consultation for the healthcare system. The total approximate fixed costs of setup was $33,400/year/spoke site. While conducting the simulation analysis we found that at least 283 patients are needed to break even for the investment costs of telestroke, with just reimbursement of consultation costs. After introducing uncertainties, the model generated a probability of 80.1% that the network would break-even its costs within the first year of operations. After accounting for increasing variable costs of operations and maintenance of the network, we concluded that the if the hub-unit sees atleast 283 patients annually, and if variable costs are kept below $35/patients, the Telestroke model would prove to be sustainable and cost effective.

Conclusion: Stroke Units and Telestroke seems to be cost effective strategies when compared to the conventional systems of care. Active collaborations between different in-hospital services to create a cohesive environment conducive to specialized care of stroke patients, and inter-hospital networks to leverage infrastructure and clinical expertise are both initiatives that should be pursued widely.

1. INTRODUCTION

Stroke is the leading cause of disability and the third leading of cause of death worldwide after heart disease and cancer. Annually, nearly 15 million people suffer from stroke worldwide of which nearly 5.3% are in the United States (U.S.) alone. [1] Leaving approximately 33% disabled, and an equal number dead worldwide, stroke remains a disease yet to be conquered. In addition to its profound physical, psychological and social impact, stroke exacts an enormous economic burden on the healthcare system. Effective treatment of stroke patients consists of a survival-chain from emergency care, acute management in a stroke unit, through the complex of neuro-rehabilitation and return to home/work environment.

Many advances have been made in stroke prevention, imaging, and treatment of stroke over the past twenty years. The advent of intravenous recombinant tissue plasminogen activator (IV rt-PA) in 1995 as a thrombolytic for ischemic stroke [2] significantly improvedpatient outcomes. Adoption of improved practices decreased the mortality rate of stroke by 34.3% between 1997-2007 in U.S. [3] Costs of stroke care have however sustained their escalating spiral. In 2007, the direct and indirect costs of stroke in U.S. were estimated to be $40.9 million. The mean lifetime cost per patient was estimated to approximate $140,048. This included the inpatient care, the rehabilitation and follow up cost [3, 4]. The estimated cost of care for patients with stroke in 2010 is $73.7 billion, for both direct and indirect costs. [1] Given the increasing prevalence of stroke in the U.S., projected costs of stroke care from 2005-2050 will exceed $2 trillion. [1]

Emergingconcepts of stroke teams, uniform treatment protocols, stroke units, primary stroke centers for the effective management of stroke patients [5] and Telestroke to expedite the diagnosis and decision making for inaccessible patients have been widely investigated as cost-effective interventions [6-12]. For the first part of this paper we concentrate on Stroke Units and in the later section we present a case for the adoption of Telestroke networks.

2. STROKE UNITS

Background

Of all the above strategies, Stroke Unit (SU) has probably remained the most analyzed, with the earliest studies dating back to the 1970s. There has been a paradigm shift in the functioning of these units over time. Earlier, SUs were specialized inpatient care units specifically designed for the sole purpose of assistive rehabilitation of stroke patients. Over the years, the goals of SUs have shifted to careof acute stroke patients, provision ofimproved diagnostic accuracy, systematic prevention of complications through specialized nursing care and appropriate monitoring with early rehabilitation [13-15].

The Joint Commission in December 1993 approved guidelines for the establishment of Primary stroke centers, listing an SU as one of its desirable features. Varied types of SUs have been described in literature. An intensive SU is a specific geographic area within the healthcare facility that caters to only specific cases or is used solely for post-operative monitoring. Acute only SU are described as units that care for acute/subacutestroke patients, with the goal of discharging them within 7-10 days. Acute andRehabilitation Stroke units (Acute + Rehab SU) are designed to provide both early acute care as well as rehabilitative facilities. SU with early supported discharge (Acute + Rehab + ESD SU) provide acute care and initial rehabilitation at the hospital that continues at home with support from other community services if needed. Their aim is to accelerate discharge of patient to home from hospital and provide the rehabilitation/support in the home setting. Arecent concept in SU is the SU with continuous monitoring that is analogous to an intensive care unit caring solely for stroke patients. In addition to these there are alsostroke units that concentrate purely on rehabilitation of stroke patients once they have survived the acute episode itself [16-18].

In the past, researchers have compared the care and services offered in a SU with that in a general medical ward or a neurology ward. [19-24] The consensus view of these studies has remained that SU significantly reduces length of stay in hospital, mortality and an increases the proportion of dischargesto home. [25, 26] But healthcare systems have remained hesitant to adopt this system of care. A survey in 2001 revealed that only 38% of Primary Stroke Centers (PSCs) in U.S. had a stroke unit [27]. Some of the main reasons cited for this reluctant implementation of SU have been the extra resources required, both human and infrastructure, and the perceived high setup costs.

Our aim in this section of the paper was to conduct a literature review comparing outcomes and costs of care for stroke patients treated in a stroke unit compared to conventional general wards or neurology units.We also compare outcomes and costs of care for patients treated in different types of stroke units. A number of researchers have studied the cost effectiveness of SU before 1996. [24, 28-30] Following FDA approval of IV rt-PA in 1996 and its gradual adoption as the standard of carefor treatment for eligible ischemic stroke since then, the outcomes and costs of care for these patients have changed drastically. [31] Thus we felt it imperative to restrict this analysis to only studies conducted in the post IV rt-PA era. To the best of our knowledge, this remains the first analysis of its kind.

Cost Effectiveness Analysis – Methods

We present a cost effectiveness analysis ofstroke units in the post rt-PA era. We compared incremental outcomes and costs for stroke patients treated in a stroke unit compared to traditional neurology or general wards. We also compared cost effectiveness ratios for different types of stroke units.

A literature search was performed using the search term "Stroke Unit" in the Pubmed database. We limited this search to manuscripts published in English from 01/01/1996 to 01/01/2011. Any studies classified as reviews were excluded. We further restricted eligible studies to those that were conducted in developed countries only. This was done because of the assumption that the stroke care costs differ substantially between developed and developing countries. We excluded any studies that initiated data collection prior to 1996, to ensure that no patients treated prior to the introduction of IV rt-PA would be included in our analysis. We also excluded studies that reported data on purely rehabilitative SUs. Once these studies were identified they were analyzed to ensure documentation of costs and outcomes. Any study that documented cost/hospital admission per patient, long term costs of care or the surrogate marker of costs - length of stay in hospital was included. Studies eligible for inclusion were also mandated to have one of the following quantifiable measures of outcomes for stroke patients - modified Rankin score (mRS), National Institute of Health Stroke Severity (NIHSS), Barthel Index (BI), modified BI, Functional Independence Measurement (FIM), Activity of Daily Living scores (ADL), Quality Adjusted Life Years (QALY).

Costs of care were documented directly from the studies wherever given. Non US$ costs were converted into US$ using historical rates of conversion. [32] These were then inflated to 2010 US$. [33] Average costs of each in-hospital day were calculated from these costs ($1049.78). For studies that reported only length of stay this average measure was used to calculate costs of in-patient care. All non-QALY outcomes were converted into QALYs using logistic regressions. [10, 34-36] These conversions are shown in the Table-1.

Table 1. Conversion of outcome measures to QALY

FIM to Barthel Index	$BI = 0.297^{*}FIM - 6.212$
Barthel Index to modified Barthel Index	$mBI = 0.579 + 0.222*BI$
ADL to Modified Barthel Index	$mBI = ADL^{*} 20/ADLitems$
Modified Barthel Index to QALY	$QALY = 0.05^{*}mBI - 0.25$
Modified Rankin Score to QALY	$QALY = mRS^{*}0.7 - 0.12$
NIHSS to QALY	$QALY = 0.2882-0.0247^{*}NIHSS$

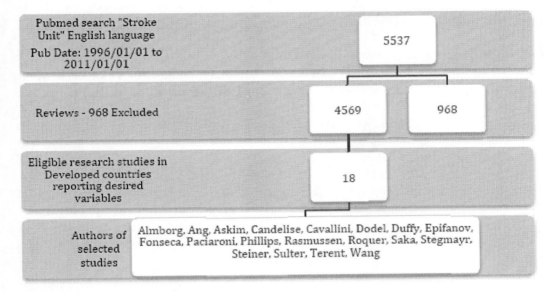

Figure 1. Inclusion of studies in review of stroke units post 1996.

For the different types of SUs we calculated costs/QALY and a weighted average of these cost-effectiveness ratios. Ratios less than \$50,000/QALY were considered as cost effective. Ratios between \$50,000/QALY and \$100,000/QALY were considered as possibly cost effective and any ratio beyond \$100,000/QALY were considered non cost effective.

Incremental cost effectiveness ratios were calculated for studies that compared stroke units to other conventional care units using the formula:

$$\frac{Costs_{SU}- Costs_{comparison}}{QALY_{SU} - QALY_{comparison}}$$

Cost Effectiveness Analysis - Results

We reviewed a total of 5537 articles in Pubmed with the pre-defined search criteria and excluded 968 review articles from them. Of the remaining 4569, only 19 met the inclusion criteria (Figure -1). There were 4 studies conducted in Sweden, 3 in Italy, 2 in Australia, 2 in Germany, 1 in US, 1 in UK, 1 in Norway, 1 in Canada, 1 in Portugal, 1 in Spain, 1 in Austria, and 1 in Netherlands.

Cost Effectiveness of Stroke Unit vs.Conventional Care Units (Table- 2)

Of all the articles included in the review, 7 studies had comparisons between SU and conventional care units. The length of stay for patients managed in a stroke unit ranged from 9.2 to 32.3 days vs. 8-35.3 days for management in a general or neurology ward. The average incremental QALY for patients admitted to SU vsconventional care was 0.0903. The average incremental cost/patient was $1,623.55. The overall average incremental cost/QALY was $41,204.37. Only one of the studies (Saka et al) studied long term outcomes and costs (10 years) after a stroke unit admission.

Cost Effectiveness of Different Types of SU

Acute only SU (Table- 3): There were a total 11 studies for this group. The average length of stay in hospital for stroke patients admitted to acute Stroke unit was 8.01 days (range 5.8-25). The average cost/QALY was $19,428.64.

Acute + rehab SU (Table- 4): There were a total of 6 studies, which reported data on this variety of SU. The average length of stay per patient was 18.2 days (range 13.6-34). The average cost/QALY was $44,228.81.

Acute + rehab +ESD SU (Table- 5): There were a total of 3 studies, which reported data regarding stroke patients admitted to Acute+rehab +ESD stroke unit.The average length of stay per patient was 11.23days (range 11-32.3). The average cost/QALY was $29,145.93.

SU with continuous monitoring (Table- 6): There were 3 studies that were reviewed for this subtype of SU. The average length of stay in hospital for stroke patients was 9.63 days (range 9.1-16). The average cost/QALY was $20,460.56.

There was no study that estimated costs of care in a SU with continuous monitoring. Costs were therefore estimated based on length of stay. However, this may underestimate costs, as it is unlikely that costs per day would remain the same when continuous monitoring is added. In order to adjust for this, we re-analyzed the data by increasing costs by 100%. The average cost per QALY with this sensitivity analysis was still $40,921.11/QALY.

The most effective of the various subtypes seems to be the Acute + Rehab + ESD SU. Patients in these units reported a QALY of 0.574 at the end of therapy. The costliest is expectedly the Acute + Rehab SU with average costs of $19,109.45 per patient. The cheapest strategy appears to be the Acute only SU ($19,428.64/QALY). On calculating incremental cost effectiveness ratios (ICER) for different subtypes of SU in comparison with acute SU (Figure 2), both SU with continuous monitoring (ICER 25,120.89) and Acute + Rehab + ESD SU (ICER $24,574.59) were cost effective alternatives. Use of Acute + Rehab SUresulted in increased costs by more than 100% while offering only minimal gains in QALYs (ICER $1,565,474) which was not cost effective.

Table 2. Cost effectiveness of stroke unit v/s conventional care units

Stroke Units in comparison with other wards
Average Incremental Cost per QALY $41,204.37

Author	Year	Country	Subjects in study		Length of Stay		Net change in LOS	Outcomes		QALY		Cost/pt		Incremental Cost/ QALY
			SU	Comparison	SU	Comparison		SU	Comparison	SU	Comparison	SU	Comparison	
Candelise	2000-2004	Italy	4936	6636	12	12	0	mRS mean 3.09	mRS mean 3.54	0.409	0.343	$12,597.36	$12,597.36	$0
Cavallini	1999-2001	Italy	134	134	9.2	17.1	7.9	mRS ≤3 85%	mRS ≤3 58%	0.4	0.55	$9657.98	$17951.24	$55,288.41
Duffy	1999-2001	Australia	536	604	10	8	-2	4 ADL mean 2.87	4 ADL mean 2.55	0.47	0.39	$10497.8	$8398.24	$26,244.50
Epifanov and Dodel	2002	Germany	314	253	10.1	11.6	-1.5	mRS mean 2	mRS mean 2.2	0.46	0.436	$4,207.75	$3,930.02	$11,572.08
Saka	2005-2006	United Kingdom	571	581	32.3	35.3	3	QALY and costs over 10 years		2.19	1.679	$83,086.08	$72,835.20	$20,060.43
Stegmayr	1996	Sweden	6563	3278	15.8	14.35	-1.45	3 ADL mean 2.20 2	3 ADL mean 2.12	0.484	0.457	$16,586.52	$15,064.34	$56,377.07
Terent	2001-2005	Sweden	79689	25354	18.4	14.7	-3.7	mRS ≤3 65.6 %	mRS ≤3 56.8%	0.427	0.377	$19,315.95	$15,431.77	$77,683.72

Table 3. Acute only stroke units – costs and outcomes

Acute Only Stroke Units
Average Cost/QALY $19,428.64

Author	Year	Country	Subjects	Length of Stay	Outcome	QALY	Cost	Cost/QALY
Almborg	2003-2005	Sweden	188	20.6	BI mean 92.3	0.804	$21,625.47	$26,897.35
Ang	1999-2000	Australia	242	10.6	FIM mean 51.38	0.475	$11,127.67	$23,426.67
Candelise	2000-2004	Italy	4936	12	mRS mean 3.09	0.409	$12,597.36	$30,800.39
Duffy	1999-2001	Australia	536	10	4 ADL mean 2.55	0.3	$10,497.80	$34,992.67
Epifanov and Dodel	2002	Germany	314	10.1	mRS mean 2	0.46	$4,207.75	$9,147.28
Fonseca	1995-1997	Portugal	103	9.4	mRS $\leq$3 34%	0.274	$9,867.93	$36,014.35
Paciaroni	2006	Italy	1921	6.44	mRS $\leq$2 56.6%	0.475	$6,760.58	$14,232.81
Roquer	2003-2006	Spain	433	13.1	mRS $\leq$2 59.8%	0.493	$13,752.12	$27,894.76
Steiner	1998-2000	Austria	2313	5.8	mRS $\leq$3 52.5%	0.37	$6,088.72	$16,456.01
Sulter	2002	Netherlands	27	25	mRS $\leq$3 51.9%	0.355	$26,244.50	$73,928.17
Wang	1997	United States	23	6	NIHSS mean 7.8	0.483	$24,213.79	$50,132.07

Table 4. Acute + rehab stroke units – costs and outcomes

Acute + Rehab Stroke Units
Average cost/QALY $44,228.81

Author	Year	Country	Subjects	Length of Stay	Outcome	QALY	Cost	Cost/QALY
Ang	1999-2000	Australia	113	34	FIM mean 83.3	0.7	$35,692.52	$50,989.31
Askim	1999-2001	Norway	31	13.6	BI mean 79	0.657	$14,277.01	$21,730.61
Phillips	1997-2000	Canada	1284	17	BI mean 69	0.545	$17,846.26	$32,745.43
Saka	2005-2006	United Kingdom	571	32.3		2.151	$94,172.25	$43,780.68
Stegmayr	1996	Sweden	6563	15.8	3 ADL mean 2.202	0.484	$16,586.52	$34,269.67
Terent	2001-2005	Sweden	79689	18.4	mRS $\leq$3 65.6%	0.427	$19,315.95	$45,236.42

Table 5. Acute + rehab + ESD stroke units – costs and outcomes

Acute + Rehab + Early Supported Discharge Stroke Units
Average Cost/QALY $29,145.93

Author	Year	Country	Subjects	Length of Stay	Outcome	QALY	Cost	Cost/QALY
Askim	1999-2001	Norway	31	12.9	BI mean 71.7	0.576	$13,542.16	$23,510.70
Rasmussen	2005-2006	Sweden	226	11	6 ADL mean 4.94	0.574	$11,547.58	$20,117.74
Saka	2005-2006	United Kingdom	167	32.3	BI 11.27	2.23	$94,573.84	$42,409.79

Table 6. Acute stroke units with continuous monitoring – costs and outcomes

Stroke Units with continuous Monitoring
Average Cost/QALY $20,460.56

Author	Year	Country	Subjects	Length of Stay	Outcome	QALY	Cost	Cost/QALY
Cavallini	1999-2001	Italy	134	9.2	mRS $\leq$3 85%	0.4	$9,657.98	$24,144.94
Roquer	2003-2006	Spain	215	9.1	mRS $\leq$2 71.6%	0.56	$9,553.00	$17,058.93
Sulter	2002	Netherlands	27	16	mRS $\leq$3 74.1%	0.574	$16796.48	$29,262.16

Table 7. Telestroke networks in the developed world

STROKE Network	Hospitals	Hubs	Patients	Thrombolysed	Duration of Study (months)	Patients per year	Thrombolysed per year	% Thrombolysed per year	Transfer percentage
Alberta (Univ. Alberta Stroke Network) [85]	7	1	210	44	24	105	22	20.95%	
Arizona (STARR) [92]	2	1	33	10	6	66.00	20.00	30.30%	45%
Arizona (STRokE DOC AZ TIME) [89]	2	1	54	16	11	59	17	29.63%	0%
Bavaria (TEMPiS) [73,86]	12	2	21000	1800	84	3000.00	257.14	8.57%	5%
Georgia (REACH) [70,79]	7	1	194	30	26	89.54	13.85	15.46%	72%
Houston (Univ. Texas) [90]	6	2	328	14	13	302.77	12.92	4.27%	0%
Illinois (OSF) [94]	20	1	900	57	30	360.00	22.80	6.33%	100%
Maryland (Maryland brain attack center) [74]	1	1	50	6	24	25.00	3.00	12.00%	24%
Massachusetts (PTC) [87]	1	1	24	6	27	10.67	2.67	25.00%	27%
Michigan (Michigan Stroke Network) [95]	22	1	149	56	12	149.00	56.00	37.58%	46%
Missouri (Mid America Brain and Stroke Institute Network) [88]	19	1	547	99	30	218.80	39.60	18.10%	100%
Ontario (Ontario Telehealth Network) [93]	2	2	88	27	34	31.06	9.53	30.68%	-
San Diego (STRokE DOC) [83,84]	4	4	222	56	42	63.43	16.00	25.23%	66%
Swabia (TESS) [80]	7	1	153	2	18	102.00	1.33	1.31%	-
TOTAL / Mean	112	20	23952	2223		4582 Mean 327	494	Mean 18.96%	Mean 44.12%
% / Std. Deviation						Sdev 776	10.79%	Sdev 0.11	Sdev 0.37

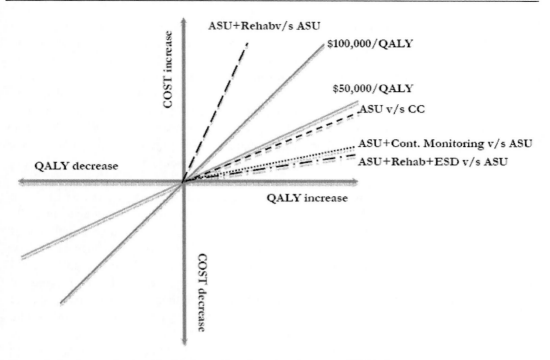

Figure 2. Incremental cost effectiveness of stroke unit subtypes on ICER plane.

Cost Effectiveness Analysis - Discussion

The results of our review reveal that patient care in a stroke unit is more effective and costlierwhen compared to conventional treatment in healthcare facilities. The incremental cost per QALY gained is below $50,000/QALY, making this strategy cost effective. Similar conclusions have been presented in an earlier review of stroke units not restricted by the pre-post IV rtPA era [37]. Studies published prior to 1996 have reported reduction in hospital length of stay by nearly 25%,with resultant cost savings exceeding $400,000 per year with the implementation of Stroke Units. [23, 38, 39] However, initial results of randomized controlled trials of Stroke Units conflicted with these findings by concluding that there was no significant difference in the outcome and cost among patients treated at SU or general ward. [28, 29] In 1997, results of a meta-analysis by Stroke unit Trialist's Collaboration were published, and they concluded that a stroke unit seemed to be a cost effective design when compared with the management of stroke patient in a general ward. These were more prominently seen for patients with severe stroke rather than those with mild stroke [25]. Stroke units have thus been effective both prior to and after adoption of thrombolytic therapy for ischemic stroke. We believe that SU not only help improve outcomes by increasing the compliance with new therapeutic protocols and treatment guidelines, but also improve overall patient management by a coordinated multidisciplinary approach.

When we analyzed costs and outcomes reported by studies of different sub-types of stroke units, we found thatcost/QALY for each of these were below $50,0000. Acute SU, Acute + Rehab + ESD SU and Acute SU with continuous monitoring appear to be feasible alternatives to conventional care systems. Early supported discharge appears to be the most favorable strategy considering that it offers the maximum QALYs at a modest increase in cost. In the past ESD has been reported as a cost effective strategy to reduce burden of care for patients with major functional limitations by Teng and his colleagues in Canada.[40]The theory behind the success of these units remains the fact that home is the best place to relearn skills needed to function. [41] But at the same time patients with significant disability resulting from stroke require a period of guided rehabilitation in a formal healthcare setting. These units succeed in finding the optimal time point amenable to transition between healthcare settings and home settings for recuperation of these patients. Continuous physiological monitoring has been thought of as being more effective than an ideal stroke unit [42], and results of our review seem to confirm these views.

Although the efficacy of stroke unit in terms of improved outcomes, decreased LOS and an increased home discharge has been concluded in each of the studies we reviewed, still the rate of implementation has been quite low. This can be attributed to the high initial cost of setting up these units and resistance-to-change on the part of healthcare managements. The brain attack coalition specified the guidelines for the establishment of a stroke unit in 2000 [5]. According to them, a stroke unit should be staffed 24x7. It should be directed by personnel (i.e physicians, nurses, speech therapist, physical therapists) who have special training and expertise in taking care of patients with cerebrovascular diseases. Among the infrastructure requirements, continuous telemetry, written care protocols and capabilities to monitor blood pressure continuously and non-invasively are essentials. They also specify the above requirements irrespective of whether there is a distinctive hospital ward or unit for carrying out the abovementioned activities. In a study from Netherlands the average start-up costs which consisted of development of uniform transfer of patient information, setting up communication and treatment protocols between care facilities and treatment disciplines, dedicated training (neurology and stroke), developing dossiers, producing news letters, organizing working conferences etc was approximately €96,000(~ $129,922.04 in 2010 US $). [43] If a hospital builds a new stroke unit with a new nursing staff, the cost could range from $50,000 to $500,000 depending on its specific structure and operations. But this is just a one time cost, and once built, the annual operating cost would depend on its size and staffing level, which was estimated to range between $0-$120,000 per year. [5] The improved outcome with projected cost savings counteracts the extra initial setup cost. What is important to understand though is that in today's scenario, setting up of a stroke unit does not mean introduction of new services to the hospital. It is just the reorganization of already established services in a streamlined fashion resulting in better care of patients and efficient use of those resources.

There are some limitations of this review, which should be acknowledged before interpreting the results. The rate of thrombolysis at each of the stroke units would differ given the different geographic locations and healthcare systems. This would also have a direct bearing on outcomes and rate of complications. These could be the sole causes of better or worse outcomes noted in stroke units. We have assumed for purposes of our analysis that all patients in stroke units, had uniform costs/day. Most of the studies reviewed here did not have cost reported in their research, so we deduced the cost from length of stay and QALY from outcome measures reported. Costs of care may vary as per geographical location and stroke severity.For our base case analysis of the Stroke units with continuous monitoring we assumed that the costs per day were same as that in a regular stroke unit. This assumption is obviously incorrect, but our sensitivity analysis shows that even a 100% increase in costs per day would keep these units cost effective. However the exact magnitude of increase in costs remains unknown.

Thus in conclusion our review of studies, conducted post 1996 revealed that stroke unit is a cost effective strategy when compared to conventional healthcare facilities for management of stroke patients.

3. TELESTROKE

The Case for Telestroke

As mentioned earlier, Acute Stroke Care requires timely clinical assessment with brain imaging to obtain an accurate diagnosis given the narrow therapeutic windows for treatment. [44] In the NINDS rt-PA Stroke trial approximately 50% of stroke patients arrived too late to be offered the benefits of therapy. [45] Despite significant efforts and educational campaigns since this initial study, progress in this domain still remains distant. Analysis of the 'Get with the Guidelines' database of the American Heart Association revealed that over 40.1% of acute ischemic stroke patients arrived beyond the 3-hour time window for intravenous thrombolysis (IV rt-PA). What was even more dismal was the fact, that of the 253,148 stroke patients only 4.95% received IV rt-PA. [46]

Multiple approaches are under investigation to overcome these challenges. Researchers and clinicians are vigorously trying to safely increase the time interval from stroke onsetfor effective and safe thrombolysis, withrecent guidelines increasing this time window to 4.5 hours from symptom onset. [47-49] New trials have also been initiated to look at the efficacy, feasibility and costs of bridging IV thrombolysis in conjunction with intra-arterial endovascular revascularization, using therapies for salvage of brain tissue well beyond these time intervals. [50, 51] New imaging techniques are also being rapidly deployed to allow clinicians to predict extent of salvageable penumbra and risk of hemorrhagic transformation to safely and effectively triage patients with acute ischemic stroke into appropriate treatment strategies. [52-54] On a more grassroots level, significant efforts have been made to increase awareness about stroke symptoms in the population, thereby empowering patients to seek early access to care in presence of stroke symptoms. [55-57]

However, each of these strategies can fail in face of the disparities that exist within the healthcare system. Access to appropriate expertise is essential to high-quality stroke care. In most cases of ischemic stroke, this means access to a neurologist and, for many hemorrhagic strokes, access to a neurosurgeon. Approximately 21% of the country's population lives in rural areas as per the results of the 2000 census. Residents within these nonurban areas have higher risks for stroke. Some reasons cited for this include that a large proportion of this rural population is comprised of the elderly and there is a higher prevalence of diabetes mellitus, cardiovascular disease, and smoking in these areas. [58, 59] Hospital Statistics in 2002, reported that of 4856 US hospitals, >50% (with less than 100 beds) were located in rural areas. [60] Rural areas in the United States often lack the resources for adequate stroke care. This lack is due to the lack of both physical diagnostic infrastructure as well as physicians trained in stroke care. [61, 62] Compounding this is the finding that evidence based guidelines for stroke care are often not adhered to in these areas. [61, 63] The Joint commission PSC

(Primary stroke center) certification is far less prevalent in rural areas than in urban hospitals (1% of rural healthcare facilities in a survey of Northwestern rural hospitals were certified PSCs, compared to 45% of urban facilities in the same area). The survey also confirmed the significant lack of neuro-imaging services, healthcare personnel trained to take care of stroke patients, acute stroke treatment protocols and community education activities in the rural areas. [64] Furthermore, outcomes for stroke patients have been significantly worse at these rural healthcare centers. [61] In each case, Telestroke networks can readily address the challenges of stroke care in such rural/isolated health care settings.

Telestroke Networks – Benefits

The importance of stroke networking systems lies in their principle of defragmenting care by facilitating transition of care from one level to another while delivering sustained excellence in care. [65] A number of successful stroke networks have been functional in the country for the past many years. [66-70] These Stroke networks have successfully improved each link in the chain of survival for acute stroke, by leveraging efficiency in care by each of the coordinating healthcare partners to achieve better outcomes. Even as early as 1999, it was suggested that reverse gate-keeping in a managed-care environment to guarantee early access to stroke care experts would be an effective model for stroke care that could be scaled on a nation-wide level. A Telestroke network is defined as a collaborative that enables sharing electronic, visual and/or audio communication to provide diagnostic consultation support to practitioners at distant sites, to assist or directly deliver medical care to stroke patients. [71]

The primary benefit of Telestroke network is that stroke experts are able to support areas with insufficient resources by means of a real-time video consultation. These directly improve the quality and processes of stroke care and increase the use of IV rt-PA in ischemic stroke patients, which has been proven to reduce long-term societal costs of stroke care. [10] Many Telestroke networks have reported better outcomes with fortified drip-and-ship protocols, wherein patients were initiated on IV rt-PA on the basis of remote evaluation, prior to transfer to higher level of care. [72] Studies have successfully demonstrated better outcomes for stroke patients treated in facilities with Telestroke capabilities compared to conventional non-expert care. [73, 74] Additional cost savings also result indirectly because of the increased compliance with protocols in acute and post stroke/TIA recommendations for medical and surgical management. [72, 75-77] Accuracy of remote clinical examination and diagnosis of stroke patients via Telestroke has been demonstrated in the past. [78] There is also an increasing body of evidence that obtaining imaging and image sharing prior to the actual execution of transport of stroke patients to tertiary care facilities improves outcomes. By effective sharing of imaging and clinical examination of patients, appropriate triage of patients requiring transfer to a higher center of care can be achieved. This itself would further cost savings by decreasing transfer costs and physician travel costs.

At the same time, Telestroke networks do have the added costs of setup and maintenance. There remains a lack of published cost effectiveness analysis of Telestroke models within the United States, and the high initial costs are often a deterrent to substantial investment in this technology. [79, 80] Most Telestroke networks remain dependant upon federal and public funding in the form of grants. An additional barrier to Telestroke networks till recently was the lack of re-imbursement for such consultations by Medicare-Medicaid and other health insurers. [74, 81, 82] Today, with the growing availability and access to video and voice over high-bandwidth internet connections, along with rapid spread of powerful handheld multimedia devices, an extensive Telestroke network becomes a more realizable project than ever before.

Telestroke Networks – Results

A Pubmed search revealed 15 Telestroke projects conducted around the globe (mostly from North America and Europe) [70, 73, 74, 79, 80, 83-94] with data on effectiveness of these networks. While a formal cost effectiveness analysis is not readily feasible at present, we analyzed the cost savings afforded by a Telestroke network, while achieving similar effectiveness (measured by thrombolysis rates) as compared to traditional care model. Table-7 presents projects around the world to date that have demonstrated the effectiveness of Telestroke towards resultant treatment of acute ischemic stroke patients.

Of almost 24,000 Telestroke consultations worldwide, nearly 10.8% patients have received thrombolysis; with each center on average seeing 327 ± 776 (mean $\pm$ SD) patients per year. The principal theory behind the success of Telestroke is empowering the local referral centers to become primary care centers for stroke, offering the all-essential thrombolytic therapy on-site, without delay. The most obvious cost savings achieved by Telestroke would therefore be a result of the execution of thrombolytic treatments at the local rural sites or hub sites themselves when needed. The NINDS rt-PA stroke study estimated that the IV rt-PA reduced in-patient length of stay (LOS) by 1.5 days on an average (average LOS for rt-PA patients – 10.9 days, average LOS for stroke patients not receiving rtPA 12.4 days). While IV rt-PA administration did increase hospitalization cost by $1700 per patient treated, this was offset by the decrease in rehabilitation costs of $1400 per patient and nursing home costs of $4800 (1996 US$) per thrombolysis eligible patient. The net savings reported in this trial reached almost $6000 (1996 US$) per patient treated with IV-rtPA. [10] If we apply these costs to the comprehensive numbers obtained after reviewing Telestroke studies, we find that the total cost savings afforded by Telestroke approximate $90,000 (2010 US$) per 100 patients who receive consultation.

The data also shows that these Telestroke systems have thus far avoided on an average 56.88% of transfers (standard deviation 0.37%), while reaching thrombolysis rates that are greater than the US national average. Many experts have suggested reducing secondary triage transfers to tertiary care hospitals for stroke patients as a way to reduce costs of healthcare. Secondary over-triage rates have been reported to be as high as 38% in the country for trauma patients. Studies for these patients, have reported recently that costs for secondary over-triage hovered around $5900 (2006 US$), which is a substantial cost when we consider that the average health care related expenditure per person in the United States is about $8000/year (2006 US$). [95] Taking precedent from these studies, one could argue that the resultant savings afforded by Telestroke by avoiding inter-hospital transfer could easily be close to $365,800 (2010 US$) per 100 patients who avail consultation.

Telestroke Networks - Revenue

Although initially Telestroke consultations were either not reimbursed, or were reimbursed only when the hospital initiating the call was actually in a rural geographic area, systems developed their own pay per use models. [74, 96] The Center for Medicare and Medicaid Services issued a new administrative V code (V45.88 "Status post administration of tPA in a different facility within the last 24 hours before admission to current facility") to permit tracking of "drip and ship" practice, and potentially address the reimbursement inequity created in this scenario in which neither the spoke nor hub hospital receives the appropriate higher diagnosis-related group payment. What is perhaps even more encouraging is the fact that Medicare now reimburses 2-way consultation by video, which allows Telestroke systems to actively generate revenue. As per these revenues generated depend upon the duration of the consultation as shown in Table- 8.

Table 8. Medicare reimbursement for 2 way teleconsultation

Duration of Consultation	Reimbursement offered
15	45.92
30	85.33
40	117.08
60	171.59
80	211.74

Table 9. Projected revenues from telestroke networks

Network	Duration of call	Patients per year	Minimum Average Revenue/ year
Bavaria (TEMPiS)	15	3000.00	137,760.00
Swabia (TESS)	15	102.00	4,683.84
San Diego (STRokE DOC)	28	63.43	5,188.92
Arizona (STARR)	55	66.00	9,737.12
Total/Average	Mean 28.25	3231.43	157,369.88

Table 10. Costs for telestroke network

Network	Fixed Costs / spoke site	Variable Costs / year	Total Costs / year including setup
Bavaria (TEMPis)		19,664.67	$33,400 adding average costs per spoke
Swabia (TESS)	$8,500.00		
Arizona (STARR)	$26,706.00	$13,011	$39,717
Georgia (REACH)	$6,000.00		
Average	$13,745.33		

In our review of research from Telestroke models, the average duration for consultations with Telestroke networks was reported as 28.25 minutes with standard deviation 18.86 minutes. If each of these calls had been reimbursed in the United States, the total revenue that could have been collected over 1 year would be $158,000, giving average revenue of $4870 per 100 consultations (Table- 9).

Telestroke Networks – Costs

From an economic perspective it is also important to consider costs for such networks. There are few if any reports that have outlined setup costs for Telestroke networks, primarily because of the high variance in installation and maintenance of the technology used to generate such networks. While estimates of these fixed costs are possible, what is even more scarcely reported is the variable costs associated with maintenance of the network and the incremental costs per consult. These costs per spoke site are shown in Table-10.

Fixed costs of setup have been reported for the hub-spoke model followed by many Telestroke networks. As reported in response to the TESS network, setup costs were reported as $8000 for a stroke network center and $500 for each network site. [12] Costs for the statewide 'STARR' network reported setup costs of $26,706 per connection at each spoke site. [92] The 'STARR' network also reported projected overhead and maintenance costs to approximate $13,011 per year per connection at each spoke site. The total budget including personnel costs for this project was nearly $231,500 in the first year per spoke site, and tripling in 5 years time. [92] The only other project that mentioned costs was 'REACH', that reported equipment setup costs to be around $6000 per spoke site. The TEMPiS study did mention costs, but it remains unclear if these were fixed/variable. So for purposes of this analysis we assumed total approximate costs of $33,400 per year per spoke site.

Table 11. Economic simulation model for telestroke networks

Costs			
	Fixed	13735	
	Variable	0	
Revenue			
	Consult	48.7	
Variables			
	Spokes	1	
	Patients	?	Analyzed Result = 282.033
Output			
	Profit	=total_revenue - total_costs	Break Even analysis – equating Profit Function to 0
		Total Costs	=spokes*fixed_cost + patients_per_spoke*spokes*variable_cost
		Total Revenue	=spokes*patients_per_spoke*consult_fee

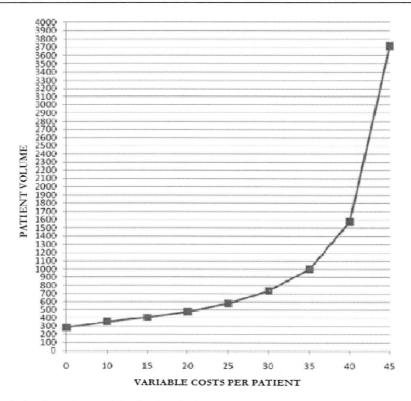

Figure 3. Variation in patients required to break even with varying variable costs.

Telestroke Networks – A Business Model

An economic analysis model, omitting uncertainty, was created as shown in Table-11. Our analysis of the above model suggests that if the network had $0 in variable costs, then each spoke would need a minimum of 283 patients to cover its investment costs by reimbursement of its consultations. If variable costs per consultation increase, then sensitivity analysis demonstrates the number of patients required at each site to increase substantially, as shown in Figure- 2. Based on this analysis, any variable costin excess of $48.70 per patient would never be profitable because it would exceed incremental revenues per patient from the consult (Ceiling Variable Cost for Telestroke Model).

Across the United States, 795,000 patients suffer an acute or recurrent stroke every year, who would then be eligible for care across the 685 PSCs in the country as of March 2010. If all these patients were seen at PSCs, then each PSC would receive 1160 patients on an average. But not all stroke patients reach a PSC as 21% of the country's population actually lives in rural areas, where PSC density is relatively low. A reasonable estimate of the number of patients seen at each spoke site in a Telestroke network might then be <1000 per year. This would correspond to a targeted Variable cost of <$35 ($34.96 Adjusted Ceiling Variable Cost, Figure 3). As previously noted, the average number of patients seen at each Telestroke site worldwide is 327/year, suggesting that the most appropriate Variable Cost for these models should approximate $5.8 per patient ($5.79 most appropriate Variable Cost to enable break-even revenue).

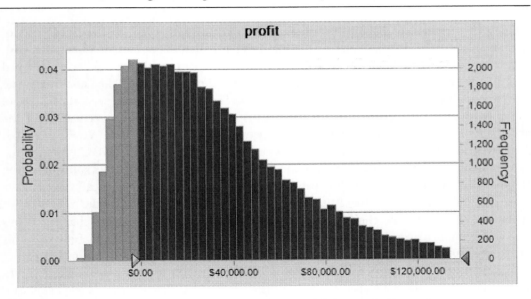

Figure 4. Probability analysis for breakeven of telestroke models in year 1 of operations.

Table 12. Sensitivity analysis simulation model for break even probability with varying variable costs

Variable	profit: Mean	probability of > break even profit: Mean
$5.79	$32,001.27	80.13%
$7.87	$30,955.95	79.50%
$9.96	$29,910.63	78.80%
$12.04	$28,865.30	78.11%
$14.12	$27,819.98	77.22%
$16.21	$26,774.66	76.40%
$18.29	$25,729.34	75.48%
$20.38	$24,684.02	74.55%
$22.46	$23,638.69	73.49%
$24.54	$22,593.37	72.29%
$26.63	$21,548.05	70.96%
$28.71	$20,502.73	69.52%
$30.79	$19,457.41	68.04%
$32.88	$18,412.08	66.33%
$34.96	$17,366.76	64.52%

We then proceeded to introduce uncertainties into the economic model, in order to generate a simulation model. This was done because we had limited data to estimate costs and revenue generation for the Telestroke models. In order to account for variability in our estimates we created probability distributions for each of the variables. The fixed costs of setup for each spoke were modeled as a triangular distribution to account for a minimum cost, maximum cost and a most likely cost. Revenue generated per consult was similarly simulated as a triangular distribution. For both of these, the most likely cost was taken as the estimate from our analyses of existing Telestroke models. The number of patients seen at each spoke site was estimated to resemble a limited normal distribution. We also accounted for the uncertainty in the number of spoke sites each network could connect with. We assumed that there was uniform probability of each network to have between 1 and 22 spokes (the maximum and minimum spoke sites seen in our review). We used simulator software to run 100,000 arbitrary trials incorporating each of these uncertainties. The statistical analysis gave us a probability of 80.1% for Telestroke models to break even within the first year of operations (Figure 4). To check the robustness of this model and possible changes to our estimates with increasing variable costs we ran a sensitivity analysis, shown in Table-12. This sensitivity analysis revealed that despite raising costs to our ceiling costs estimated earlier ($35/patient), the probability for the model to break even with costs still exceeded 60%.We can reasonably conclude that Telestroke is a sustainable and effective business and healthcare model, provided each of the hub units sees atleast 283 patients annually and if the variable costs are kept below $35/patient.

CONCLUSION

Stroke remains one of the most debilitating diseases both worldwide and across the USA, with considerable impact upon its victims and society at large. Despite introduction of intravenous thrombolytic therapy with rTPA for acute stroke more than a decade and a half ago, treatment rates hover < 5%. There has therefore been a growing shift in (relatively scarce) health-care resources towards increased neuro-imaging and invasive intervention in patients with stroke, in hopes of identifying candidates who might benefit from treatment amongst the > 95% who don't/can't receive IV rTPA. However, rate-limiting steps for any emergent therapy for acute stroke (including IV rTPA) continue to exist within the "stroke survival chain", in particular the (a) early identification of patients eligible for treatment and (b) the subsequent care of stroke patients after treatment is delivered. Telestroke networks and Stroke Units have been previously shown to be efficacious in addressing these two rate-limiting steps. We believe that the analysis presented in this chapter further supports enhanced use of Stroke Units and Telestroke networks to address these rate-limiting steps, by additionally demonstrating their cost-effectiveness and sustainability as a business model in delivery of health care to patients with stroke.

REFERENCES

[1]   Lloyd-Jones D, Adams RJ, Brown TM, Carnethon M, Dai S, De Simone G, et al. Heart disease and stroke statistics--2010 update: a report from the American Heart Association. *Circulation*. 2010; 121(7): e46-e215.

[2]   Adams HP, Jr., del Zoppo G, Alberts MJ, Bhatt DL, Brass L, Furlan A, et al. Guidelines for the early management of adults with ischemic stroke: a guideline from the American Heart Association/American Stroke Association Stroke Council, Clinical Cardiology Council, Cardiovascular Radiology and Intervention Council, and the Atherosclerotic Peripheral Vascular Disease and Quality of Care Outcomes in Research Interdisciplinary Working Groups: the American Academy of Neurology affirms the value of this guideline as an educational tool for neurologists. *Stroke*. 2007; 38(5): 1655-711.

[3]   Roger VL, Go AS, Lloyd-Jones DM, Adams RJ, Berry JD, Brown TM, et al. Heart Disease and Stroke Statistics--2011 Update: A Report From the American Heart Association. *Circulation*. 2010.

[4]   Taylor TN, Davis PH, Torner JC, Holmes J, Meyer JW, Jacobson MF. Lifetime cost of stroke in the United States. *Stroke*. 1996; 27(9): 1459-66.

[5]   Alberts MJ, Hademenos G, Latchaw RE, Jagoda A, Marler JR, Mayberg MR, et al. Recommendations for the establishment of primary stroke centers. Brain Attack Coalition. *JAMA* 2000; 283(23): 3102-9.

[6]   Demaerschalk BM, Yip TR. Economic benefit of increasing utilization of intravenous tissue plasminogen activator for acute ischemic stroke in the United States. *Stroke*. 2005; 36(11): 2500-3.

[7]   Demaerschalk BM, Durocher DL. How diagnosis-related group 559 will change the US Medicare cost reimbursement ratio for stroke centers. *Stroke*. 2007; 38(4): 1309-12.

[8]   Scott PA, Silbergleit R. Economic benefit of increasing utilization of intravenous tissue plasminogen activator for acute ischemic stroke in the United States. *Stroke*. 2006; 37(4): 943-4; author reply 4.

[9]   Stahl JE, Furie KL, Gleason S, Gazelle GS. Stroke: Effect of implementing an evaluation and treatment protocol compliant with NINDS recommendations. *Radiology*. 2003; 228(3): 659-68.

[10]   Fagan SC, Morgenstern LB, Petitta A, Ward RE, Tilley BC, Marler JR, et al. Cost-effectiveness of tissue plasminogen activator for acute ischemic stroke. NINDS rt-PA Stroke Study Group. *Neurology*. 1998; 50(4): 883-90.

[11]   Lattimore SU, Chalela J, Davis L, DeGraba T, Ezzeddine M, Haymore J, et al. Impact of establishing a primary stroke center at a community hospital on the use of thrombolytic therapy: the NINDS Suburban Hospital Stroke Center experience. *Stroke*. 2003; 34(6): e55-7.

[12]   Wang DZ. Editorial comment-- telemedicine: the solution to provide rural stroke coverage and the answer to the shortage of stroke neurologists and radiologists. *Stroke*. 2003; 34(12): 2957.

[13]   Jorgensen HS, Kammersgaard LP, Nakayama H, Raaschou HO, Larsen K, Hubbe P, et al. Treatment and rehabilitation on a stroke unit improves 5-year survival. A community-based study. *Stroke*. 1999; 30(5): 930-3.

[14]   Nikolaus T, Jamour M. [Effectiveness of special stroke units in treatment of acute stroke]. *Z. Gerontol. Geriatr*. 2000; 33(2): 96-101.

[15]   Barreiro Tella P, Diez Tejedor E, Frank Garcia A, Lara Lara M, Fuentes B. [The organization of health care for stroke. The stroke units make the difference]. *Rev. Neurol*. 2001; 32(2): 101-6.

[16] Roquer J, Rodriguez-Campello A, Gomis M, Jimenez-Conde J, Cuadrado-Godia E, Vivanco R, et al. Acute stroke unit care and early neurological deterioration in ischemic stroke. *J. Neurol.* 2008; 255(7): 1012-7.

[17] Sulter G, Elting JW, Langedijk M, Maurits NM, De Keyser J. Admitting acute ischemic stroke patients to a stroke care monitoring unit versus a conventional stroke unit: a randomized pilot study. *Stroke.* 2003; 34(1): 101-4.

[18] Cavallini A, Micieli G, Marcheselli S, Quaglini S. Role of monitoring in management of acute ischemic stroke patients. *Stroke.* 2003; 34(11): 2599-603.

[19] Candelise L, Gattinoni M, Bersano A, Micieli G, Sterzi R, Morabito A. Stroke-unit care for acute stroke patients: an observational follow-up study. *Lancet.* 2007; 369(9558): 299-305.

[20] Strand T, Asplund K, Eriksson S, Hagg E, Lithner F, Wester PO. A non-intensive stroke unit reduces functional disability and the need for long-term hospitalization. *Stroke.* 1985; 16(1): 29-34.

[21] Kalra L, Dale P, Crome P. Improving stroke rehabilitation. A controlled study. *Stroke.* 1993; 24(10): 1462-7.

[22] Kaste M, Palomaki H, Sarna S. Where and how should elderly stroke patients be treated? A randomized trial. *Stroke.* 1995; 26(2): 249-53.

[23] Jorgensen HS, Nakayama H, Raaschou HO, Larsen K, Hubbe P, Olsen TS. The effect of a stroke unit: reductions in mortality, discharge rate to nursing home, length of hospital stay, and cost. A community-based study. *Stroke.* 1995; 26(7): 1178-82.

[24] Indredavik B, Bakke F, Solberg R, Rokseth R, Haaheim LL, Holme I. Benefit of a stroke unit: a randomized controlled trial. *Stroke.* 1991; 22(8): 1026-31.

[25] Collaborative systematic review of the randomised trials of organised inpatient (stroke unit) care after stroke. Stroke Unit Trialists' Collaboration. *BMJ.* 1997; 314(7088): 1151-9.

[26] Organised inpatient (stroke unit) care for stroke. Stroke Unit Trialists' Collaboration. *Cochrane Database Syst. Rev.* 2000; (2): CD000197.

[27] Kidwell CS, Shephard T, Tonn S, Lawyer B, Murdock M, Koroshetz W, et al. Establishment of primary stroke centers: a survey of physician attitudes and hospital resources. *Neurology.* 2003; 60(9): 1452-6.

[28] Claesson L, Gosman-Hedstrom G, Johannesson M, Fagerberg B, Blomstrand C. Resource utilization and costs of stroke unit care integrated in a care continuum: A 1-year controlled, prospective, randomized study in elderly patients: the Goteborg 70+ Stroke Study. *Stroke.* 2000; 31(11): 2569-77.

[29] Fagerberg B, Claesson L, Gosman-Hedstrom G, Blomstrand C. Effect of acute stroke unit care integrated with care continuum versus conventional treatment: A randomized 1-year study of elderly patients: the Goteborg 70+ Stroke Study. *Stroke.* 2000; 31(11): 2578-84.

[30] Cabral NL, Moro C, Silva GR, Scola RH, Werneck LC. Study comparing the stroke unit outcome and conventional ward treatment: a randomized study in Joinville, Brazil. *Arq. Neuropsiquiatr.* 2003; 61(2A): 188-93.

[31] Tissue plasminogen activator for acute ischemic stroke. The National Institute of Neurological Disorders and Stroke rt-PA Stroke Study Group. *N. Engl. J. Med.* 1995; 333(24): 1581-7.

[32] OANDA. http://wwwoandacom/currency/historical-rates?date_fmt=usanddate=07/01/04anddate1=06/30/04andexch=EURandexpr=USDandformat=HTMLandmargin_fixed=0.

[33] US Inflation Calculator. http://wwwusinflationcalculatorcom/.

[34] van Exel NJ, Scholte op Reimer WJ, Koopmanschap MA. Assessment of post-stroke quality of life in cost-effectiveness studies: the usefulness of the Barthel Index and the EuroQoL-5D. *Qual. Life Res.* 2004; 13(2): 427-33.

[35] Mortimer D, Segal L, Sturm J. Can we derive an 'exchange rate' between descriptive and preference-based outcome measures for stroke? Results from the transfer to utility (TTU) technique. *Health Qual. Life Outcomes.* 2009; 7: 33.

[36] Darzins P, Robyn S, Bremner F. Outcome measures in rehabilitation. http://wwwhealthvicgovau/subacute/outcomefinalpdf. 2002.

[37] Fuentes B, Diez Tejedor E. [Stroke unit: a cost-effective care need]. *Neurologia.* 2007; 22(7): 456-66.

[38] Wentworth DA, Atkinson RP. Implementation of an acute stroke program decreases hospitalization costs and length of stay. *Stroke.* 1996; 27(6): 1040-3.

[39] Summers D, Soper PA. Implementation and evaluation of stroke clinical pathways and the impact on cost of stroke care. *J. Cardiovasc. Nurs.* 1998; 13(1): 69-87.

[40] Teng J, Mayo NE, Latimer E, Hanley J, Wood-Dauphinee S, Cote R, et al. Costs and caregiver consequences of early supported discharge for stroke patients. *Stroke.* 2003; 34(2): 528-36.

[41] Langhorne P. Editorial comment--Early supported discharge: an idea whose time has come? *Stroke.* 2003; 34(11): 2691-2.

[42] Steiner T. Stroke unit design: intensive monitoring should be a routine procedure. *Stroke.* 2004; 35(4): 1018-9.

[43] Van Exel J, Koopmanschap MA, Van Wijngaarden JD, Scholte Op Reimer WJ. Costs of stroke and stroke services: Determinants of patient costs and a comparison of costs of regular care and care organised in stroke services. *Cost Eff. Resour. Alloc.* 2003; 1(1): 2.

[44] Marler JR, Tilley BC, Lu M, Brott TG, Lyden PC, Grotta JC, et al. Early stroke treatment associated with better outcome: the NINDS rt-PA stroke study. *Neurology.* 2000; 55(11): 1649-55.

[45] Tilley BC, Lyden PD, Brott TG, Lu M, Levine SR, Welch KM. Total quality improvement method for reduction of delays between emergency department admission and treatment of acute ischemic stroke. The National Institute of Neurological Disorders and Stroke rt-PA Stroke Study Group. *Arch. Neurol.* 1997; 54(12): 1466-74.

[46] Saver JL, Smith EE, Fonarow GC, Reeves MJ, Zhao X, Olson DM, et al. The "golden hour" and acute brain ischemia: presenting features and lytic therapy in >30,000 patients arriving within 60 minutes of stroke onset. *Stroke.* 2010; 41(7): 1431-9.

[47] Shobha N, Buchan AM, Hill MD. Thrombolysis at 3-4.5 Hours after Acute Ischemic Stroke Onset - Evidence from the Canadian Alteplase for Stroke Effectiveness Study (CASES) Registry. *Cerebrovasc. Dis.* 2010; 31(3): 223-8.

[48] Hacke W, Kaste M, Bluhmki E, Brozman M, Davalos A, Guidetti D, et al. Thrombolysis with alteplase 3 to 4.5 hours after acute ischemic stroke. *N. Engl. J. Med.* 2008; 359(13): 1317-29.

[49] Wahlgren N, Ahmed N, Davalos A, Hacke W, Millan M, Muir K, et al. Thrombolysis with alteplase 3-4.5 h after acute ischaemic stroke (SITS-ISTR): an observational study. *Lancet*. 2008; 372(9646): 1303-9.

[50] Khatri P, Hill MD, Palesch YY, Spilker J, Jauch EC, Carrozzella JA, et al. Methodology of the Interventional Management of Stroke III Trial. *Int. J. Stroke*. 2008; 3(2): 130-7.

[51] Donnan GA, Davis SM. IV and IA thrombolytic stroke strategies are complementary. *Stroke*. 2009; 40(7): 2615.

[52] Sims J, Schwamm LH. The evolving role of acute stroke imaging in intravenous thrombolytic therapy: patient selection and outcomes assessment. *Neuroimaging Clin. N. Am.* 2005; 15(2): 421-40, xii.

[53] Schellinger PD. The evolving role of advanced MR imaging as a management tool for adult ischemic stroke: a Western-European perspective. *Neuroimaging Clin. N. Am.* 2005; 15(2): 245-58, ix.

[54] Tong DC, Adami A, Moseley ME, Marks MP. Prediction of hemorrhagic transformation following acute stroke: role of diffusion- and perfusion-weighted magnetic resonance imaging. *Arch. Neurol*. 2001; 58(4): 587-93.

[55] Brice JH, Griswell JK, Delbridge TR, Key CB. Stroke: from recognition by the public to management by emergency medical services. *Prehosp. Emerg. Care*. 2002; 6(1): 99-106.

[56] Stern EB, Berman M, Thomas JJ, Klassen AC. Community education for stroke awareness: An efficacy study. *Stroke*. 1999; 30(4): 720-3.

[57] York KA. Rural case management for stroke: the development of a community-based screening and education program. *Lippincotts Case Manag*. 2003; 8(3): 98-114; quiz 5-6.

[58] Eberhardt MS, Pamuk ER. The importance of place of residence: examining health in rural and nonrural areas. *Am. J. Public Health*. 2004; 94(10): 1682-6.

[59] Pearson TA, Lewis C. Rural epidemiology: insights from a rural population laboratory. *Am. J. Epidemiol*. 1998; 148(10): 949-57.

[60] Facilities and Services in the U.S. Census Divisions and States. Hospital Statistics. Chicago, Ill. Health Forum LLC, an affiliate of the American Hospital Association. 2002.

[61] Leira EC, Hess DC, Torner JC, Adams HP, Jr. Rural-urban differences in acute stroke management practices: a modifiable disparity. *Arch. Neurol*. 2008; 65(7): 887-91.

[62] Ruland S, Gorelick PB, Schneck M, Kim D, Moore CG, Leurgans S. Acute stroke care in Illinois: a statewide assessment of diagnostic and treatment capabilities. Stroke. 2002; 33(5): 1334-9.

[63] Burgin WS, Staub L, Chan W, Wein TH, Felberg RA, Grotta JC, et al. Acute stroke care in non-urban emergency departments. *Neurology*. 2001; 57(11): 2006-12.

[64] Shultis W, Graff R, Chamie C, Hart C, Louangketh P, McNamara M, et al. Striking rural-urban disparities observed in acute stroke care capacity and services in the pacific northwest: implications and recommendations. *Stroke*. 2010; 41(10): 2278-82.

[65] NINDS. Improving the Chain of Recovery for Acute Stroke in Your Community. . http://wwwnindsnihgov/news_and_events/proceedings/acute_stroke_workshoppdf. National Institute of Neurological Disorders and Stroke.

[66] Katzan IL, Furlan AJ, Lloyd LE, Frank JI, Harper DL, Hinchey JA, et al. Use of tissue-type plasminogen activator for acute ischemic stroke: the Cleveland area experience. *JAMA* 2000; 283(9): 1151-8.

[67] Grotta JC, Burgin WS, El-Mitwalli A, Long M, Campbell M, Morgenstern LB, et al. Intravenous tissue-type plasminogen activator therapy for ischemic stroke: Houston experience 1996 to 2000. *Arch. Neurol.* 2001; 58(12): 2009-13.

[68] Goldstein LB, Hey LA, Laney R. North Carolina stroke prevention and treatment facilities survey. Statewide availability of programs and services. *Stroke.* 2000; 31(1): 66-70.

[69] Morgenstern LB, Staub L, Chan W, Wein TH, Bartholomew LK, King M, et al. Improving delivery of acute stroke therapy: The TLL Temple Foundation Stroke Project. *Stroke.* 2002; 33(1): 160-6.

[70] Wang S, Lee SB, Pardue C, Ramsingh D, Waller J, Gross H, et al. Remote evaluation of acute ischemic stroke: reliability of National Institutes of Health Stroke Scale via telestroke. *Stroke.* 2003; 34(10): e188-91.

[71] Levine SR, Gorman M. "Telestroke" : the application of telemedicine for stroke. *Stroke.* 1999; 30(2): 464-9.

[72] Uchino K, Massaro L, Jovin TG, Hammer MD, Wechsler LR. Protocol adherence and safety of intravenous thrombolysis after telephone consultation with a stroke center. *J. Stroke Cerebrovasc. Dis.* 2010; 19(6): 417-23.

[73] Audebert HJ, Schultes K, Tietz V, Heuschmann PU, Bogdahn U, Haberl RL, et al. Long-term effects of specialized stroke care with telemedicine support in community hospitals on behalf of the Telemedical Project for Integrative Stroke Care (TEMPiS). *Stroke.* 2009; 40(3): 902-8.

[74] LaMonte MP, Bahouth MN, Xiao Y, Hu P, Baquet CR, Mackenzie CF. Outcomes from a comprehensive stroke telemedicine program. Telemed J E Health. 2008; 14(4): 339-44.

[75] Amarenco P, Bogousslavsky J, Callahan A, 3rd, Goldstein LB, Hennerici M, Rudolph AE, et al. High-dose atorvastatin after stroke or transient ischemic attack. *N. Engl. J. Med.* 2006; 355(6): 549-59.

[76] Gage BF, Cardinalli AB, Albers GW, Owens DK. Cost-effectiveness of warfarin and aspirin for prophylaxis of stroke in patients with nonvalvular atrial fibrillation. *JAMA* 1995; 274(23): 1839-45.

[77] Young KC, Holloway RG, Burgin WS, Benesch CG. A cost-effectiveness analysis of carotid artery stenting compared with endarterectomy. *J. Stroke Cerebrovasc. Dis.* 2010; 19(5): 404-9.

[78] Shafqat S, Kvedar JC, Guanci MM, Chang Y, Schwamm LH. Role for telemedicine in acute stroke. Feasibility and reliability of remote administration of the NIH stroke scale. *Stroke.* 1999; 30(10): 2141-5.

[79] Hess DC, Wang S, Hamilton W, Lee S, Pardue C, Waller JL, et al. REACH: clinical feasibility of a rural telestroke network. *Stroke.* 2005; 36(9): 2018-20.

[80] Wiborg A, Widder B. Teleneurology to improve stroke care in rural areas: The Telemedicine in Stroke in Swabia (TESS) Project. *Stroke.* 2003; 34(12): 2951-6.

[81] Cho S, Khasanshina EV, Mathiassen L, Hess DC, Wang S, Stachura ME. An analysis of business issues in a telestroke project. *J. Telemed. Telecare.* 2007; 13(5): 257-62.

[82] Hess DC, Wang S, Gross H, Nichols FT, Hall CE, Adams RJ. Telestroke: extending stroke expertise into underserved areas. *Lancet Neurol.* 2006; 5(3): 275-8.

[83] Meyer BC, Raman R, Chacon MR, Jensen M, Werner JD. Reliability of site-independent telemedicine when assessed by telemedicine-naive stroke practitioners. *J. Stroke Cerebrovasc. Dis.* 2008; 17(4): 181-6.

[84] Meyer BC, Raman R, Ernstrom K, Tafreshi GM, Huisa B, Stemer AB, et al. Assessment of Long-Term Outcomes for the STRokE DOC Telemedicine Trial. *J. Stroke Cerebrovasc. Dis.* 2010.

[85] Khan K, Shuaib A, Whittaker T, Saqqur M, Jeerakathil T, Butcher K, et al. Telestroke in Northern Alberta: a two year experience with remote hospitals. *Can. J. Neurol. Sci.* 2010; 37(6): 808-13.

[86] Audebert HJ, Kukla C, Clarmann von Claranau S, Kuhn J, Vatankhah B, Schenkel J, et al. Telemedicine for safe and extended use of thrombolysis in stroke: the Telemedic Pilot Project for Integrative Stroke Care (TEMPiS) in Bavaria. *Stroke.* 2005; 36(2): 287-91.

[87] Pervez MA, Silva G, Masrur S, Betensky RA, Furie KL, Hidalgo R, et al. Remote supervision of IV-tPA for acute ischemic stroke by telemedicine or telephone before transfer to a regional stroke center is feasible and safe. *Stroke.* 2010; 41(1): e18-24.

[88] Rymer MM, Thurtchley D, Summers D. Expanded modes of tissue plasminogen activator delivery in a comprehensive stroke center increases regional acute stroke interventions. *Stroke.* 2003; 34(6): e58-60.

[89] Demaerschalk BM, Miley ML, Kiernan TE, Bobrow BJ, Corday DA, Wellik KE, et al. Stroke telemedicine. *Mayo Clin. Proc.* 2009; 84(1): 53-64.

[90] Choi JY, Porche NA, Albright KC, Khaja AM, Ho VS, Grotta JC. Using telemedicine to facilitate thrombolytic therapy for patients with acute stroke. *Jt. Comm. J. Qual. Patient Saf.* 2006; 32(4): 199-205.

[91] Morgenstern LB, Lisabeth LD, Mecozzi AC, Smith MA, Longwell PJ, McFarling DA, et al. A population-based study of acute stroke and TIA diagnosis. *Neurology.* 2004; 62(6): 895-900.

[92] Miley ML, Demaerschalk BM, Olmstead NL, Kiernan TE, Corday DA, Chikani V, et al. The state of emergency stroke resources and care in rural Arizona: a platform for telemedicine. *Telemed. J. E. Health.* 2009; 15(7): 691-9.

[93] Waite K, Silver F, Jaigobin C, Black S, Lee L, Murray B, et al. Telestroke: a multi-site, emergency-based telemedicine service in Ontario. *J. Telemed. Telecare.* 2006; 12(3): 141-5.

[94] Wang DZ, Rose JA, Honings DS, Garwacki DJ, Milbrandt JC. Treating acute stroke patients with intravenous tPA. The OSF stroke network experience. *Stroke.* 2000; 31(1): 77-81.

[95] Osen HB, Bass RR, Abdullah F, Chang DC. Rapid discharge after transfer: risk factors, incidence, and implications for trauma systems. *J. Trauma.* 2010; 69(3): 602-6.

[96] Medicare Guide to Rural health services information for providers, suppliers and physicians. The Medicare Learning Network. http://www.cms.hhs.gov/Medlearn Products/downloads/MedRuralGuide.pdf.

In: Toward Healthcare Resource Stewardship
Editors: J. S.Robinson, M. S.Walid et al.

ISBN: 978-1-62100-182-9
© 2012 Nova Science Publishers, Inc.

Chapter 6

STRATEGIES TO IMPROVE COST-EFFICIENCY OF STROKE CARE: INTEGRATING AUTOMATED PROMPTS INTO STANDARD PHYSICAL ASSESSMENTS TO REDUCE ASPIRATION RISK IN DYSPHAGIC STROKE PATIENTS[♦]

Brandi S. Rambo, Kimberly F. Mancin, Aaron C. M. Barth,
M. Sami Walid,* Patricia Bertram-Arnett, Laura Yarbrough,
Sheri Leslein, Margaret Boltja and Delanor D. Doyle
Medical Center of Central Georgia, Macon, GA, US

BACKGROUND

Dysphagia occurs in approximately half of stroke patients and is usually associated with longer hospital stay and worse outcome [1]. Dysphagia frequently leads to aspiration pneumonia – a serious complication that is estimated to be the cause of death in a third of patients who expire within the first month after stroke [2,3]. This is usually related to absence of the reflex of coughing, severe impairment of consciousness in the acute phase of stroke and poor functional outcome in the chronic phase [4]. Dysphagia apparently facilitates silent aspiration of intranasal bacteria which in the presence of chronic obstructive pulmonary disease and stroke-induced immunodepression (by overactivation of the sympathetic nervous system) leads to the propagation of bacterial aspiration to pneumonia [5-7]. The Joint Commission asserts in its Specifications Manual for Joint Commission National Quality Core Measures (2010B) that *"Stroke patients should be screened for dysphagia before being given any oral intake including food, fluids, or medications"* [8]. In this paper, we present our

---

♦ The current paper was presented at the International Stroke Conference 2010 Nursing Symposium February 23, San Antonio, TX.

* Corresponding Author: M. Sami Walid, PhD. 840 Pine Street, Suite 880, Medical Center of Central Georgia, Macon, GA 331201. Email: mswalid@yahoo.com.

experience with dysphagia screening in stroke patients according to the Joint Commission guidelines.

MATERIALS AND METHODS

In August 2007, a standardized dyphagia screen was created for use in our hospital where nurses are required to screen all stroke and transient ischemic accident (TIA) patients prior to any oral intake (including medications). The screen has been integrated into the hospital's existing electronic documentation system where nurses are automatically prompted with question "Is this a possible stroke or TIA patient?" (Figure 1).

A Dysphagia Screen prompt was added to the physical assessment form and the staff was educated about its requirements (Figure 2). In May 2008 a nurse practitioner was hired as the Stroke Program Clinical Coordinator to further monitor compliance and educate the staff.

Data collection began in October of 2006. Thirty (30) random charts reviewed each month to monitor compliance and improvement. The initial compliance rate was only 16.7%. We aimed to raise compliance rate to at least 85% of stroke patients in accordance with the goals set forth by the Joint Commission.

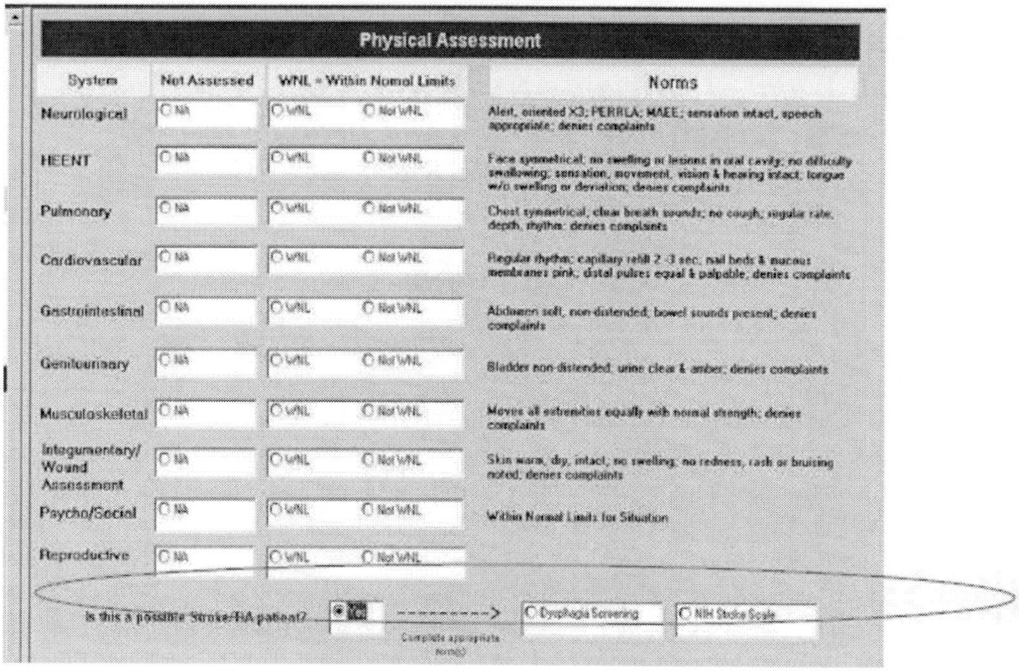

Figure 1. A snapshot of the automated prompt "Is this a possible stroke or TIA patient?"

Dysphagia Screening

If you answer "Yes" to all of the patient assessments below, the patient may have PO intake as ordered.

If you answer "No" to any of the patient assessments below, keep the Patient NPO. If the patient is awake and able to participate, a referral will automatically be made to Speech Therapy for a swallow evaluation.

	Yes	No
Is the patient able to participate?		
Is the patient able to manage own secretions?		
Is the patient's speech understandable?		
Does the patient have pharyngeal sensation?		
Can the patient swallow 50 ml of water without difficulty?		

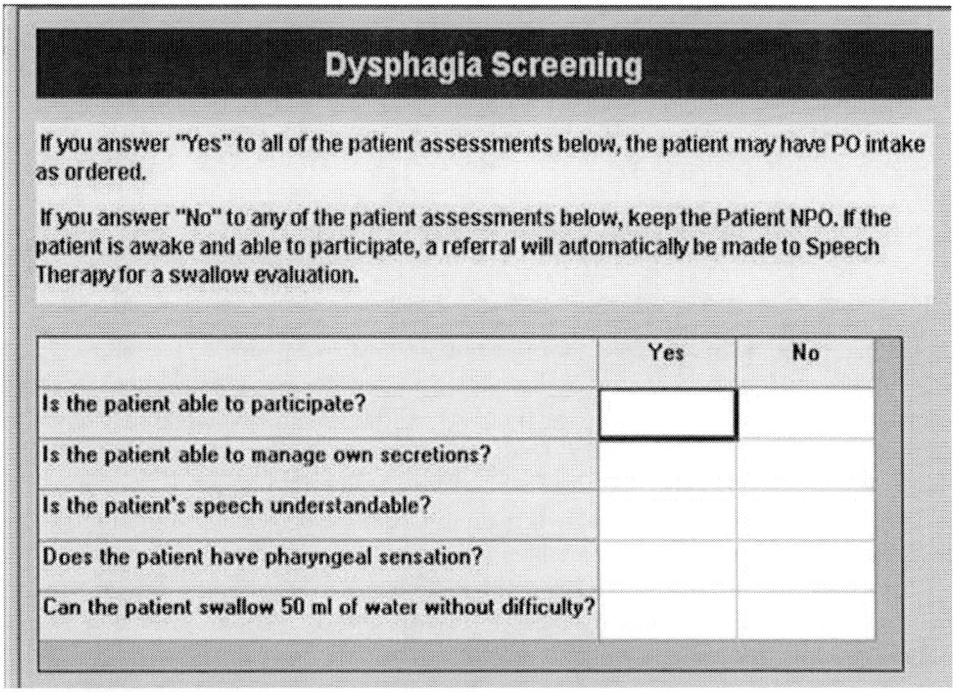

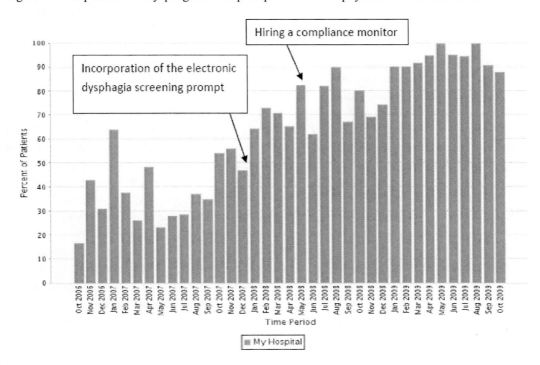

Figure 2. A snapshot of the dysphagia screen prompt added to the physical examination form.

Figure 3. Monthly dysphagia screen compliance from October 2006 to October 2009.

RESULTS

By May 2008 the compliance rate for the dysphagia screening had improved to 82.4%. Between January and October 2009 compliance with the dysphagia screen was consistently maintained at over 85% (Figure 3).

DISCUSSION

Dysphagia is the main risk factor for pneumonia in stroke patients. Therefore, dysphagia screening is essential in this category of patients. In a recent study, dysphagia screening was not associated with reduction of in-hospital deaths [9]. However, several studies have pointed to the fact that dysphagia screening leads to significant decreases in stroke-associated pneumonia regardless of stroke severity [9-11]. The pneumonia rate can be cut in half (2.4% versus 5.4%, P<.01) if formal dysphagia screening is applied [10]. This would logically affect hospital stay and consumption of hospital resources in stroke admissions.

In this study we sought to improve nursing compliance with the administration and documentation of the integrated dysphagia screen. Our hypothesis was that integrating automated prompts into the hospital's existing computer documentation system would improve compliance with performing and documenting the dysphagia screen for all stroke patients and would thus decrease the risk of aspiration pneumonia in the stroke population.

In our model, the simple integration of the screen into the nurse physical assessment has significantly improved compliance with dysphagia screening. Automating prompts into standard physical assessments has served as a useful way to remind the nurse to complete the dysphagia screen immediately at the moment of assessment so that it is less likely to be overlooked. This system, in combination with ongoing monitoring, helps improve outcome in regards to dysphagia in stroke patients.

Managing dysphagia in the acute phase of stroke is a challenging task [12]. Several concepts have been proposed recently to deal with this problem. Ickenstein et al (2010) proposed a stepwise model to be used by both trained nursing staff as well as swallowing therapists and physicians to identify patients with neurogenic oropharyngeal dysphagia at an early stage and so enable an appropriate therapy to be started [13]. Their intervention led to low rates of pneumonia and in-house mortality [13]. Others have suggested videofluoroscopy and more recently videoendoscopy as objective methods for evaluating swallowing disorders [14-17]. Video fluoroscopic evaluation showed the highest rates of silent aspiration in stroke patients, whether in the hemispheres or brainstem" [12]. Videoendoscopy is increasingly becoming a useful tool in the evaluation and treatment of oropharyngeal dysphagia, particularly in patients who may be unable to tolerate videofluoroscopy [18]. Recently, noninvasive brain stimulation in combination with swallowing maneuvers showed promising results in facilitating swallowing recovery in dysphagic stroke patients during early stroke convalescence [19].

REFERENCES

[1] Guyomard V, Fulcher RA, Redmayne O, Metcalf AK, Potter JF, Myint PK. Effect of dysphasia and dysphagia on inpatient mortality and hospital length of stay: a database study. *J. Am. Geriatr. Soc.* 2009 Nov;57(11):2101-6.

[2] Martino R, Foley N, Bhogal S, Diamant N, Speechley M, Teasell R. Dysphagia after stroke: incidence, diagnosis, and pulmonary complications. *Stroke.* 2005 Dec;36(12): 2756-63.

[3] Ickenstein, G.W., et al., Predictors of survival after severe dysphagic stroke. *J. Neurol,* 2005. 252(12): p. 1510-6.

[4] Masiero, S., et al., Pneumonia in stroke patients with oropharyngeal dysphagia: a six-month follow-up study. *Neurol. Sci,* 2008. 29(3): p. 139-45.

[5] Prass, K., et al., Stroke propagates bacterial aspiration to pneumonia in a model of cerebral ischemia. *Stroke,* 2006. 37(10): p. 2607-12.

[6] Emsley, H.C. and S.J. Hopkins, Post-Stroke Immunodepression and Infection: An Emerging Concept. *Infect. Disord. Drug Targets.* 9(5).

[7] Garon, B.R., T. Sierzant, and C. Ormiston, Silent aspiration: results of 2,000 video fluoroscopic evaluations. *J. Neurosci. Nurs,* 2009. 41(4): p. 178-85; quiz 186-7.

[8] Dysphagia Screen. Specifications Manual for Joint Commission National Quality Core Measures (2010B). Available online at: http://manual.jointcommission.org/releases/ Archive/TJC2010B1/DataElem0205.html

[9] Yeh SJ, Huang KY, Wang TG, Chen YC, Chen CH, Tang SC, Tsai LK, Yip PK, Jeng JS. Dysphagia screening decreases pneumonia in acute stroke patients admitted to the stroke intensive care unit. *J. Neurol. Sci.* 2011 May 4. [Epub ahead of print]

[10] Hinchey JA, Shephard T, Furie K, Smith D, Wang D, Tonn S; Stroke Practice Improvement Network Investigators. Formal dysphagia screening protocols prevent pneumonia. *Stroke.* 2005 Sep;36(9):1972-6.

[11] Lakshminarayan K, Tsai AW, Tong X, Vazquez G, Peacock JM, George MG, Luepker RV, Anderson DC. Utility of dysphagia screening results in predicting poststroke pneumonia. Stroke. 2010 Dec;41(12):2849-54.

[12] Tippett DC. Clinical challenges in the evaluation and treatment of individuals with poststroke dysphagia. *Top Stroke Rehabil.* 2011 Mar-Apr;18(2):120-33.

[13] Ickenstein, G.W., et al., Pneumonia and in-hospital mortality in the context of neurogenic oropharyngeal dysphagia (NOD) in stroke and a new NOD step-wise concept. *J. Neurol.*

[14] Allen, J.E., et al., Prevalence of penetration and aspiration on videofluoroscopy in normal individuals without dysphagia. Otolaryngol Head Neck Surg. 142(2): p. 208-13.

[15] Bingjie, L., et al., Quantitative videofluoroscopic analysis of penetration-aspiration in post-stroke patients. *Neurol. India.* 58(1): p. 42-7.

[16] Rugiu, M.G., Role of videofluoroscopy in evaluation of neurologic dysphagia. *Acta Otorhinolaryngol. Ital,* 2007. 27(6): p. 306-16.

[17] Sordi, M., et al., Interdisciplinary evaluation of dysphagia: clinical swallowing evaluation and videoendoscopy of swallowing. *Braz. J. Otorhinolaryngol,* 2009. 75(6): p. 776-87.

[18] Staff, D.M. and R. Shaker, Videoendoscopic evaluation of supraesophageal dysphagia. *Curr. Gastroenterol. Rep*, 2001. 3(3): p. 200-5.

[19] Kumar S, Wagner CW, Frayne C, Zhu L, Selim M, Feng W, Schlaug G. Noninvasive brain stimulation may improve stroke-related dysphagia: a pilot study. *Stroke*. 2011 Apr;42(4):1035-40.

In: Toward Healthcare Resource Stewardship
Editors: J. S.Robinson, M. S.Walid et al.

ISBN: 978-1-62100-182-9
© 2012 Nova Science Publishers, Inc.

Chapter 7

HOSPITALIST AND PERIOPERATIVE CARE

M. Sami Walid[1] and Joe Sam Robinson Jr.[1,2,3]*

[1]Medical Center of Central Georgia, Macon, Georgia, US
[2]Georgia Neurosurgical Institute, Macon, Georgia, US
[3]Mercer University School of Medicine, Macon, Georgia, US

The American society places a high value on human life, and methodically demands and expects quality medical care. But quality care comes with an increasingly high cost. The national healthcare expenditures, estimated at $2.3 trillion in 2008, exceeded 16% of the gross national product (GDP) [1]. The same amount of money stands between the whole gross national product of such countries as France and England. The healthcare spending increased to $2.5 trillion in 2009 or 17.3% of the GDP and is expected according to the predictions of the Centers for Medicare and Medicaid Services to reach 19.3% of the nation's total economic output by 2019 [1]. In view of this, *"The trajectory our nation is on is one that is unsustainable"* said Dr. Richard Carmona, the Surgeon General of the United States between 2002 and 2006 [3].

With the economic recession and rising healthcare cost, the results of American healthcare are being challenged. For example, longevity in the United States (79 years) is lower than in Japan (83 years) despite the higher healthcare expenses in our country (>14% of GDP in USA vs. <8% in Japan) [2]. Considering this fact, less and less money is available for healthcare a good illustration of which is the Medicare physician reimbursement cuts that took place in January 2011 [4].

How to decrease healthcare cost is a big dilemma. There are two options with different views of the problem and degrees of effectiveness: Either to impose healthcare rationing on the population or to increase efficiency in the healthcare system itself. Physicians have a great potential in improving the efficiency of healthcare system. Several difficulties, however, marginalize physician role as an active participant in healthcare reform including government regulations, lack of access to cost information, bureaucratic control, rupture of doctor-patient covenant and the debasing transformation of physicians into healthcare providers.

---

* Corresponding Author: M. Sami Walid, PhD. 840 Pine Street, Suite 880, Medical Center of Central Georgia, Macon, GA 331201. E-mail: mswalid@yahoo.com.

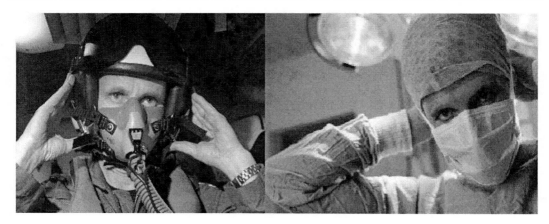

Figure 1. Physician's and pilot's paradigm: *Make no mistake no matter what the cost.*

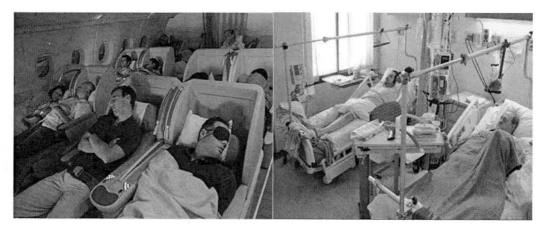

Figure 2. Flight passengers and hospital patients.

The healthcare system is complex with different parties have a say in its structure and functioning including insurance companies, hospitals, physicians and patients. The core element in this system is the doctor-patient relationship which has always been one of trust and physical salvation. The physician's role consists of providing the patient with medical services in form of screening, diagnosing and treating physical and mental illnesses and making decisions regarding proper discharge and follow-up. In the middle of this, the physician, like a pilot (Figures 1-2), has no right to error in his human profession. As a result of this, defensive medicine has become a norm of medical practice in the United States leading to excessive costs emanating from extra diagnostic orders and therapeutic interventions. Malpractice costs in the U.S. are estimated at $55.6 billion a year, mostly in form of "defensive" medical practices [5].

PREOPERATIVE ROLE OF HOSPITALIST

When patients are admitted to hospital to undergo a certain procedure they often have comorbidities that increase the burden of disease. The physician's role is very important in screening and treating these conditions. In a recently published study, we have conducted research on the factors that affect cost in each phase of hospital care – screening, operation and discharge. We found that the average age of spine surgery patients is 55 years many of whom suffer from chronic systemic diseases that significantly affect cost [6]. The following comorbidities were the most notable:

- Hypertension: 78 percent
- History of diabetes mellitus or an elevated glycosylated hemoglobin: 35 percent
- High cholesterol: 31 percent
- Coronary heart disease: 20 percent
- History of hypothyroidism: 10 percent
- History of chronic obstructive pulmonary disease: 8 percent
- An active malignant disease: 2.5 percent
- Epilepsy: 1.6 percent
- Rheumatoid arthritis or lupus erythematosis: 1.4 percent
- Advanced or chronic renal disease: 1.4 percent
- Additionally, 25.4 percent of all patients were on antidepressants.

In that paper we found that half of spine surgery patients had a Charlson Comorbidity Index Score of zero and 11.3 percent had a ≥5 score. Patients come from different backgrounds so do their comorbidities. The prevalence of comorbidities differs significantly between patients per age, body mass index, employment status, and other factors leading to differences in the cost of care [7, 8]. Some comorbidities may be insidious which emphases the importance of preoperative screening in prediabetic, hypothyroid patients and patients with less common occult conditions [9].

Generally, patients are triaged to inpatient and outpatient categories [10]. Patients with less severe comorbidities can undergo outpatient (ambulatory) surgery. Surgery is an outpatient setting consumes less hospital resources and is therefore less costly than inpatient surgery. For example, the cost of outpatient anterior cervical decompression and fusion (ACDF) is $10,201 vs. $17,989 for inpatient ACDF.

In the following chapter we will discuss the importance of preoperative screening by an experienced hospitalist for spine surgery candidates. Hospitalists-internists serves as an essential member of surgical teams as he helps manage high-risk spine surgery patients and improve surgery outcome as well as generate hospital cost savings. Such cooperative efforts between internists and surgeons are vital for the viability of tertiary care centers as cost of hospitalization continue to rise.

INTRAOPERATIVE ROLE OF HOSPITALIST

Intrahospital factors also play a role in cost fluctuation and can be more modifiable than chronological (age), physical (body mass index) and medical factors (comorbidities). Different operation instruments, materials or treatment protocols significantly affect cost. In a following chapter we present a study involving patients undergoing 1-2 level anterior cervical decompression and fusion (ACDF). We found that for 1-level patients, allograft usage yielded a shorter length of hospital stay with comparable hospital charges as autograft. However, for 2-level patients undergoing ACDF, allograft yielded higher hospital charges at a statistically significant rate, without resulting in statistically significant reductions in length of stay. The decision as to which graft type to use for ACDF procedures is a multi-factorial issue in which short and long term cost considerations must be weighed.

Other factors like drain use at the end of surgery may also affect cost in a negative or positive way. In a recent paper accepted for publication in World Neurosurgery we investigated how drain use affects the outcome of lumbar fusion. We found that drain use did not increase the risk of wound infection but had some influence on the prevalence of postoperative fever and significant association with posthemorrhagic anemia and allo-blood transfusion. Despite this, drain use did not have significant impact on hospital length of stay and charges except in cases of ≥3 level lateral procedures [11].

POSTOPERATIVE ROLE OF HOSPITALIST

The hospitalist has a crucial role in dealing with postoperative complications. Postoperative complications may either be general or specific to the type of surgery undertaken, and should be managed with consideration of the patient's history.

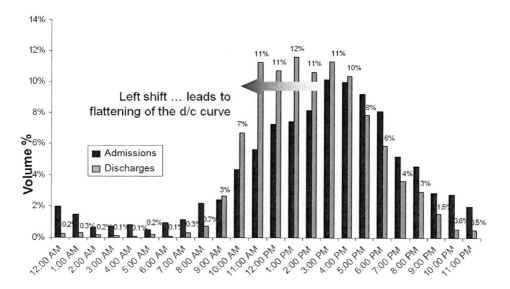

Figure 3. Improving discharge process makes beds available for new admissions. Data from the Medical Center of Central Georgia.

Common general post-operative complications include post-operative fever, posthemorrhagic anemia, atelectasis, wound infection, embolism and deep vein thrombosis. The highest incidence of postoperative complications occurs between 1 and 3 days after the operation.

Discharge is the last phase of hospitalization and incurs significant pressure from many hospital and patient-related factors. In a recent paper we sought to identify and address the causes for discharge delays in neurological patients. Discharge delays from the moment of writing of the discharge order to actual patient discharge from the neurosurgical floor were investigated. Among the 395 patients for whom discharge took more than two hours, the three most prevalent reasons for delay were related to securing rides or addressing family issues, obtaining needed patient medications or equipment, and general delays that could not be specified [12]. Most discharges from hospital took place between 11 am and 3 pm. Shifting the discharge curve to early morning hours (Figure 3) would enable the hospital to create significant savings in hospital resources and generate income through new admissions that is necessary for hospital financial stability.

From another perspective, practice guidelines imposed by the goverment on tertiary care centers contribute in some way to prolonged length of stay of hospitalized patients. For example, prohibiting discharge of patients with postoperative temperatures as subtle as 100° Fahrenheit leads to waste of enormous amount of hospital resources that are mobilized to take care of benignly febrile patients whereas a same-quality care can be delivered in an outpatient service or even at home for a large percentage of these patients [13]. When the Congress established professional standards review organizations in 1993 to oversee decisions regarding the appropriateness and quality of treatment rendered to hospitalized patients commendable guidelines were developed to facilitate and improve patient care. These guidelines provided a balance role against a possible abuse of the diagnosis-related group (DRG) system which could be exploited when patients are prematurely discharged from hospital care for the purpose of institutional financial benefit. On the contrary, these propagated guidelines have encouraged the discharge of patients in a nonfebrile state.

It is important to note that savings from expeditious discharge is negated if readmission does occur due to complications that might have been prevented with close observation. Any patient who is discharged and rehospitalized within 30 days results in substantial financial loss for the institution [14]. Having said this, the oath-driven *Patient First* clinical responsibility of physicians should remain above bureaucratic dictations. Parallel to this, the role of physicians in preserving healthcare resources is important in a time of economic retraction by raising awareness about value-based cost-efficient care [15,16].

REFERENCES

[1]   Medical expenses have 'very steep rate of growth'. USAToday. 2/4/2010.

[2]   Chronic Disease Costs "Staggering" - Illnesses Such As Diabetes And Heart Disease Cost Economy $1.3 Trillion, Report Shows. CBS News. 10/3/2007.

[3]   Friedman M. How to cure health care. The Public Interest. Winter 2001. http://www.thepublicinterest.com/archives/2001winter/article1.html

[4]   Cuts to doctor Medicare payments delayed - Doctors could face a payment cut of almost 25 percent on Jan. 1. Healthcare on msnbc.com. 11/29/2010.

[5]   Malpractice liability costs U.S. $55.6 billion: Study. *Reuters.* 9/7/2010.

[6]   Walid MS, Zaytseva N. How does chronic endocrine disease affect cost in spine surgery? *World Neurosurg.* 2010 May;73(5):578-81.

[7]   Walid MS, Sanoufa M, Robinson JS. The Impact of Age and Body Mass Index on Cost of Spine Surgery. *J. Clin. Neuroscience* (in press).

[8]   Walid MS, Robinson EC, Robinson JS. Higher Comorbidity Rates in Unemployed Patients May Significantly Impact Cost of Spine Surgery. *J. Clin. Neuroscience* (in press).

[9]   Walid MS, Newman BF, Yelverton JC, Nutter JP, Ajjan M, Robinson JS Jr. Prevalence of previously unknown elevation of glycosylated hemoglobin in spine surgery patients and impact on length of stay and total cost. *J. Hosp. Med.* 2010 Jan;5(1):E10-4.

[10] Walid MS, Robinson JS 3rd, Robinson ER, Brannick BB, Ajjan M, Robinson JS Jr. Comparison of outpatient and inpatient spine surgery patients with regards to obesity, comorbidities and readmission for infection. *J. Clin. Neurosci.* 2010 Dec;17(12):1497-8.

[11] Walid MS. The Role of Drains in Lumbar Spine Fusions. Oral presentation at the Georgia Neurosurgical Society 2010 Annual Fall Meeting, Atlanta, GA.

[12] Barth ACM, Walid MS, Mancin KF, Faircloth LR, Robinson JS. Benefits of Improved Efficiency in the Process of Discharging Patients. *AANS Neurosurgeon* 2010;19(3):36-39.

[13] Walid MS, Sahiner G, Robinson C, Robinson JS III, Ajjan M, Robinson JS. Postoperative Fever Discharge Guidelines Increase Hospital Charges Associated with Spine Surgery. *Neurosurgery* (In Press).

[14] Lawrence D: Get out--and stay out. With readmission penalties on the horizon, CIOs are laying the groundwork for post-discharge solutions. *Healthc Inform* 26(7):30–32, 2009.

[15] LG Nikolakakos, JS Robinson III, C Sevin, MA Kassam, CH Feltes, KN Fountas, JS Robinson Jr., EO Richter. Absence Of Economic Analysis In Neurosurgical Literature. Presented at AANS Annual Meeting 2007, Washington, DC.

[16] Porter ME. What is value in health care? *N. Engl. J. Med.* 2010 Dec 23;363(26):2477-81.

In: Toward Healthcare Resource Stewardship
Editors: J. S.Robinson, M. S.Walid et al.

ISBN: 978-1-62100-182-9
© 2012 Nova Science Publishers, Inc.

Chapter 8

THE EFFECT OF COMORBIDITIES ON LENGTH OF STAY AND HOSPITAL CHARGES OF SPINE SURGERY PATIENTS

M. Sami Walid[1] and Tracey Blalock[2]*
[1]Medical Center of Central Georgia, Macon, GA, US
[2]Patient Care Services Administration,
Medical Center of Central Georgia, Macon, GA, US

ABSTRACT

Background: Chronic back pain is a known risk factor for spine surgical intervention concomitant with comorbidities that may affect outcome and cost.

Methods: In order to investigate the interaction of comorbidities and hospital cost of spine surgery the charts of 816 spine surgery patients between 14 and 92 years old were retrospectively reviewed and data on their comorbidities were collected. Three types of spine surgery were studied: Lumbar microdiskectomy, anterior cervical decompression and fusion and lumbar decompression and fusion. Length of hospital stay and hospital cost (charges) were the outcome variables.

Results: Overall, the Charlson index assumed a two-peaked distribution at zero and three with half of the patients (49.4%) having a Charlson score of zero. However, when looking inside age groups, the first peak seemed to decrease with older age and the second peak shifted to the right with more comorbidities.

Subcategorizing patients by age group and type of surgery, significant correlations were detected between Charlson index score on one side and length of stay and hospital cost on the other side especially in the middle age group and in LDF patients of older age.

Conclusion: Comorbidities impact length of stay and hospital cost of spine surgery.

---

* Corresponding Author: M. Sami Walid. Medical Center of Central Georgia, 840 Pine Street, Suite 880, Macon, GA 331201. Email: mswalid@yahoo.com.

INTRODUCTION

Chronic back pain is a known risk factor for spine surgical intervention concomitant with comorbidities that may affect outcome and cost. With over a million spine surgical procedures performed annually in the United States at over $20 billion cost [1], it is useful to investigate the interaction of comorbidities, length of stay and hospital cost of spine surgery.

MATERIALS AND METHODS

In order to investigate the interaction of comorbidities and hospital cost of spine surgery the charts of 816 spine surgery patients between 14 and 92 years old with an average of 54.5 years were retrospectively reviewed and data on their comorbidities and consumption of hospital resources were collected. Three types of spine surgery were studied: Lumbar microdiskectomy (LMD), anterior cervical decompression and fusion (ACDF) and lumbar decompression and fusion (LDF).

Comorbid conditions were coded using the Charlson comorbidity Index [2]. This scale measures comorbidity level based on 19 pre-defined comorbid conditions weighted according to their impact on the general health of the individual. It is often used as an adjusting variable in multivariate analyses. Correlations with length of hospital stay and hospital cost (charges) were studied using SPSS v16.

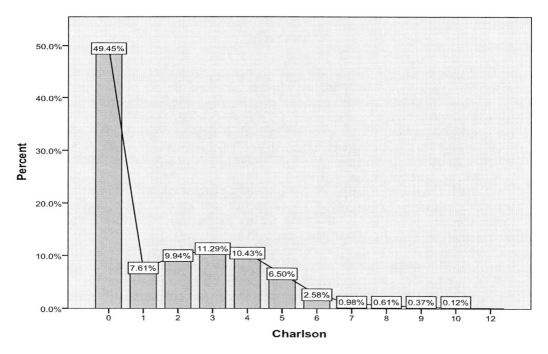

Figure 1. Charlson comorbidity index distribution in a cohort of spine surgery candidates.

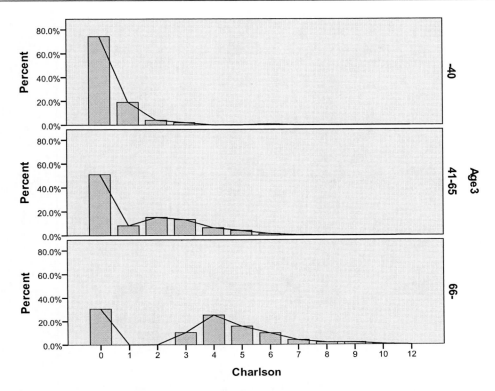

Figure 2. Charlson comorbidity index shifting with age in a cohort of spine surgery candidates.

RESULTS

Overall, the Charlson index assumed a two-peaked distribution at zero and three with half of the patients (49.4%) having a Charlson score of zero (Figure 1). However, when looking inside age groups, the first peak seemed to decrease with older age and the second peak shifted to the right with more comorbidities (Figure 2).

Subcategorizing patients by age group and type of surgery (Figure 3), significant correlations were detected between Charlson index score on one side and length of stay and hospital cost on the other side especially in the middle age group and in LDF patients of older age (Tables 1-3).

DISCUSSION

Patients come from different backgrounds to hospital to undergo spine surgery with often concomitant comorbidities that may increase the burden of disease. The prevalence of comorbidities differs significantly between patients based on age, body mass index, employment status, and other factors leading to differences in the cost of care. But age is considered the most important determinant of physical status and comorbidities in the general and spine surgery populations. These comorbidities evidently increase with age and do not follow a normal distribution as scored by the Charlson comorbidity index.

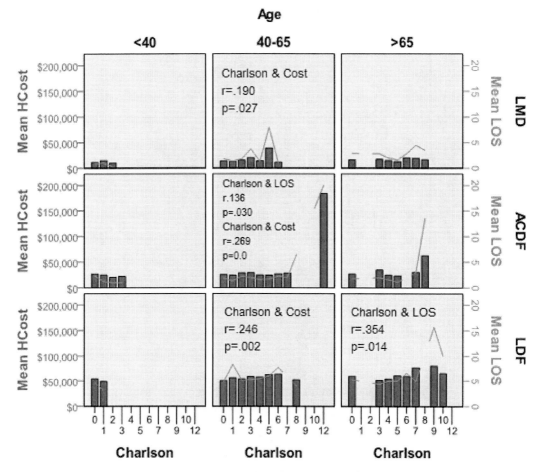

Figure 3. the correlation between Charlson comorbidity score and length of stay and hospital cost in a cohort of spine surgery candidates.

In previous studies, we demonstrated the impact of individual comorbidities on length of stay and hospital cost of spine surgery [3-5]. In this study, comorbidities summated on a single scale correlated with the cost of hospitalization of spine surgery patients. Specifically, comorbidities seem to have a notable effect on length of stay and hospital cost in middle-aged patients.

In a time of economic recession and soaring healthcare expenditures it is important to study the factors that impact the utilization of healthcare resources in an effort to improve hospital efficiency. Physicians have an important role in preoperative screening necessary to indentify and treat high-risk patients prone to a complicated postoperative course. Payors, on the other hand, should consider comorbidities in the reimbursement plans of spine procedures in order not to marginalize patients with chronic diseases. In the clinical research arena, peer-reviewed journals should encourage the inclusion of comorbidities as a confounding variable and cost as an outcome measure in the cost-benefit analysis of spine surgical interventions.

REFERENCES

[1]   Deyo RA: Back surgery--who needs it? N Engl J Med 356:2239-2243, 2007. 4. Emanuel EJ, Fuchs VR: The perfect storm of overutilization. *JAMA* 299:2789-2791, 2008.

[2]   Charlson ME, Pompei P, Ales KL, MacKenzie CR. A new method of classifying prognostic comorbidity in longitudinal studies: development and validation. *J. Chronic. Dis.* 1987;40(5):373-83.

[3]   Walid MS, Robinson JS. Economic impact of comorbidities in spine surgery. *J. Neurosurg. Spine.* 2011 Mar;14(3):318-21.

[4]   Walid MS, Zaytseva N. How does chronic endocrine disease affect cost in spine surgery? *World Neurosurg.* 2010 May;73(5):578-81.

[5]   Walid MS, Robinson EC, Robinson JS Jr. Higher comorbidity rates in unemployed patients may significantly impact the cost of spine surgery. *J. Clin. Neurosci.* 2011 May;18(5):640-4.

In: Toward Healthcare Resource Stewardship
Editors: J. S.Robinson, M. S.Walid et al.

ISBN: 978-1-62100-182-9
© 2012 Nova Science Publishers, Inc.

Chapter 9

THE IMPACT OF PREOPERATIVE SCREENING ON SPINE SURGERY COST

Mohammed Ajjan,[1]* Aaron C. M. Barth,[2] M. Sami Walid,[2] Vicki L. Conlon,[1] Kimberly F. Mancin[2] and Joe Sam Robinson Jr.[1]

[1]Georgia Neurosurgical Institute, Macon, GA, US
[2]The Georgia Neuro Center at the Medical Center of Central Georgia, Macon, GA, US

ABSTRACT

This is a prospective study whereby the neurosurgical internist was tasked with covering the medical aspects of care for spine surgery patients. Preoperatively, the internist was responsible for performing consultations, triaging, and preparing patients for surgery. Postoperatively the neurosurgical internist directly managed their care during hospital stay. Eighty five spine surgery candidates with two or more comorbidities were studied. Sixty (71%) patients received internist consultation and management. The rest made a control/comparison group of 25 patients (29%) who did not receive internist consultation during this period. Reductions in length of stay amounted to hospital direct cost savings of $340/case and total direct cost savings of $30,600 over a six-month period. Indirect cost savings were also generated through bed availability for new patients. Neurosurgical internists can serve as a vital component of neurosurgical teams as they help manage high-risk spine surgery patients and improve patient throughput and generate hospital cost savings.

INTRODUCTION

As medicine becomes increasingly complicated, hospitalist specialties have emerged with the aim of improving medical treatment of patients during their hospital stays. Owing to the

---

* Corresponding Author: Mohammed Ajjan. 840 Pine Street, Suite 880, Macon, GA 31201. E-mail: tarabajjan@yahoo.com.

fact that neurosurgery medical complications can differ dramatically from those in other fields, the need for a hospitalist specializing in care of neurosurgical patients is apparent.

The aim of this prospective study was to analyze the effect of preoperatively consulting and managing "high-risk" spine surgery patients using a neurosurgical internist.

METHODS

Hospital administrators and an affiliated neurosurgery group made a concerted effort to prospectively utilize the primary author, a neurosurgical internist, in the consultation and management of spine surgery candidates with specific medical comorbid conditions.

The neurosurgical internist was tasked with covering the medical aspects of care for surgical inpatients. Preoperatively, the internist was responsible for performing consultations, triaging, and preparing patients for surgery. Postoperatively the neurosurgical internist treated patients and directly managed their care during their hospital stay.

Criteria were established to define "high-risk" spine surgery candidates: two or more comorbidities, diabetes mellitus, chronic obstructive pulmonary disease, anesthesia problems, morbid obesity, sleep apnea, etc.

During preoperative evaluations, nurses ordered internist consultation if patients met high-risk criteria. Further evaluation and tests were administered as necessary and the internist aided in the postoperative management of the patient [1, 2]. Hospital length of stay (LOS) and financial data were evaluated. Outpatient surgery data was excluded.

RESULTS

From April-November 2006, 85 spine surgery candidates met high-risk criteria including 60 (71%) who received internist consultation and management. A control/comparison group of 25 patients (29%) did not receive internist consultation during this period.

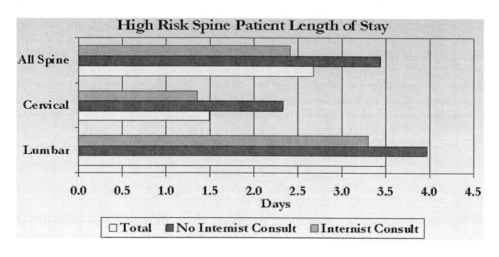

Among high-risk lumbar patients with internist consultation LOS was 3.37 days vs. 3.62 days. For cervical patients with internist consultation LOS was 1.22 days vs. 2.00 days (see graph).

These reductions in LOS amounted to hospital direct cost savings of $340/case and total direct cost savings of $30,600 over a six-month period. Indirect cost savings were also generated through bed availability for new patients.

DISCUSSION

The medical field is a perpetually evolving field where human factors and technological developments play significant roles in impacting healthcare costs. Mechanisms such as MRI, MRA, CT, PET Scan, and navigator guided brain surgery, serve as examples of how technological advances can improve health but lead to steep increases in medical expenditure. Further, longer human life expectancy often results in more medical complications, more sophisticated patients, and higher cost to maintain health.

The medical profession has often reacted to changes in market and medical field by moving towards more specialized healthcare providers. The practice of Medicine is generally complicated and each specialty has its requirements. Neurosurgery complications differ vastly from those in other fields and specialized knowledge is required to treat these conditions. The use of a primary care clinician with expertise in the management of neurosurgical complications can be invaluable. A dedicated hospital-based Internal Medicine physician with this type of training can greatly assist with the medical aspects of these patients. Prior to surgery the physician can handle consultations, triage, and preparations for surgery. The hospitalist can not only manage patients directly before surgery, but also during their hospital stays.

Our study shows that neurosurgical internist care can result in immediate financial savings for both patients and hospitals. Over a six-month period, the average hospitalization time was reduced for all spine surgery patients who received neurosurgical internist consultation by 0.58 days (13.92 hours). Average hospital direct cost savings of $344/patient were realized. These findings suggest that a hospitalist in a neurosurgical ward could:

1) Improve clinical outcome by:
    -   treating complications and comorbidities,
    -   Assuring safe discharge,
    -   Making decisions regarding patient's recovery.
2) Improve financial outcome by:
    -   reducing hospitalization time (length of stay),
    -   Preventing complications and further illness.

As hospitalist specialties become an engrained part of medical care in the USA, further specialized training of these physicians will be necessary for optimal neurosurgical care. Addressing preexisting medical comorbidity concerns preoperatively enables physicians to anticipate postoperative needs and ensure that patients do not remain longer than necessary in the hospital.

Neurosurgical internist consultation may also bring indirect savings as they work to improve both clinical and financial outcomes. Clinical improvements may include successful decreases in complications and comorbidities, assurance of safe discharge, and prevention of complications and further illness. Indirect financial improvements also include increases in bed availability for new patients as existing patients are discharged appropriately. Neurosurgical internists may also be able to make decisions that benefit patients in terms of long term costs and recovery.

Neurosurgical internists can serve as a vital component of neurosurgical teams as they help manage high-risk spine surgery patients and improve patient throughput and generate hospital cost savings. Such cooperative efforts are vital for the viability of the national healthcare system as costs continue to rise.

REFERENCES

[1]   Walid MS, Newman BF, Yelverton JC, et al. Prevalence of previously unknown elevation of glycosylated hemoglobin in spine surgery patients and impact on length of stay and total cost. *J. Hosp. Med*;5:E10-4.

[2]   Walid MS, Woodall MN, Nutter JP, et al. Causes and risk factors for postoperative fever in spine surgery patients. *South Med. J.* 2009;102:283-6.

In: Toward Healthcare Resource Stewardship
Editors: J. S.Robinson, M. S.Walid et al.

ISBN: 978-1-62100-182-9
© 2012 Nova Science Publishers, Inc.

Chapter 10

THE IMPACT OF SURGICAL MATERIAL ON HOSPITAL COST: ECONOMIC ANALYSIS OF ALLOGRAFT VS. AUTOGRAFT FOR ELECTIVE ONE- AND TWO-LEVEL ANTERIOR CERVICAL DECOMPRESSION AND FUSION SURGERY[♦]

Aaron C. M. Barth,[1] Robert A. Lummus,[1] M. Sami Walid,[1][*]
Kostas N. Fountas,[2] Aleksandar Tomic,[3]
Joe Sam Robinson III[4] and Joe Sam Robinson Jr.[1,4,5]

[1]The Medical Center of Central Georgia, Macon, GA, US
[2]University of Thessaly School of Medicine, Larissa, Greece
[3]Department of Business and Economics,
Wesleyan College, Macon, GA, US
[4]Mercer University School of Medicine, Macon, GA, US
[5]Georgia Neurosurgical Institute (GNI), Macon, GA, US

ABSTRACT

Background Context: Studies demonstrate comparable clinical results with the use of either autogenous hip bone (autograft) or cadaver bone (allograft) for both single and multilevel anterior cervical decompression and fusion (ACDF) with rigid plate fixation.

Purpose: Very few studies, however, have analyzed the economic implications of these two ACDF variations. We analyze the short-term hospital economic impact of these alternatives.

Study Design and Setting: A retrospective study in a tertiary care center in central Georgia.

[♦] The paper was presented by Aaron Barth at the 2007 American Association of Neurological Surgeons Annual Meeting, Washington, DC.

[*] Corresponding Author: M. Sami Walid, MD, PhD. 840 Pine St., Suite 880, Macon, GA 31201. E-mail: mswalid@yahoo.com.

Patient Sample: 550 consecutive elective 1- or 2-level ACDF patients met inclusion criteria for our study. 305 consecutive patients undergoing 1-level ACDF with rigid plate fixation (mean age 50.5 years) and 245 consecutive 2-level patients (mean age 52.6 years) received allograft implants (1-level n=86, 2-level n=33) or autograft (1 level n=219, 2-level n=212) bone. 32 patients were treated in an outpatient setting.

Outcome Measures: Hospital charges were reviewed for cost factors such as procedure time, hospital supplies, labor, and length of stay.

Methods: T-tests were used to establish statistical significance of any differences between the studied variables with respect to the choice of allograft vs. autograft.

Results: Allograft usage led to statistically insignificant faster average procedure times for both 1-level (80.9 vs. 83.3 min, $p>0.05$) and 2-level patients (97.6 vs. 99.8 min, $p>0.05$). Allograft resulted in significant reductions in average length of stay (LOS) for 1-level patients (0.78 vs. 1.37 days, $p<0.01$), but insignificant reductions in average LOS for 2-level patients (1.21 vs. 1.42 days, $p>0.05$). For hospital charges, allograft usage resulted in insignificantly higher mean hospital charges for 1-level patients (allograft $17,243, autograft $16,969, $p>0.05$), but significantly increased hospital charges for 2-level patients (allograft $21,240, autograft $19,056, $p<0.01$). Significant variances in cost included allograft implants in allograft procedures 1 s and pain pumps in autograft procedures.

Conclusion: In 1-level patients undergoing ACDF, allograft usage yielded a shorter length of hospital stay with comparable hospital charges as autograft. However, for 2-level patients undergoing ACDF, allograft yielded higher hospital charges at a statistically significant rate, without yielding statistically significant reductions in LOS. As with many issues, the decision as to which graft type to use for ACDF procedures is a multi-factorial issue. Both short and long term cost considerations must be heavily weighed. The limitations of our study must also be weighed against our conclusions.

I. INTRODUCTION

Anterior Cervical Decompression and Fusion (ACDF) is one operation that was introduced in 1958 and allows for the decompression and stabilization of the cervical spine to relieve pressure from the spinal cord or to secure access to the spinal cord in order to remove certain respectable pathologies [1]. The benefits of utilizing a patient's own bone (autograft) or a cadaver bone (allograft) for this procedure is a topic that is still widely discussed [2]. Deutsch, et al report that while allograft has begun to outpace autograft usage, the three considerations of clinical efficacy, graft harvest morbidity, and cost and availability remain contentious [2].

Table 1. ACDF Patient Characteristics

# Levels	Graft Type	# Pts	Age	Range	Male/Female
1-Level	Allograft	86	46.9	29-78	40/46
	Autograft	219	51.9	26-82	102/117
2-level	Allograft	33	52.4	27-87	12/21
	Autograft	212	53.5	28-79	100/112
Total / Average		550	52.2	26-87	254/296

Within the literature, autograft is generally considered as the "gold standard" for bone grafting [3-4]. Autograft from the iliac crest is the preferred fusion material and reported to be used in 76% of cases [5]. Allograft bone, however, may be used as an alternative to the patient's own bone although healing and fusion is not as predictable as with the previous. Allograft does not require a separate incision to take the patient's own bone for grafting, and therefore is associated with less postoperative pain. Smoking, medications, and other health factors can affect the rate of healing and fusion [6].

Several clinical studies have demonstrated that the use of either autograft or allograft produces comparable results in terms of efficacy and graft harvest morbidity [3, 7-8]. Very few studies [8-13], however, have analyzed the economic implications of these two ACDF variations. As the American healthcare system has become increasingly cost-conscious, a responsibility has been placed on health care providers to become attuned to the costs associated with delivering care. The primary aim of this study is to analyze the short-term economic impact for anterior cervical decompression and fusion (ACDF) when autogenus bone graft is harvested from a patient's iliac crest as compared to the utilization of allograft bone taken from a cadaver.

II. MATERIALS AND METHODS

Our study included a total of 550 consecutive patients from 2005-2007 undergoing elective one or two-level ACDF with plate fixation in either an inpatient or outpatient setting. Surgeries were performed primarily for degenerative disc disease and/or cervical spondylosis. Patients and physicians discussed a variety of clinical considerations before making final determinations as to which graft types and surgical settings would be utilized. It is important to note that for cases requiring the harvest of autograft bone at our institution, a second surgeon or surgical assistant aided the primary surgeon by harvesting the graft from the iliac crest of the patient's hip during surgery. In cases that used allograft bone, only one surgeon was involved.

Patients were initially divided into 1- and 2-level surgery categories, and into subsequent allograft and autograft subsets. 86 consecutive patients undergoing one-level ACDF received allograft implants while 219 received autograft implants. Regarding two-level patients, 33 consecutive received allograft implants while 212 received autograft implants. In an outpatient setting, 32 patients underwent 1-level ACDF with allograft. No patients were treated in an outpatient setting with 1-level autograft or 2-level autograft or allograft. Patients were nearly equally divided by gender (254 males and 296 females) and their ages ranged between 26 and 87 years (Table 1).

Patient accounts were retrospectively reviewed for cost factors such as procedure time, hospital supplies, labor, and length of stay (LOS). T-tests were used to establish statistical significance of differences in costs resulting from graft choice.

Table 2. Comparison of Procedure time, LOS and charges between 1-level ACDF patients (n=305)

Variable	Autograft (n=219)				Allograft(n=86)			
	Mean	Std. Dev.	Min	Max	Mean	Std. Dev.	Min	Max
Age[***]	51.93	11.19	26	82	46.90	10.77	29	78
Procedure Minutes	83.26	20.57	33	178	80.86	20.04	28	143
Avg LOS[***]	1.37	1.07	0	9	0.78	0.74	0	5
Hospital Charges	16,969.05	3,935.18	9,214.00	48,642.00	17,243.08	2,763.99	11,922.00	24,664.00
Direct Cost	6,275.83	1,246.53	3,395.53	15,276.32	6,373.50	1,159.45	1,750.44	8,873.15
Indirect Cost	1,902.09	674.49	1,078.23	6,221.39	1,840.52	411.09	796.34	3,858.32
Total Cost	8,177.92	1,869.98	4,473.76	21,497.71	8,214.02	1,459.13	2,546.78	12,575.68
Direct Anesthesia Cost/Case	379.07	82.07	0.00	876.32	368.25	101.40	0.00	720.36
Direct Lab and Blood Bank Cost/Case	113.45	46.69	11.20	334.75	102.62	27.61	0.00	226.85
Direct Pharmacy Cost/Case[***]	428.04	149.73	210.33	1961.41	357.14	104.87	208.04	965.99
Direct Respiratory Therapy Cost/Case[**]	19.90	27.42	0.00	354.19	13.74	7.77	0.00	34.96
Direct Radiology Cost/Case	45.63	58.53	0.00	530.81	42.90	31.49	0.00	299.87
Direct Physical/Occupational Therapy Cost/Case[*]	8.58	34.83	0.00	355.01	1.42	9.30	0.00	64.69
Other Direct Routine Cost/Case[**]	365.39	550.86	0.00	7364.39	214.76	320.28	0.00	2655.78
Direct O.R. Labor Cost/Case	1,387.12	745.74	259.10	8698.23	1,283.65	504.04	321.84	3713.20
Direct O.R. Supply Cost/Case[***]	2,630.95	570.71	0.00	4262.91	2,870.03	813.25	69.09	4477.72

[***]significant at 1% (p-value<.01); [**]significant at 5% (p-value<.05); [*]significant at 10% (p-value<.10)

III. RESULTS

Surgical and Hospitalization Costs

The mean surgical procedure time for 1-level ACDF with allograft was 80.9 minutes (1 standard deviation STD 20.0, range 28-143) compared to 83.3 minutes for 1-level ACDF with autograft (STD 20.6, range 33-178) (Table 2). The mean procedure time for 2-level ACDF with allograft was 97.6 minutes (STD 19.2, range 60-143) compared to 99.8 minutes for 2-level ACDF with autograft (STD 22.8, range 48-181) (Table 3). This did not reach statistical significance (p>0.05). One-level patients with allograft remained in the hospital 0.78 days (STD 0.74, range 0-5) compared to 1.37 days for 1-level patients with autograft (STD 1.07, range 0-9) (see Figure), a statistically significant difference of 0.59 days (p<0.01) (Table 2). Two-level patients with allograft remained in the hospital 1.21 days (STD 0.82; range 1-5) compared to 1.42 for 2-level patients with autograph (STD 1.34, range 1-14). This did not reach statistical significance (p>0.05) (Table 3).

Among 1-level ACDF patients mean hospital charges for allograft were $17,243 (STD $2,764, Range $11,922-$24,664) compared to $16,969 for 1-level autograft (STD $3,935, range $9,214-$48,642) (see Figure), a statistically insignificant difference of $274 (p>0.05) (Table 2). Among 2-level patients, the mean hospital charges associated with allograft were $21,240 (STD $3,639, range $15,932-$35,057) compared to $19,056 for 2-level patients with autograft (STD $6,142, range $6,350-$93,590). This was statistically significant (p<0.01) difference (Table 3). A regression model serving as a predictor of hospital charges (Table 4) was calculated as follows:

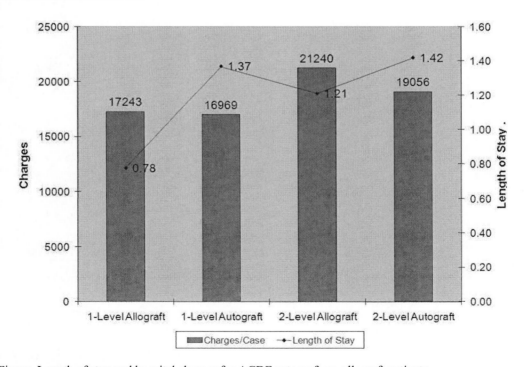

Figure. Length of stay and hospital charges for ACDF autograft vs. allograft patients.

**Table 3. Comparison of Procedure time, LOS and charges between
2-level ACDF patients (n=245)**

Variable	Autograft (n=212)				Allograft (n=33)			
	Mean	Std. Dev.	Min	Max	Mean	Std. Dev.	Min	Max
Age	52.43	9.41	28	79	53.55	12.87	27	87
Procedure Minutes	99.76	22.75	48	181	97.58	19.17	60	143
Avg. LOS	1.42	1.34	0	14	1.21	0.82	0	5
Hospital Charges***	19,056.32	6,142.37	6,350.00	93,590.00	21,239.85	3,639.25	15,932.00	35,057.00
Direct Cost***	7,043.04	1,697.44	1,643.33	23,052.83	8,353.13	1,450.29	6,256.31	14,923.33
Indirect Cost	2,113.04	985.63	803.03	12,649.70	2,270.32	824.85	1,698.46	6,616.85
Total Cost***	9,156.08	2,622.91	2,446.36	35,702.54	10,623.45	2,227.70	7,954.77	21,540.18
Direct Anesthesia Cost/Case	418.84	76.73	0.00	654.97	426.80	92.60	0.00	580.56
Direct Lab and Blood Bank Cost/Case	113.94	68.13	0.00	899.71	104.39	39.01	25.33	231.58
Direct Pharmacy Cost/Case	439.86	176.36	285.99	2,530.69	394.48	53.44	294.13	547.01
Direct Respiratory Therapy Cost/ Case	28.68	141.67	0.00	2,036.34	16.29	7.44	0.00	37.96
Direct Radiology Cost/Case	42.44	48.40	0.00	708.21	58.73	125.26	0.00	738.32
Direct Physical/ Occupational Therapy Cost/Case	8.59	34.38	0.00	370.39	16.80	51.26	0.00	243.40
Other Direct Routine Cost/Case	419.37	739.73	0.00	7,234.06	377.11	663.30	0.00	4,020.68
Direct O.R. Labor Cost/Case	1,517.01	852.38	0.00	8,601.91	1,507.83	530.51	1,125.08	4,384.64
Direct O.R. Supply Cost/Case***	3,103.79	678.47	0.00	4,822.28	4,331.77	679.43	2,645.39	5,758.25

***significant at 1% (p-value<.01); **significant at 5% (p-value<.05); *significant at 10% (p-value<.10)

Breakdown of Hospital Costs

Both indirect and direct costs are factored into the total hospital charges ascribed to a patient. In order to determine which factors varied or contributed most to the differences in charges between patients receiving allograft or autograft bones, we examined a variety of direct cost factors over the course of the patients' operations and hospital stays. These direct cost values are presented separately from the indirect costs associated with ACDF surgical procedures and post operative hospitalization in order to better evaluate variations expenses directly related to the procedures. Costs were grouped into broad categories in order to observe any statistically significant differences (Tables 2-3).

The cost category that presented the greatest difference in costs was the operating room (O.R.) supply cost per case (p<0.01) (Tables 2-3). O.R. supply costs included any necessary equipment utilized during surgery ranging from expensive items such as surgical tools to inexpensive items such as sutures. Among 1-level allograft patients average O.R. supply costs were $2,870 compared to $2,631 for autograft, a difference of $239 that was not statistically significant (p>0.05). The difference was statistically significant (p<0.01) among 2-level patients where mean direct costs associated with allograft were $4,332 compared to $3,104 for autograft, a difference of $1,228.

In order to study the difference in O.R. Supply costs between patients receiving allograft and autograft, the costs associated with every O.R. supply item were analyzed. While most supply costs were similar regardless of graft type, two O.R. supply costs accounted for substantial difference between the allograft and autograft groupings. Among all 88 of the 119 (100%) allograft patients, there was an average additional hospital direct cost of $1,196 that correlated to the cost of the allograft implant (Table 5). Among autograft patients, 137 of the 431 (31.7%) received a pain pump system to reduce post-operative pain on their donor graft sites. For these 137 patients, the pain pumps resulted in an additional direct hospital cost of $306 (Table 5).

Table 4. Regression Results

Variable	Hospital Charges	
	Coefficient	Std. Dev.
Age	57.3793***	18.8276
Male	394.1214	401.3315
level 2	1763.7220***	437.6495
autograft	-1150.6290**	496.4544
length of procedure	35.1837***	9.4388
Constant	11885.42	1248.713
N	550	
R squared	0.0939	
***significant at 1% (p-value<.01); **significant at 5% (p-value<.05); *significant at 10% (p-value<.10)		

Table 5. Noteworthy Operating Room Supply Costs

Noteworthy O.R. Costs	N	% of pts in group	% of total pts	Direct Hospital Cost
Allograft Implant	119	100% (119 of 119 allograft pts)	21.6% (119 of 550 pts)	$1,196
Pain Pump System for autograft harvest site	137	31.7% (137 of 431 autograft pts)	24.9% (137 of 550 pts)	$306

IV. DISCUSSION

Patient Characteristics

There was a statistically significant difference ($p<0.01$) in the age of 1-level allograft patients (46.9 years) compared to the mean for all patients (51.4 years). This may be related to the supposition that llografts, with their reportedly higher rates of nonunion [14], may be better indicated for younger patients better able to incorporate the allograft in their system.

A larger percentage of patients in our study received autograft implants (78%) similar to what Picket et. al reported, 76% [5]. However, trends nationally and internationally may vary. According to Deutsch et al, in the United States, unlike the rest of the world, the use of allograft in ACDF has expanded so much that a deficit in allografts appeared in the market [2]. Although autograft remains the standard in many countries, allograft procedures have also gained footholds in the United States and different parts of the world [15-19]. Options such as peak cages and the use of bone morphogenic proteins (BMP) have become more prevalent in enhancing or displacing these traditional graft options [31].

Procedure Time and LOS

Our results showed that the use of allograft did not lead to statistically significant changes in surgical procedure time ($p>0.05$). This is consistent with the study of Bai et al who found longer time on operation with the use of autograft ($P < 0.001$) [8]. Unfortunately, our study provides an imperfect comparison of procedure time. During our study, a second party harvested the graft and closed the site while the primary surgeon performed the procedure. The fact that two surgeons are working simultaneously likely reduced the operating time for autograft. One might expect to see an increase in procedure time if one surgeon performs both the ACDF procedure and the harvesting of the autograft bone.

Allograft usage for 1-level patients in our cohort did result in a statistically significant ($p<0.01$) reduction in average length of stay of 0.59 days compared to 1-level autograft. This could largely be attributed to the outpatient subgroup of the 1-level allograft patients who were able to return home on the same day of surgery. This is also consistent with the results of Bai et al reporting significant increase in length of stay after autograft ($P < 0.001$) [8]. The difference in length of stay for allograft and autograft in 2-level patients did not reach statistical significance ($p>0.05$).

Costs

Looking at hospital charges there was a statistically significant $2,184 increase for 2-level ACDF patients receiving allograft ($p<0.01$). Although most hospital cost categories analyzed yielded comparable results regardless of graft types, OR supply costs created a statistically significant increase ($p<0.01$) in direct costs for 2-level allograft patients. This increase was largely due to the expense of obtaining allograft implants at a rate of $1,196 per implant. While 1-level allograft patients also incurred this additional implant cost, these expenses were offset for this group by the direct hospital savings that resulted from a decreased length in hospitalization time of 0.59 days compared to 1-level autograft patients.

Several studies have analyzed cost differences between allograft and autograft usage [8-13]. Angevine et al study measured the long term economic benefit of autograft versus allograft in quality-adjusted life years (QALYs) [10]. The use of allograft for 1 ACDF without plating offered an improvement in quality of life compared to ACDF with autograft, at a cost of $496 per QALY. They further determined that ACDF with plating had a benefit relative to ACDF without plating at an approximate cost of $32,560 dollars per QALY. The results were most sensitive to assumptions regarding differences in the length of the postoperative recovery period.

Long-Term Efficacy Considerations

Length of Stay, operating time and hospital expenses are important factors to consider when making a decision between graft types. However, these are only small segments of a larger economic picture from a patient care standpoint. Secondary economic factors such as quality of life issues, ability to return to work, long-term pain and disability, and home medication costs are considerations that have not been addressed in our paper and are a part of the larger picture.

Furthermore, total patient costs may vary widely between countries, states, and even from one region to another within the same state. For meaningful discussions of the long-term economic advantages of one graft type over another, it is important to recognize that clinical outcomes as these have a large bearing on long term economic implications. Although this study does not seek to delve into a discussion of the clinical advantages of either allograft or autograft bone, it is worth noting the results of other studies that address these issues. Clinically, autograft and allograft have demonstrated comparable clinical results for ACDF in previous studies [3, 7-8, 15].

As with any surgical procedure, a patient always faces a risk of infection. In cases of ACDF with autograft, two surgical sites exist, and thus the risk of infection may be doubled. While concern is primarily directed toward the surgical site on the spine, donor site infections can pose additional problem that may complicate postoperative recovery of the patient [8, 16].

Several long-term follow up studies have studied chronic pain in patients with autograft due to the fact that harvesting bone from the iliac crest can create ambulation difficulties [17]. Silber et al report ambulation difficulties in 50% of cases [18]. Pain has been recorded in 14-26% of cases [18-19]. Steiber et al also note that as a result of these minor complications ACDF, patients receiving autograft experience an increased average length of hospital stay [19], a finding consistent with our 1-level patients. Polly and Kuklo report that donor site pain decreases over time and plateaus at 3 months, while the percentage of patients experiencing pain decreases until about 12 months and then appears to remain stable [20]. With the use of allograft bone in ACDF procedures, donor site morbidity is avoided and hospital stay has been reported as shorter than with autograft [8, 21], a finding also consistent with the results for 1-level patients in our study.

Although some concerns have been raised regarding the safety of allograft, there does not appear to be an overt risk associated with the use of allograft bone for spine surgery [22-23].

ACDF as an Outpatient Procedure

In our study, 32 of our 550 patients (5.8%) underwent surgery in an outpatient setting. Although some surgeons feel comfortable performing ACDF in an outpatient setting, there are very few studies in the literature analyzing its cost and safety [24]. Steiber et al studied the efficacy of ACDF with plate fixation in an outpatient setting and determined that the outpatient group had a lower complication rate compared with the controls [19]. However, the authors note that this variance may have been the result of selection bias that limited outpatient inclusion criteria to one or two level involvement at C4-5 or lower, absence of myelopathy, and subjective neck size.

In general, outpatient procedures tend to reduce costs to both a patient and hospital, and therefore, inquiries into the clinical feasibility of outpatient ACDF procedures may also be worthwhile from an economic perspective.

Study Limitations

As noted earlier, one of the limitations of our study was the imperfect comparison of Procedure Times between allograft and autograft owing to the manner in which the graft is harvested by a second surgeon at our institutions. Also, our study was a retrospective study, which is not as ideal as a prospective randomized study. In regards to graft comparisons, we did not have an equal representation between allograft and autograft patients. Further, our study only analyzes autograft and allograft usage in ACDF procedures from 2005-2007, even though options such as peak cages and bone morphogenic proteins (BMP) have begun to enhance or displace these traditional graft options. In regards to costs, this study was a snapshot of a larger economic picture and only considered costs from a hospital perspective. It is important to mention that the numbers used in this paper reflect the cost levels at one Medical Center within the broader United States healthcare system. As a result, caution should be taken in projecting or comparing our findings to other national institutions or healthcare systems in the world.

Future Studies

There are advantages to both allograft and autograft usage for ACDF when comparing the two graft options to one another. Although allograft may yield shorter hospitalization periods, it may also increase costs. Conversely, though autograft usage may result in short-term hospital cost savings, it is unclear as to whether it will yield greater benefits from a patient's long-term recovery and economic standpoint as it carries an association of donor site complication and morbidity issues. It would be beneficial to study long term costs to the patient in future studies so as to evaluate if the short term cost savings for autograft outweigh the morbidity and complication issues described in literature.

The feasibility of performing ACDF in an outpatient setting is also worthy of further analysis both from a safety and economic standpoint. Outpatient procedures may reduce the risk of hospital infection and eliminate the costs associated with the hospitalization period. Case studies and review articles that discuss complications associated with ACDF provide important cautions that may bring into question appropriateness of performing procedure in outpatient setting. The risk of hematoma as a complication associated with ACDF is of significant concern, and has been previously reported by Fountas et al. at a 5% rate of occurrence [22]. Its incidence among previously reported series varies between 1% to 11% [22]. While new technologies continue to develop as alternatives to traditional graft materials [23-25], autograft is still represented as the gold standard in literature [3]. Jeong et al predict that BMP will eventually become the most practical option in spinal surgery with expectations for lower complication rates and greater cost effectiveness [30]. However, in a more recent retrospective analysis, Cahill et al found that BMP usage resulted in more frequent complications for ACDF procedures and resulted in higher hospital charges for all categories of fusions [26].

Studies that analyze emerging graft-related technologies such as these should continually be conducted to validate these projections and to analyze improvements in patient care. Once the efficacy and safety of new technologies have been proven there is a further obligation to weigh the improvements from a socioeconomic standpoint.

CONCLUSION

Two findings emerge from our study. First, in 1-level patients undergoing ACDF, allograft usage yields a shorter length of hospital stay at a comparable rate of hospital charges to autograft. However, for 2-level patients undergoing ACDF, allograft resulted in higher hospital charges at a statistically significant rate, without yielding statistically significant reductions in LOS.

American and international healthcare systems have become increasingly cost-conscious, placing a demand on healthcare providers to become attuned with the costs associated with delivering healthcare. While excellent clinical care must remain the highest priority, it is vital that clinicians and patients are informed about the economic impact of their decisions. Our study provides a brief analysis of economic components associated with allograft and autograft usage for ACDF during the surgical and hospitalization period. By undertaking this study we did not attempt to draw large-scale conclusions. Rather, we analyzed only the costs of ACDF surgery and subsequent hospitalization. It must be emphasized that these costs are only one segment of the larger economic picture, and the limitations of our study must also be weighed against our conclusions. As with many issues, the decision as to which graft type to use for ACDF procedures is multi-factorial. Both short and long term cost and efficacy considerations must be considered.

REFERENCES

[1]   Cloward RB. The anterior approach for removal of ruptured cervical disks. *J. Neurosurg.* 1958 Nov;15(6):602-17.

[2]   Deutsch H, Haid R, Rodts G, Jr., Mummaneni PV. The decision-making process: allograft versus autograft. *Neurosurgery.* 2007 Jan;60(1 Suppl 1):S98-102.

[3]   Samartzis D, Shen FH, Goldberg EJ, An HS. Is autograft the gold standard in achieving radiographic fusion in one-level anterior cervical discectomy and fusion with rigid anterior plate fixation? *Spine* (Phila Pa 1976). 2005 Aug 1;30(15):1756-61.

[4]   Zigler JE, Anderson PA, Boden SD, Bridwell KH, Vaccaro AR. What's new in spine surgery. *J. Bone Joint Surg. Am.* 2003 Aug;85-A(8):1626-36.

[5]   Pickett GE, Van Soelen J, Duggal N. Controversies in cervical discectomy and fusion: practice patterns among Canadian surgeons. *Can. J. Neurol. Sci.* 2004 Nov;31(4):478-83.

[6]   Peolsson A, Peolsson M. Predictive factors for long-term outcome of anterior cervical decompression and fusion: a multivariate data analysis. *Eur. Spine J.* 2008 Mar;17(3): 406-14.

[7]   Yue WM, Tay BK, Kasinathan ST. Patellar allografts in anterior cervical fusion - a two-year clinical and radiographic study. *Singapore Med. J.* 2003 Oct;44(10):521-5.

[8]   Bai YB, Wang Y, Zhang YG. [Is allograft a procedure with high-risk in anterior cervical fusion]. Zhonghua Liu Xing Bing Xue Za Zhi. 2004 Jul;25(7):620-2.

[9]   Castro FP, Jr., Holt RT, Majd M, Whitecloud TS, 3rd. A cost analysis of two anterior cervical fusion procedures. *J. Spinal Disord.* 2000 Dec;13(6):511-4.

[10] Angevine PD, Zivin JG, McCormick PC. Cost-effectiveness of single-level anterior cervical discectomy and fusion for cervical spondylosis. *Spine* (Phila Pa 1976). 2005 Sep 1;30(17):1989-97.

[11] Ramnarain A, Govender S. Fibular allograft and anterior plating for dislocations/fractures of the cervical spine. *Indian J. Orthop.* 2008 Jan;42(1):83-6.

[12] Buttermann GR. Prospective nonrandomized comparison of an allograft with bone morphogenic protein versus an iliac-crest autograft in anterior cervical discectomy and fusion. *Spine J.* 2008 May-Jun;8(3):426-35.

[13] Vaidya R, Carp J, Sethi A, Bartol S, Craig J, Les CM. Complications of anterior cervical discectomy and fusion using recombinant human bone morphogenetic protein-2. *Eur. Spine J.* 2007 Aug;16(8):1257-65.

[14] Malloy KM, Hilibrand AS. Autograft versus allograft in degenerative cervical disease. *Clin. Orthop. Relat. Res.* 2002 Jan(394):27-38.

[15] Floyd T, Ohnmeiss D. A meta-analysis of autograft versus allograft in anterior cervical fusion. *Eur. Spine J.* 2000 Oct;9(5):398-403.

[16] Rawlinson JN. Morbidity after anterior cervical decompression and fusion. The influence of the donor site on recovery, and the results of a trial of surgibone compared to autologous bone. *Acta Neurochir.* (Wien). 1994;131(1-2):106-18.

[17] Mizuno J, Nakagawa H. Outcome analysis of anterior decompressive surgery and fusion for cervical ossification of the posterior longitudinal ligament: report of 107 cases and review of the literature. *Neurosurg. Focus.* 2001;10(4):E6.

[18] Silber JS, Anderson DG, Daffner SD, Brislin BT, Leland JM, Hilibrand AS, et al. Donor site morbidity after anterior iliac crest bone harvest for single-level anterior cervical discectomy and fusion. *Spine* (Phila Pa 1976). 2003 Jan 15;28(2):134-9.

[19] Stieber JR, Brown K, Donald GD, Cohen JD. Anterior cervical decompression and fusion with plate fixation as an outpatient procedure. *Spine J.* 2005 Sep-Oct;5(5):503-7.

[20] Polly DW, Kuklo TR. Bone graft donor site pain. 39th Annual Meeting of the Scoliosis Research Society; September 18–21; Seattle, WA2002.

[21] Sarwat AM, O'Brien JP, Renton P, Sutcliffe JC. The use of allograft (and avoidance of autograft) in anterior lumbar interbody fusion: a critical analysis. *Eur. Spine J.* 2001 Jun;10(3):237-41.

[22] Fountas KN, Kapsalaki EZ, Nikolakakos LG, Smisson HF, Johnston KW, Grigorian AA, et al. Anterior cervical discectomy and fusion associated complications. *Spine* (Phila Pa 1976). 2007 Oct 1;32(21):2310-7.

[23] Mroz TE, Joyce MJ, Lieberman IH, Steinmetz MP, Benzel EC, Wang JC. The use of allograft bone in spine surgery: is it safe? *Spine J.* 2009 Apr;9(4):303-8.

[24] Rosen VB, Hobbs LW, Spector M. The ultrastructure of anorganic bovine bone and selected synthetic hyroxyapatites used as bone graft substitute materials. *Biomaterials.* 2002 Feb;23(3):921-8.

[25] Block JE. Potential effectiveness of novel bone graft substitute materials. *Spine* (Phila Pa 1976). 1995 Oct 15;20(20):2261-2.

[26] Cahill KS, Chi JH, Day A, Claus EB. Prevalence, complications, and hospital charges associated with use of bone-morphogenetic proteins in spinal fusion procedures. *JAMA.* 2009 Jul 1;302(1):58-66.

In: Toward Healthcare Resource Stewardship   ISBN: 978-1-62100-182-9
Editors: J. S.Robinson, M. S.Walid et al.   © 2012 Nova Science Publishers, Inc.

Chapter 11

PREVALENCE AND ECONOMIC IMPACT OF POSTOPERATIVE ANEMIA FOLLOWING LUMBAR SPINE FUSION

M. Sami Walid[1] and Nadezhda Zaytseva*

[1]Medical Center of Central Georgia, Macon, GA, US
[2]Kuban State Medical University, Krasnodar, Russia

ABSTRACT

Introduction: Postoperative/posthemorrhagic anemia frequently occurs after typical spine surgery procedures; however; no concrete data are published on this subject. In this paper, we study the prevalence of this complication in spine fusion patients and its impact on hospital cost.

Methods: The hospital records of 1535 spine surgery patients operated between 2003 and 2008 were retrospectively reviewed and their secondary diagnosis ICD-9 codes were filtered for posthemorrhagic anemia. The cohort included patients who underwent one of two most common fusion procedures (81.07 and 81.08).

Results: Posthemorrhagic anemia was more common after procedure 81.07 lumbar/lumbosacral fusion lateral (16.4%) compared with procedure 81.08 lumbar/lumbosacral fusion posterior (12.2%) without statistical significance (p=.57). However, significant differences in hospital charges were noted between patients with and without posthemorrhagic anemia in the lateral fusion group ($53,285.98 vs. $48,509.24). No statistically significant difference in hospital charges were recorded in the poster fusion group.

Conclusion: Posthemorrhagic anemia is more common in lateral fusions and appears to be statistically associated with increased hospital charges in this category of patients. It is important to pay attention to secondary diagnoses that may impact cost, such as posthemorrhagic anemia.

* Corresponding Author: M. Sami Walid, Medical Center of Central Georgia, 840 Pine Street, Suite 880, Medical Center of Central Georgia, Macon, GA 331201. E-mail: mswalid@yahoo.com.

Posthemorrhagic anemia refers to a physiological state where reduction in the number of red blood cells in the body occurs as a result of acute loss of blood following trauma or surgical intervention. With blood loss, blood volume diminishes, hemodilution occurs, and oxygenation of tissue declines. This manifests with hypoxemic and hemodynamic symptoms and signs that include dizziness; faintness; weakness; pallor; thirst; sweating; rapid, weak pulse; rapid respiration; and orthostatic hypotension. Erythrocytes are usually normocytic; agranulocytosis may be seen on peripheral smear; and coagulation time becomes reduced. This anemia is classified as normochromic, normocytic, regenerative type of anemia.

From our experience, posthemorrhagic anemia does occur after typical spine surgery procedures; however; no concrete data are published on this subject. In this paper, we study the prevalence of postoperative/posthemorrhagic anemia in spine fusion patients and its impact on hospital cost.

METHODS

The hospital records of 1535 spine surgery patients operated between 2003 and 2008 were retrospectively reviewed and their secondary diagnosis ICD-9 codes were filtered for posthemorrhagic anemia. The cohort included patients who underwent one of two most common fusion procedures:

- 81.07 Lumbar or lumbo-sacral lateral fusion (N=1183).
- 81.08 Lumbar or lumbo-sacral posterior fusion (N=352).

Demographically, the average age of the cohort was 55 years; 57% were females and 77% were Caucasians. The prevalence of posthemorrhagic anemia was compared using chi-square test. Differences in hospital length of stay and charges in association with posthemorrhagic anemia were studied using T-test.

RESULTS

Posthemorrhagic anemia was more common after procedure 81.07 lumbar/lumbosacral fusion lateral (16.4%) compared with procedure 81.08 lumbar/lumbosacral fusion posterior (12.2%) without statistical significance (p=.57). However, significant differences in hospital charges were noted between patients with and without posthemorrhagic anemia in the lateral fusion group (Table 1). The average charges were \$53,285.98 for patients with posthemorrhagic anemia versus \$48,509.24 for patients without anemia. No statistically significant difference in hospital charges were recorded in the posterior fusion group (Table 2).

Table 1. Average length of stay (days) and hospital charges ($) per posthemorrhagic anemia in lateral fusion patients

			DAYS	TOTAL CHARGES
	No	Mean	5.0	$48,509
		N	989	989
		Std. Deviation	3.9	$22,090
	Yes	Mean	5.5	$53,286
		N	194	194
Posthemorrhagic Anemia		Std. Deviation	3.3	$18,186

Table 2. Average length of stay (days) and hospital charges ($) per posthemorrhagic anemia in posterior fusion patients

			DAYS	TOTAL CHARGES
	No	Mean	5.6	$54,184
		N	309	309
		Std. Deviation	5.2	$31,931
	Yes	Mean	5.9	$62,127
		N	43	43
Posthemorrhagic Anemia		Std. Deviation	3.7	$30,809

DISCUSSION

The prevalence of posthemorrhagic anemia has, to our knowledge, never been studied in patients undergoing different spine fusion procedures. These procedures differ in their invasiveness and therefore carry different risk of posthemorrhagic anemia. We used hospital data to study the prevalence of this complication in this cohort of patients. The results, as expected, show significant differences in posthemorrhagic anemia rates. Our study quantified this observation by calculating prevalence rates per procedure, which has not been done before. Additionally, we investigated the impact of posthemorrhagic anemia on cost as reflected by hospital charges and length of stay. We found that posthemorrhagic anemia was more common in lateral fusions and was statistically associated with increased hospital charges in lateral fusions as well. This is probably related to the cost of blood transfusion and increased length of stay as shown in the tables.

Posthemorrhagic anemia can be easily missed especially if no blood transfusion has been performed. This diagnosis may therefore be undercoded in administrative data, a possible criticism of the study [1,2]. Nevertheless, this does not affect the strength of the paper since undercoding diminishes the actual size of the problem.

The finding of an economic impact from posthmorrhagic anemia is important as hospital costs are becoming a burden on the healthcare system and patients. Cost awareness requires us, clinicians, to explore postoperative factors that significantly affect cost including such secondary diagnoses as posthemorrhagic anemia.

REFERENCES

[1]   Romano PS, S. M. (2002). Can administrative data be used to ascertain clinically significant postoperative complications? *Am. J. Med. Qual.* 2002 Jul-Aug;17(4): , 145-54.

[2]   Campbell PG, Malone J, Yadla S, Chitale R, Nasser R, Maltenfort MG, Vaccaro A, Ratliff JK. Comparison of ICD-9-based, retrospective, and prospective assessments of perioperative complications: assessment of accuracy in reporting. *J. Neurosurg. Spine.* 2010 Dec 8.

In: Toward Healthcare Resource Stewardship
Editors: J.S.Robinson, M.S.Walid and A.C.M.Barth

ISBN: 978-1-62100-182-9
© 2012 Nova Science Publishers, Inc.

Chapter 12

A NEW CONCEPT OF INPATIENT CARE: ACUITY-ADAPTABLE PATIENT ROOM DECREASES LENGTH OF STAY AND COST – RESULTS OF A PILOT STUDY[♦]

Nena Bonuel,[1][*] Alma deGracia[2] and Sandra Cesario[3]

[1]Center for Professional Excellence, The Methodist Hospital, Texas, US
[2]Multi-Organ Transplant Unit, The Methodist Hospital, Texas, US
[3]Texas Woman's University, Texas, US

ABSTRACT

The acuity-adaptable patient room concept is an emerging care model where patient is cared for in the same room from admission through discharge regardless of the patient level of acuity. After implementation of the care cluster strategy to support the implementation of an acuity-adaptable patient room, a descriptive study was conducted looking at so whether there will be a decreased length of stay and cost on patient cared for in the acuity-adaptable patient room compared to patients cared for in a transitional care process. Result of the study showed decreased length of stay of kidney transplant patients from 9.6 (11.0) days (before acuity-adaptable patient room) to 4.1 (1.3) days (acuity-adaptable patient room). Not only that the acuity-adaptable patient room improves patient outcome and cost but with the nursing competency preparation to support the implementation of the acuity-adaptable patient room, a hybrid *nurse* was created who possessed both critical care and medical-surgical skills. This can be a potential trend in the professional nurse model to address the health care challenges we face today in terms of nursing shortage, abbreviated plan of care, and facility operation efficiency.

[♦] The study was supported by The Methodist Hospital Research Institute CTSA Award, 2007, for Acuity-Adaptable Renal Transplant Pilot Study.

[*] Corresponding Author: Nena Bonuel, MSN, RN, CCRN, CNS,ACNS-BC. The Methodist Hospital, The Center for Professional Excellence, 6565 Fannin St, Houston, TX 77030. E-mail: nbonuel@tmhs.org.

INTRODUCTION

Today, with the exponential changes in clinical services, operational trends, and new technologies, any patient room hailed as state-of-the-art 20 or even 10 years ago is becoming obsolete long before its physical life is spent. The acuity-adaptable patient room concept is an emerging care model where patient is cared for in the same room from admission through discharge regardless of the patient level of acuity. Unlike the current standard care delivery, where the patient is required to move from unit to unit, hence from room to room depending on the level of care acuity, in the acuity-adaptable patient room concept, the care is brought to the patient. In the highly competitive, complex, and challenging healthcare environment, one has to examine the impact of agency operations on its clientele: the patient, families and visitors, and the health care team. Improving patient outcomes through evidence-based practice and transdisciplinary collaboration using an acuity-adaptable patient room is a novel approach to clinical practice in the 21st century.

The acuity-adaptable patient room is a private room concept designed to support the complete range of care to adapt to patients' changing needs. The rooms are larger in size than a regular hospital room to accommodate various patient needs as their condition changes, such as critical-care equipment, additional staff, procedures, and family members. Patient visibility from the corridor is possible, and space is provided for the visitors. Acuity-adaptable rooms are expected to reduce transport costs, decrease errors, minimize bottlenecks, and delay patient flow. With acuity-adaptable care delivery, nursing staff competency will also be addressed to include hybrid nurses who possess critical-care and acute-care skills. However, the patient population that fits the acuity-adaptable room are homogenous and with predictable outcomes (Brown and Gallant, 2006; Gallant, 2006; Hill-Rom, 2002; Gallant and Lanning, 2001).

Specific Aims

1. Improve patient outcomes and satisfaction through the implementation of a single-room, acuity adaptable patient room to provide care following renal transplantation.
2. Provide a healing environment by minimizing patient care interruptions and eliminate errors, injuries, and inefficient use of time related to patient transfers.
3. Support future patient care delivery while investigating and resolving patient flow issues.

Background and Significance

Kidney transplantation is the hope for quality of life and long term survival for patients with end-stage renal disease. The care of a patient undergoing renal transplantation is complex and centered on critically assessing renal function, administering immunosuppressive therapy, observing the function of the newly transplanted kidney, monitoring fluid and electrolyte balance, preventing sources of infection, detecting early signs of complications and rejection, managing and supporting the patient and family through the recovery phase (Holechek and Armstrong, 2008). In a population of long-term dialysis patients, Wolfe found that dialysis patients on the transplant waiting list had a lower mortality rate than did nonlisted dialysis patients, reflecting that healthier patients are placed on the waiting list. A significant long-term survival benefit was detected in patients who received their first deceased-donor kidney transplant on the other hand. Even though the mortality rate in these recipients was higher initially after transplant surgery than in patients who remained on the waiting list, long term mortality was 48% to 82% lower.

With the lightning fast technological changes, creation of a global village, seeking transparency of information has reached a fever pitch. There is an almost incomprehensible list of trends that the health-care industry must face and that it is worth exploring the need for the acuity-adaptable patient room is worth exploring. To top the list is the prediction that the inpatient population over the next 25 years will dramatically increase due to the aging baby-boom generation, increased life expectancy, increased fertility rates, and continued immigration (Shactman, Altman, Eilat, Thorpe, and Doonan, 2003; Solucient, 2003). With the advancement of technology, the patients of the future are predicted to be well-informed, diverse and educated, more acute with co-morbidities, obese and will require more intensive interventions. It has been forecasted that there will be 87 million Latin Americans by the year 2060, with the Caucasian population constituting 50% (U.S. Census Bureau, 2000). There are 76 million Americans over the age of 50 with a trillion of dollars of spending power in their hands. The baby boomers (a person between the age range of 40-60 year old) have higher expectations and are forcing hospitals to abandon the traditional conveyor-belt approach to care, where patients are transferred from unit to unit in search of the proper level of care (Brown and Gallant, 2006).

It is important to note that imbedded in the boomer generation is the nurse who is also aging. Currently, the projected average age of the nurse is 45.4; it is expected to increase to 47 by 2010 (Buerhaus, Steiger, and Auerback, 2000; National Sample Survey of Registered Nurses, 2004). A survey in 2003 by the Center for American Nurse Mature Nurse claimed that 37% of the mature nurses plan to retire between 2015 and 2020. There will be at least 12% shortfall of nurses of the RN required to those that are available (JAMA, 2000). In the light of this projection, the U.S. Bureau of Labor Statistics (2004) claimed, the challenge lies in replacing those retiring and meeting the demand for 1 million nurses by the year 2012.

In the practice setting, bottlenecks in the patient flow have reached an alarming proportion. The occupancy of most hospitals at midnight hovers at 80% to 90%; by midday all the inpatient beds are usually filled when admissions and surgical volumes peak. With the inability to move patients in a timely manner, delayed discharges from the unit, new admissions' frequent demands, and patients being diverted from at-capacity hospitals and emergency departments adversely affect patient care and compromise patient safety (Hendrich, Fay, and Sorrells, 2004).

The combination of high-acuity patients, including the renal transplant patient, shrinking pool of the aging caregiver (Buerhaus et al., 2000), shortage of nurses (Cho, Ketefian, Barkauskas, and Smith, 2003), patient bottlenecks, and demands on infrastructure paint a bleak landscape. To survive this gloomy forecast, the technology, facilities, and infrastructure have to be more flexible than ever before. Energy should be focused on creating flexibility to the patient room where most of the nursing activity occurs.

Research Hypothesis

- Patients cared for in the Acuity-Adaptable Patient Room will have decreased costs for their total care experience to patient cared for in a transitional care process.
- Patients cared for in the Acuity-Adaptable patient Room will have decreased lengths of stay in comparison to patients cared for in a transitional care process.
- There will be no difference in patient satisfaction, nursing care, patient comfort, physiologic measures and nosocomial infection between those patients cared for in the Acuity-Adaptable Patient Room and those cared for in a transitional care process.

Definition of Terms

Length of Stay -The number of days of care counted from the admission date to the separation date for residents within a healthcare facility.(Doupe, Brownel, Kozyrskyi, Dik, Burnhill,Dahl,Chateau,De Coster,Hinds, and Bodnarchuk, (2006).

Costs – refer to the total amount of money spent for goods or services in the care management of the renal transplant patient in the ICU and on the floor. It also includes labor and direct costs, supply costs and total OR cost.

Nursing Care – refers to the nursing activity that promotes prevention of pressure ulcer formation, medication errors and patient falls and prevention of deep vein thrombosis.

Patient Comfort level – refers to patient's score on the validated pain scale including degree of discomfort with foley catheter.

Physiologic Measures – refers to the negative shift of biological parameters such as:

- Systolic pressure >180 mg/Hg or <100 mmgHg
- Diastolic pressure >110 or <60 mmgHg
- Urine output of less than 200 cc in 8 hour
- Glucose level of greater than 110
- Heart rate of greater than 110 or less than 60
- Temperature of greater than 100.
- CVP < 6 or greater than 15 cm. (TMH Renal order set, 2006)

Nosocomial infection – refers to hospital acquired infections common to a hospitalized patient such as urinary tract infection, pneumonia and central line infection.

Literature Review

Loma Linda University Medical Center in California pioneered the acuity-adaptable concept in the 1970s (Brown and Gallant, 2006). In 1999, Loma Linda was able to decrease the length of stay of its cardiothoracic patients with diagnosis-related groups (DRGs) of 104, 105, 106, 107, and 109 from 9.5 days, which is the California average, to 5.4 days; and 30% of its patients were discharged within 4 days (The Advisory Board, 2001). Hendrich and Lee(2005) provided a strong case for using the acuity-adaptable room concept when they analyzed intrahospital patient-transfer process time, the activity of the personnel, and cost of the transport procedure. According to Hendrich and Lee, 87% of the wasted time occurred in pretransport, and the common delays were administrative delays, bed control delays, and delays due to communication breakdown.

MedCath, a physician-owned specialty hospital, garnered positive recognition from national health-rating agencies and augmented the hospital's patient base because of its acuity-adaptable patient-room design based on the survey conducted by The Advisory Board (The Advisory Board, 2002; Brown and Gallant, 2006).

In 1999, Clarian Health System's Methodist Hospital, a tertiary-level care facility in Indiana, published the first clinical outcomes data on the effects of the acuity-adaptable room concept. Pioneered by Hendrich et al. (2004), a 3-year study done using a pre-post method compared the effects of the acuity-adaptable rooms proved that there was a significant decrease in clinician handoffs and transfer (90%), reduction of medication error (70%), and that the patient-fall index moved to a national benchmark of 2 falls per 1,000 patient days, which is a huge stride for patient safety, improvement in patient satisfaction, decrease in number of hours per patient days, increase in availability of nursing time for direct care without added cost, and increase in patient days per bed with a smaller bed base. This study made a significant impact in the health-care design industry to get the buy-in of the hospital management by showing outcomes that truly impact patient recovery and patient safety.

A 1997 nonexperimental survey by Janssen, Klein, Harris, Soolsma, and Seymour (2000) in B.C. Women's Hospital involving 205 maternity patients claimed patients were very satisfied in a single-room maternity care citing less exposure to multiple caregivers showed respect to patient privacy. A descriptive study done by Douglas, Steele, Tood, and Douglas (2002) interviewed 50 inpatients and surveyed 785 previous patients and found an increase in patient satisfaction with the care in a single room.

A similar outcome was noted in Ohio State University (OSU) Medical Center, the first academic institution to design its patient rooms with the acuity-adaptable concept. A joint survey by OSU and Corazon Consulting reported a 67% increase in patient satisfaction by the study participants compared to the competitors that did not use the acuity-adaptable room concept (Bush, Reisman, Anstine, Gallaher, and Davis, 2005; Brown and Gallant, 2006).

An abstract presentation at the National Teaching Institute (NTI) of the American Association of Critical Care Nurses in 2001 from North Memorial Medical Center in Robbinsdale, MN, claimed after 1-year collection of data of cardiac patients with DRGs of 104, 105, 106, 107, and 109, the length of stay of the patients was reduced from 6.2 days to 5.4 days and 56% of the patients were discharged within 3 to 4 days (NTI Presentation, 2001).

Walsh, McCullough, and White (2006) found that 9 months after moving to the single-room unit, noise level decreased from an average of 63 to 56 decibels. A similar outcome was obtained by Brown and Taquino (2001) upon move-in in a newly designed infant intensive care unit (ICU) with a single-room concept design where the sound measurement was decreased to an average Leq of 42.4 decibels in staff work areas with sound burst to 60 decibels. The recommended standard for noise controls in newborn ICUs state that continuous background and transient sound should not exceed an hourly Leq average of 50 decibels (a weighted scale), with peak sounds not to exceed an Lmax of 70 decibels.

A study done by Rashid (2006) on the physical design characteristics of sets of adult ICUs built between 1993 and 2003 has proven that single rooms consistently help reduce noise, improve privacy, enhance patients' quality sleep, and increase patient and nurse satisfaction. In addition, patients in single ICU rooms have lower nosocomial infection rates because of improved airflow, better ventilation, and more accessible hand-washing facilities.

Thompson, Meredith, and Molnar (2002) studied the effects of single rooms on patients with burn wound infections by reviewing burn patients during the temporary closure of the burn unit in 1999. The authors found that patients transferred to the ICU and the private ward had a significant incidence of infection (47%) compared to prior closure of the burn unit (10.8%) and after two months stay on the newly renovated burn unit (23%). Ulrich, Quan, Zimring, Joseph, and Choudhary (2004) combed 600 peer-reviewed journals and found that patients who stay in single rooms have lower nosocomial infection rates, fewer patient transfers and associated medical errors, less noise level, better patient privacy and confidentiality, better communication from the staff to patients and from patients to staff, superior accommodation of family, and consistently higher satisfaction with overall quality of care.

A nonexperimental cohort design study of 173 burn patients and a later study of 213 burn patients by Shirani et al. (1986); Passweg et al. (1998); and Cheng and Nelson (2000) found that infection was reduced from 58.1% to 30.4% in the later cohort. Providencia and pseudomonas species, endemic in the early cohort, was absent on the late cohort. Walsh et al. (2006) found a highly significant reduction of catheter-associated bloodstream infections from 10.1 per 1,000 device days to 3.3 per 1,000 device days in 9 months after the move to single-patient rooms in a newborn ICU.

Janssen, Harris, Soolsma, Klein, and Seymour (2001) made a follow-up study involving 26 delivery suite nurses' and 26 postpartum nurses' response to a single-unit patient room. The study group described their single rooms as significantly more spacious and with a more consistent room setup compared to nurses working in other areas. The nurses felt they were better able to respond to patients' physical, emotional, and spiritual needs, and they felt autonomous to practice family-centered care.

Walsh et al. (2006) did a survey involving 127 nurses in newborn intensive care and claimed that the single-room concept is superior for patient care and parent satisfaction compared to the large open unit, but emphasized that the success of the single-room care model primarily depends on sufficient staffing due to the decreased visibility between patients and greater distances between patients.

Chadbury, Mahmood, and Valente (2006) surveyed 77 nurses' perception of the advantages and disadvantages of single-room occupancy versus multioccupancy patient rooms in medical-surgical units in four hospitals. Nurses rated the single room as helpful and favored the single-room occupancy more than the multioccupancy patient room in 15 categories to include flexibility in accommodating family, suitability for examination of patients by health-care personnel, patients' comfort level, patient recovery rate, less probability of medication errors, and less probability of diet mix-ups.

Anecdotal report from Clark, Roberts, and Traylor (2004) reported that since the single-unit patient room was implemented in a 518-bed community-based hospital there has been a decrease for the first time electives from 4.2% to 0% during the past 6 years, postoperative median extubation times were reduced from 9.9 to 5.5 hours, deep sternal wound infection rates were reduced from 4.2% in 1994 to 0.9% in 2002, length of stay of open heart patients decreased from 7.5 days to 5.3 days during the first quarter of the new delivery model and the third quarter decrease to 4.0 days in 2003, patient satisfaction was 100% per National

Research Corp., improved satisfaction of staff was evident by increased staff retention, and staff turnover decreased from 28.3 % to 1.7%.

Corazon Consulting (2004) studied hospitals across the country and examined the cardiac universal bed (CUB) model and its benefits. Sixty-seven percent of the patients studied rated their hospital experience with higher patient satisfaction compared to those who do not use CUB. Further, in the CUB model, the nurses were available to rapidly assess the patient and initiate therapy during an emergency with no delay, and the complication rates of patients who had coronary artery bypass graft averaged 5.6 postoperative days compared to 6.5 postoperative days based on report of the Society of Thoracic Surgeons that year.

Gaps of the Literature Review

According to the literature review, acuity-adaptable rooms have measurable outcomes in terms of lowering infection rates, decreasing length of stay, improving care efficiency, and increasing patient and nurse satisfaction. However, there are gaps as well as opportunities to explore before one can build a strong support of the relevance and the feasibility of this novel approach.

For example, the research methods used in many of the studies described in the literature review are not randomized studies. Most of the studies used a pre- and post method, a questionnaire survey, a retrospective review, and nonexperimental methods. To build a strong study, randomization is important because it controls all possible sources of extraneous variation. It could be that randomized control studies are not be feasible in this particular research focus because it is dealing with an outcome of health-care services such as operational process and care delivery. Outcome research would be more appropriate because it is feasible and convenient. Randomization might not be the best method for this kind of study because patient perception of quality of care would be a concern, especially when most patients favor single-room status when they are admitted. It would be challenging for the researcher to approach that family for consent to take a multioccupancy room rather than a private room.

Another area of concern is the definition of a true acuity-adaptable room. Numerous studies address the concept in many different terms, for example *single-unit patient room*, *cardiac universal room*, *single-room maternity room*, and *LDRP* (labor, delivery, recovery, postpartum) *room*. These rooms are defined according to individual institution criteria. There are no set standardized criteria for these rooms. Standardization is important so this can be built into the National Healthcare Building Guideline.

The acuity-adaptable patient room is suggested to be large—approximately 400 square feet—to accommodate for the fluctuation of the patient condition. The regular patient room is about 130 square feet. Thus, health-care institutions planning a new building or future renovation will need to think carefully about nearly tripling the size of each room, especially considering that many of the studies previously mentioned examined a very few specialized patient populations (cardiac, maternity, surgical patients, intensive-care patients). What about the rest of the patient populations? For stakeholders, tripling the size of the room—and it's inherent costs— will have to be weighed heavily against the need to design rooms for a generic patient population, that is, rooms that accommodate all types of patients. The research showed that the acuity-adaptable patient room concept is highly successful with the maternity patients, cardiac patients, some surgical patients, and the patients need to be a homogeneous population for the concept to be successful. Certainly, more research is needed to address other patient populations. In the practice setting, looking at the every-day need for beds due to growing number of patient admissions, there are times that, due to shortage of beds, patients are placed wherever there is a bed available. The need for homogeneity of patients is not often possible in the real-world setting—so this is an area that needs to be explored in terms of the acuity-adaptable patient room concept being successful in a large range of patient populations.

Another need to be addressed is the nursing competency of the caregiver. What kind of education or competency skills would the staff need to work in an acuity-adaptable room? Should all staff be critical-care nurses? Should the staff be medical-surgical nurses with critical-care training? Or should the nurses be a hybrid group of critical-care nurses and medical surgical nurses? How would nurses be assigned to these patients? Given the problem of staffing shortage, what would be the nurse:patient staffing ratio? Would it be 2:1, 3:1, or 4:1? Currently, there is nothing in the literature that addresses this important piece. Ideally, all nurses who are currently working in the area where this type of patient-care delivery will be implemented should be given a needs assessment survey of their educational needs. It would be helpful for the unit management to meet with each individual nurse to allow the nurses to express their feelings and concerns about the new care delivery. The unit management should plant the seeds of support and pledge of availability for any of their concerns regarding the new care approach. Because the rationale behind the acuity-adaptable bed is for nurses to be able to take care of patients' potential fluctuation of health condition, nurses need to learn critical-care skills such as advance cardiac life support. Certification of basic life support is a given, but how about learning how to identify lethal arrhythmias and interpreting advance electrovardiographic abnormalities? Or learning how to interpret arterial blood gases? The unit management needs to collaborate with the education department to develop a curriculum that addresses these educational needs.

For staffing ratio concerns, it would be best for the staff nurses to be included in the discussion allowing them some autonomy in resolving this issue. Staff nurses most often have creative ideas of how to solve the staffing ratio. The staff nurses are most often closer to the problem than the manager, and most of the time, they have ideas of how to solve the problem. The key is to instill with the nurses the importance of good working relationships and self-governance.

Another complicated and often-complex process is how to charge for patients who stay in acuity-adaptable beds. Most institutions have a set standard of level of care criteria used to determine the appropriateness of admission, continued services, and discharge, across the continuum of care. Currently, patients are charged for staying in the ICU, med-surg unit, intermediate-care unit, or skilled nursing facility and rehabilitation. There is a need to discuss this and transdisciplinary collaboration to include appropriate charging for patient in an acuity-adaptable patient room.

Another area that needs attention is nurse pay—should nurses be compensated for working in such a highly stressful environment?

Adequate staffing is a concern in one of the studies. Further compounding this concern is the isolation that nurses might feel when other patients or coworkers are not visible. Visibility of nurses as well as of patients is vital during time of emergent conditions. One way to solve this problem is the use of technology. Currently, many nurses use cell phones to communicate, and some wear locator tracers on their shoulders so the location of each nurse is known. Technology is helpful, but then again, nurses are very social people and they would like to see each other for support and comfort. A good investment is a creation of a centralized and decentralized nurses' station combined so the nurse can be near the patient and also have an area that they can socially congregate.

Physician buy-in will be another challenge. Most physicians tend to send patients to the ICU if they consider their patients to be semi-acute and need to be closely observed. Physicians often transfer this kind of patient to the ICU because of the perception that critical-care nurses are the best nurses with excellent critical-thinking skills because of the severity and the intensity of their work environment. The way to get physicians' buy-in to the idea of putting their patients in an acuity-adaptable patient room is to engage them from the get go. Persuade one of the medical leaders to be the medical champion of the initiative so he or she can influence her or his peers to admit their patients in the acuity-adaptable patient rooms. Another recommendation is to share information with the physicians of the competency of the nurses in the unit, the appropriate educational preparation completed by the nurses to gain competency to care for the patient, and plan for the nurses' continuing education to hone their critical-care skills. With this plan of action, physicians will take comfort and be reassured that their patients will get the best care.

Conclusion of Literature Review

There are several studies regarding favorable outcomes on patient and staff satisfaction on the acuity-adaptable rooms, but the studies are very few to count; again this area truly needs to be explored to strengthen and support the previous studies and add to the body of knowledge. Empirical studies have proven that patients placed in an acuity-adaptable room have significant outcomes to patient safety, patient and family healing, staff stress and effectiveness, and improved overall health-care quality and cost. Significant clinical outcomes of the patient addressing length of stay, infection, medication errors, and reports of falls are strong evidence that this body of science needs to be pursued and examined. While it is difficult to conduct rigorous research on the impact of the acuity-adaptable patient room because the hospital system is so complex and it is difficult to isolate the impact of a single entity, several studies on acuity-adaptable care delivery model heralding effects of impact on patient outcomes make considerable progress in developing a knowledge base of evidence that this research area is relevant and it made a significant contribution to patient safety and quality of care.

Exploring New Care Direction

With the relentless pursuit of patient care quality and patient safety, one has to explore every possible avenue to transform and redesign care delivery to remain solvent and meet the health care needs of patients in the future. One institution embraced the challenge to innovate by providing care to the renal transplant patient through the use of the acuity-adaptable patient room concept. The approach was forward thinking because under the new health care reform, specifically *The Patient Protection and Affordable Care Act of 2010* (PPACA) incentivize organization that focuses on value of care rather than the volume through investment in infrastructure and redesigned care processes for high quality and efficient service delivery. Exploring the acuity-adaptable patient room concept would be fitting to demonstrate care process redesign that is relevant to support the patient room of the future.

An opportunity to explore a novel approach to care delivery was presented in our 30-bed multi-organ transplant unit in a twice Magnetdesignated1500-bed tertiary hospital in Houston area with a goal of improving patient outcomes and satisfaction through implementation of a single-room, acuity-adaptable patient room to provide care following renal transplantation. The single room conforms to the acuity-adaptable concept where patients are cared for in the same room throughout the entire hospitalization period. The care is brought to the patient rather than moving the patient to the next level of care (Brown, Gallant, 2006, Galant. 2006, and Gallant, and Lanning, K. 2001). By adapting this concept, the patient is provided with a healing environment by minimizing patient care interruptions and eliminating errors, injuries, and inefficient use of time-related patient transfers(Hendrich., Fay, and Sorrells, 2004) and Hendrich and Lee, 2005). By caring for the patient in the same room throughout hospitalization, consistency of care is increased resulting in increased nurse satisfaction (Janssen, Harris, Soolsma, Klein, and Seymour,2001) and improved work environment resulting in decreased nurse turnover. In the 30-bed multiorgan transplant unit, we were able to convert 4 patient rooms to acuity-adaptable patient rooms. The rooms are equipped with a cardiac monitor that is capable of electrocardiographic (ECG) monitoring, pulse oximetry, and hemodynamic monitoring. The room is also equipped with medical gas capability where a ventilator, a left ventricular assist device, and an oxygen administration tube can be hooked up should patient condition warrant the use of these devices. The kidney transplant patient requires the complex care coordination. To successfully care for the patient in an acuity-adaptable patient room, a cluster of care bundles needs to be set in place and nurses must be equipped with knowledge and skills needed to provide safe, high-quality effective and respectful care.

THE STRATEGY

A transdisciplinary planning team comprising the associate chief of nursing, the nursing director, a clinical nurse specialist, managers, the clinical leader, and a nurse educator was convened to develop strategy for successful implementation of the acuity-adaptable care delivery. Benchmarking was sought with likeminded academic institutions of the nation for evidence-based practices on how to care for patient in an acuity-adaptable setting. The result of benchmarking yields no 1 benchmark that has an acuity-adaptable care setting to our knowledge. Fully supported by the hospital leadership, the logistics of creating the acuity adaptable room was operationalized. Multiorgan transplant nurse-driven admission, discharge, and transfer criteria were developed and approved by the Transplant Care Management Performance Improvement Committee and the institution's Policy and Procedure Committee. A communication strategy was implemented to address patient admission from all entry points, and the coordination of the postoperative patient flow from operating theatre to the acuity-adaptable patient room was explained. Nursing competency is paramount to the success of this kind of care delivery. To be able to prepare for the sudden change in patient conditions, take appropriate actions, and successfully manage the patient undergoing renal transplantation, the nurse must possess good clinical judgment and excellent critical thinking skills and must be knowledgeable to communicate and articulate relevant information to the patient and the family with a goal of keeping them informed of the patient status and care management. According to the descriptive qualitative study by Wysong and Driver (2009) patients' perception of a nurse skill is measured by their interpersonal relationship and their critical thinking skills.

SUPPORTING NURSING COMPETENCY

Led by a clinical nurse specialist, a transdisciplinary team comprising a transplant clinical pharmacist, an intensive care pharmacist, an intensive care clinical leader, a transplant physician assistant, a nursing director, and a clinical development specialist as faculty developed a kidney transplant nursing core curriculum to address the competency of the transplant nurses. The primary focus of the educational program was to infuse critical care concepts to the transplant nurses to provide them with complex critical care skills necessary to function independently and competently in an acuity-adaptable setting. With critical thinking skills permeated through the whole curriculum, the 1-week didactic includes the following:

1. 2006 Advance Cardiac Life Support certification guidelines,
2. 12 lead ECG,
3. The kidney transplant patient,
4. Acute renal failure,
5. Treatment options for acute renal failure,
6. Treatment consideration of end-stage renal disease,
7. Ethical consideration of renal transplantation,
8. Hemodynamic monitoring,
9. Hemodynamic monitoring pressure monitoring setup exercise,
10. Physiologic roles of fluid and electrolytes,
11. Arterial blood gas interpretation,
12. Glucose control in transplant patients,
13. Postoperative management of patient undergoing renal transplantation,
14. Transplant pharmacology and immunosuppressive therapy,
15. Chronic allograft nephropathy,
16. Complication of renal transplant, and
17. Transplant infectious diseases.

Twelve seasoned transplant nurses, 4 of which were certified transplant RNs, completed the 1-week didactic "critical care immersion" education/orientation program. Having certified nurses in the multiorgan transplant unit validated the knowledge, skills, and abilities of nurses in providing safe care to patients and as well as safeguarding the nursing profession (AACN, 2003).The 2-day Advance Cardiac Life Support based on 2006 guidelines was required for the transplant nurses. The nurses simulated different scenario of successful rescue, and each nurse was tested to demonstrate successfully how to be a team leader of the emergency situation (ACLS, 2006). A basic requirement to be in the multiorgan transplant unit is to be proficient in basic ECG,so advance 12 lead ECG interpretation was offered, emphasizing the different common ECG abnormalities and the nurses' role in the treatment modalities of the patient with such abnormalities. Current evaluation of a kidney transplant candidate is presented and the advantages of living donors compared with the cadaveric donors are discussed in light of long-term patient outcomes. Different scenarios, ranging from monetary compensation to rules and laws in kidney allocation process, were presented in discussing the ethical issues involving renal transplantation, as well as cultural aspect that impact kidney transplant. Management of acute renal failure focuses the different causes of acute renal failure in transplant patients, the different diagnostic procedures to rule out failure, and the prevention and management of acute renal failure. Case studies were used in assessing the critical thinking ability of the transplant nurse on the knowledge content presented (Holechek and Armstrong 2008).Nurses learned the difference between dialysis, continuous renal replacement therapies, and plasmapheresis. The different supplies needed to perform dialysis resulted in an enthusiastic discussion from the group on the importance of access care.(ANNA,2001, Barone, Martin-Watson, Barone , 2004, Gutch, Stoner, Corea.,1999, Gutch, Stoner, Corea, 1999, andWallace, 2003). The physiologic roles of fluid and electrolytes and how the kidneys maintain homoeostasis provided the nurses important clinical clues on what to look for in the kidney transplant patient if an electrolyte imbalance is present(Ohler and Cupples (2008).Focus assessment of the postoperative kidney transplant was extremely important lesson for the transplant nurses to learn since the patient is going back directly to the acuity-adaptable patient room after surgery (Barone, Martin-Watson ,and Barone, 2004).Nurses must use critical thinking skills in assessing the airway, breathing, and circulation post anesthesia; hence, knowledge of arterial blood gas interpretation is a core critical care skill needed to care for the patient in the acuity-adaptable setting. Nurses must be equipped with knowledge on assessing the renal function by knowing the different diagnostic studies. Nurses also reviewed on the core transplantation classes: transplant infectious disease, immunosuppressive therapy, surgical complication of kidney transplantation, and chronic nephropathy allograft—the most common cause of late allograft failure (Ohler and Cupples (2008). A core critical care skill is the knowledge of hemodynamic monitoring, pressure monitoring preparation, setup, and removal. The transplant nurses avail themselves with the PACEP modules. The PACEP is a free Web based, state-of-the-art educational program on monitoring hemodynamic parameters and using the pulmonary artery catheters. Modules presented in the kidney transplant core curriculum were delivered by different transdisciplinary faculty members. A posttest after each module tested the staff understanding of the subject matter presented. A final "closed-book" examination at the end of the week reinforced the lessons learned and validated knowledge content. All the posttests and the final test were collected and filed for safekeeping and are readily available for easy access if requested. After the 1-week didactic classroom presentation of knowledge content, the 12 transplant nurses rotated to the different intensive care units (ICUs) to have an actual "hands-on "in taking care of a critical care patient for 3 months. The transplant nurse was guided by an ICU nurse as a preceptor to gain a sense of confidence in practicing the knowledge gained from the classroom to the real-life situations. A graduated program allowed the transplant nurses to complete their identified ICU competencies verified by the ICU preceptors. The completed ICU competency checklist is also collected and put on for safekeeping. After the competency training of the 12 transplant nurses was completed, the acuity adaptable patient rooms were opened for admission. The transplant nurse eagerly tested their newly learned skills to the patients undergoing renal transplantation.

THE PILOT STUDY

A pilot study using descriptive method. The author who is also the principal investigator conducted a retrospective chart review of 100 renal transplant patients from January 2006 – March 2007, and prospective review of the renal transplant patient starting October, 2007. The principal investigator gathered data on demographics and the following outcome variables: length of stay, costs, nursing care, patient comfort, physiologic measures, nosocomial infections, patient satisfaction and ICU readmission.

A randomized control design was considered in the discussion of this pilot and upon the deliberation of the team of the knowledge that the study will be conducted in a span of 9 months; it would not yield a good sample that is appropriate for the intended outcome. Hence, the nonexperimental descriptive design was most appropriate in terms of study sample to produce a meaningful analysis of study outcome.

The principal investigator was fortunate to be funded and was able to utilize two transplant nurses from the Multi-Organ Transplant unit who will be involved in obtaining patient consent as data collectors. The data collectors were briefed on the data collection tool; the data was entered through a password-protective mechanism on a laptop provided specifically for the study. Data collection was done in a span of 9 months. The strategy process will involve approaching all renal transplant patients to the study which the teams expect to enroll 100% of the potential renal patient and this will provide the study with a sample of at least 35- 45 patients.

SETTING

This study will be conducted in a designated magnet facility. This is a 1500 bed tertiary hospital in the Houston area with a 30- bed Multi-Organ Transplant unit located near the renal transplantation surgery floor. The 30-bed Multi-Organ Transplant unit has 4- acuity-adaptable patient rooms. These 4- acuity adaptable patient rooms are equipped with a cardiac monitor that is capable of monitoring ECG, pulse oximetry, and hemodynamic monitoring. The room is also equipped with medical gas capability where a ventilator, left ventricular assist device (LVAD) and oxygen administration can be connected should the patient condition warrant these devices.

POPULATION AND SAMPLE

The sample will be taken from all patients admitted for renal transplant in Methodist Hospital. Inclusion criteria would be:

- Renal patient with a primary diagnosis of end-stage renal disease
- Must be able to read and write at a 3rd grade level
- Must be 18-75 years of age.
- Post-transplant patients with an American Society of Anesthesiologist (ASA) score of III or IV.

The exclusion criteria of the sample would be:

- Renal patient who are intubated post-renal transplant
- Renal transplant patient who developed severe hemorrhage in the immediate post-operative period.
- Renal transplant patients who develop cardiac problems immediate post-operative period.
- Renal transplant patient who develop other kind of emergent condition immediate post-operative period.

PROCEDURE

The pilot study involves a retrospective review of renal transplant that were cared for in the traditional practice in comparison to the renal transplant patients admitted to the acuity-adaptable patient room. The traditional practice was to send renal transplant patients to the Intensive Care Unit (ICU) post-operatively patients while on the acuity-adaptable care delivery, renal transplant patients go directly to the 4 acuity-adaptable patient rooms after post-anesthesia care unit (PACU) care. A prospective review will be done on renal transplant admitted in the 4 acuity-adaptable patient room as well as those renal transplant patients that are not admitted in the acuity-adaptable patient room.

In order for the study to be successful, the competency of the staff was immediately addressed. A Kidney Transplant Nursing CORE Curriculum (KTNCC) was developed by the principal investigator in collaboration with the VP of Operation, Multi-Organ Transplant Unit director, an ICU clinical leader, a physician assistant (PA), two pharmacists one of which is a transplant pharmacist. Eleven transplant nurses completed the curriculum. The content of that curriculum was mentioned in the earlier discussion.

After the one-week didactic, the 11 transplant nurses oriented to the Cardiovascular ICU, Surgical ICU and the Coronary Care ICU. A graduated program allowed the nurse to complete identifies ICU competencies.

The pilot study was presented by the research team members to the medical director of the Department of Transplantation for recommendations. Plan for pilot study was also presented to the study to the Kidney Transplant Research Committee, Transplant Executive Committee, Multi-Organ Transplant CMPI (Care Management Performance Committee) and the Renal Transplant Care Management Performance Committee in order to get the physician's support for the study. A presentation to the nursing leadership was also done to get the nursing leadership support for the study. Educational in-services to increase staff awareness regarding the Pilot study were presented to several nursing units and departments to capture potential renal transplant patient's entry points. Educational in-services about the pilot study and the study process was also presented to the pre-transplant kidney coordinators in the Multi-Organ Transplant Center to increase patient enrollment in the study.

Nursing staff in the Multi-Organ Transplant unit was instructed to call the principal investigator or co-investigator immediately when a potential patient is identified. The investigators clearly explained the consent to the potential study patient and allow time for the potential participants to ask questions. The risk and benefits of the study was explained thoroughly to the patients in compliance to the current rules and regulation of the Institutional Review Board on human subject's protection. The identified two nursing staff in the Multi-Organ Transplant unit was educated them in obtaining consent of potential renal patients should that patient happen to be admitted in the evening or nights or when the principal investigator is not available.

Patients who met the inclusion criteria was transferred to the 4 acuity-adaptable patient rooms in the Multi-Organ Transplant unit immediately post recovery from the Post Anesthesia Care Unit (PACU). A trained transplant nurse will be responsible to care of the patient using the Renal Transplant Clinical pathway and Order set approved by the Medical Staff.

DATA COLLECTION

A data collection tool (a survey instrument) was developed by the principal investigator to reflect the demographic of the sample population as well as the outcome variables that are to be measured in the study.

- The average length of stay was measured through prospective chart reviews using a survey instrument developed by the principal investigator.
- Costs data was gathered from the hospital operating data system.
- Nursing Care was measured through prospective chart review using the survey instrument developed by the principal investigator.
- Patient comfort was measured through prospective chart review using a survey instrument developed by the principal investigator.
- Physiologic measures will be measured through prospective chart review using a survey instrument developed by the principal investigator.
- Nosocomial infections will measured through prospective chart review using a survey instrument developed by the principal investigator.
- Patient satisfaction will be measured through a survey instrument developed by the principal investigator.

STATISTICAL ANALYSIS

Student's t-test and Mann-Whitney tests were performed to determine significant differences in the average length of stay (ALOS) and cost. Differences in nursing care, patient comfort, physiologic measures and nosocomial infection will be determined using chi-square and McNemar tests.

Table 1. Baseline characteristics

	Acuity-adaptable care		p-value
	Yes	No	
Age (years)	44.5 ± 2.4	48.7 ± 1.2	0.10
Male	17 (47.2)	68 (63.5)	0.12
Race			
White	17 (47.22)	45 (42.1)	
Black or African American	9 (25.0)	24 (22.4)	
Hispanic or Latino	9 (25.0)	31 (29.0)	
Other	1 (2.8)	7 (6.5)	0.87
Body mass index (kg/m^2)	27.8 ± 5.7	25.9 ± 4.7	0.05
ASA			*<0.0001*
2	0 (0)	1 (1.0)	
3	22 (71.0)	29 (29.3)	
4	9 (29.0)	69 (69.7)	
Duration of surgery (min)	38.7 ± 21.2	41.1 ± 21.6	0.57
Length of stay (days)	4.1 ± 1.3	9.6 ± 11.0	*0.004*
Cost			
Total	61291 ± 11508	82859 ± 24882	*<0.0001*
Labor	10146 ± 3477	12126 ± 7128	0.12
Direct	21489 ± 4755	26308 ± 9760	*0.006*
Medical condition			
Hypertension	31 (86.1)	98 (93.3)	0.18
Diabetes	32 (30.8)	6 (16.7)	0.13
Anemia	22 (61.1)	71 (67.0)	0.55
TB	2 (5.6)	2 (1.9)	0.27
Pulmonary disease	3 (8.3)	13 (12.3)	0.76
Peptic ulcer disease	3 (8.3)	6 (5.7)	0.69
Hepatitis	3 (8.3)	9 (8.5)	1.0
Bone disease	2 (5.6)	7 (6.7)	1.0
HIV	0 (0)	2 (2.1)	1.0
Family history			
Kidney disease	11 (30.6)	40 (38.8)	0.43
Hypertension	28 (77.8)	75 (70.7)	0.52
Diabetes	15 (41.7)	58 (54.2)	0.25
Cancer	14 (38.9)	34 (32.1)	0.54
Cardiac	11 (30.6)	35 (32.7)	1.0

RESULTS OF THE PILOT STUDY

The baseline characteristics are presented in Table 1. There were significant differences between acuity-adaptable care and traditional care in ASA, length of stay, and total costs (mainly from direct cost).

Table 2.

	Day 0		Day 1		Day 2		Day 3	
	Acuity-adaptable care		Acuity-adaptable care		Acuity-adaptable care		Acuity-adaptable care	
	Yes	No	Yes	No	Yes	No	Yes	No
Nursing care								
Pressure ulcer	0/36	0/102	0/36	0/102	0/36	0/102	0/26	0/101
Reported medication error	0/36	0/101	0/36	0/102	0/36	0/102	0/26	0/102
Reported patient fall	0/36	0/102	0/36	0/102	0/36	0/102	0/26	0/102
DVT	0/36	0/102	0/36	0/102	0/36	0/102	0/26	0/102
Patient comfort								
Pain scale								
Average	$1.2 \pm 1.9^{*}$	1.8 ± 1.8	$1.4 \pm 1.7^{*}$	1.6 ± 1.2	$1.1 \pm 1.6^{*}$	1.2 ± 0.5	$0.7 \pm 1.2^{*}$	1.2 ± 0.6
Maximum	3 ± 2.7	3.9 ± 3.9	3.9 ± 2.5	4.2 ± 3.2	4.0 ± 2.5	4.5 ± 3.0	3.3 ± 3.0	4.1 ± 3.5
Catheter obstruction	0/36	0/102	0/36	0/102	0/35	1/100	0/25	1/90
Physiological measures								
Hypertensive episodes	2/34*	43/57	3/33*	43/56	3/33†	28/72	2/24	20/79
Urine output<200 in 8 hr	0/36	3/95	1/35	5/96	0/35	5/96	0/26	3/98
Glucose level>110	30/6	73/15	34/2	72/17	34/1¶	66/23	23/3†	61/32
Heart rate <110 or <60	9/22	33/68	8/23	32/69	8/22	21/80	2/21	17/84
Temperature >100	2/29	12/89	6/25	18/83	6/25	10/91	2/21	5/96
Nosocomial infections								
Urinary tract infection	0/31	0/102	0/31	0/102	0/31	1/101	0/23	2/100
Pneumonia	0/30	0/102	0/30	1/101	0/30	1/101	0/22	1/101
Central line infection	0/29	0/102	0/29	0/102	0/29	0/102	0/21	0/102

Data was presented as yes/no for categorical variables or mean ± SD for continuous variables.

[*] P<0.0001 for comparison between acuity-adaptable care and no acuity-adaptable care at each day based on Kolmogorov-Smirnov test for continuous variables or Chi-square test for categorical variables.

[†] P<0.05 for comparison between acuity-adaptable care and no acuity-adaptable care at each day based on Chi-square test.

P<0.01 for comparison between acuity-adaptable care and no acuity-adaptable care at each day based on Chi-square test.

In the univariate linear regression model, care type (acuity-adaptable care vs. tradition care), age at the transplantation, diabetes, male sex, and hepatitis were significant associated with length of stay, and care type, age at the transplantation, and diabetes were significant associated with total cost (Table 3). In the multivariate linear regression model, only care type and hepatitis were significant associated with length of stay.

Table 3. Percent change (95% CI) of length of stay and total cost from univariate and multivariate linear regression models

	AAC vs. non AAC	Age (per 5 years)	Diabetes (yes vs no)	Male vs Female	Hepatitis (yes vs no)
Length of stay					
Univariate					
Percent change (95% CI)	-66.7 (-86.6, -46.9)	3.8 (0.2, 7.4)	24.9 (4.1, 45.6)	24.8 (5.3, 44.2)	(9.4, 79.5)
p-value	<0.0001	0.04	0.02	0.01	0.01
Multivariate					
Percent change (95% CI)	-59.7 (-78.5, -40.9)	1.5 (-1.7, 4.6)	7.7 (-11.3, 26.7)	12.8 (-3.8, 29.3)	35.4 (5.3, 65.5)
p-value	<0.0001	0.35	0.42	0.13	0.02
Total costs					
Univariate					
Percent change (95% CI)	-28.1 (-37.8, -18.3)	0.4 (0.05, 0.7)	14.8 (4.2, 25.4)		
p-value	<0.0001	0.03	0.007		
Multivariate					
Percent change (95% CI)	-25.7 (-35.4, -16.0)	1.1 (-0.5, 2.7)	10.1 (0.3, 19.9, 16.5)		
p-value	<0.0001	0.19	0.04		

AAC: acuity-adaptable care. Both length of stay and total costs were log-transformed before the analyses.

Compared with traditional care, acuity-adaptable care would result in a 59.7% decrease in the average length of stay, and having hepatitis would result in a 35.4% increase in the average length of stay. Care type and diabetes were significant associated with total cost. Compared with traditional care, acuity-adaptable care would result in a 25.7% decrease in the average total cost, but diabetic patients would yield a 10.1% increase in the average total cost.

DISCUSSION

After 6 months of operation, the acuity-adaptable care delivery has shown improvement in the length of stay and cost in renal transplantation outcomes. This pioneering pilot study conducted using descriptive method, which resulted in decreased length of stay of kidney transplant patients from 9.6 (11.0) days (before acuity-adaptable patient room) to 4.1 (1.3) days (acuity-adaptable patient room) clearly demonstrated improvement in patient care outcomes and ultimately cost. The combination of the care cluster, the critical care skill preparation of the transplant nurses, and the acuity-adaptable patient room has shown promise in a new direction looking at this kind of care delivery for the future to support efficient care coordination. Not only that the acuity-adaptable patient room improve patient outcome and cost, but with the nursing competency strategies that we implemented to support the implementation of the acuity-adaptable patient room, a hybrid *nurse* was created who possessed both critical care and medical-surgical skills.

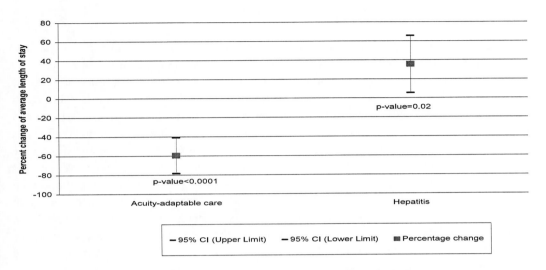

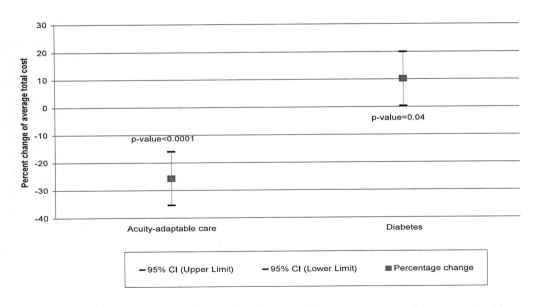

This can be a potential trend in the professional nurse model to address the health care challenges we face today in terms of nursing shortage, abbreviated plan of care, and facility operation efficiency. The transplant nurses confident after 6 months in operation serve as mentors and trainers of the junior and new nurses in the transplant floor. Transplant nurses gain increasing confidence in their nursing skills with the added knowledge of critical care concepts and skills. Transplant floor nurses are consistently recognized in the honor rolls for patient satisfaction in the organization.

CONCLUSION

There are several studies regarding favorable outcomes on patient and staff satisfaction on the acuity-adaptable rooms, but the studies are very few to count; again this area truly needs to be explored to strengthen and support the previous studies and add to the body of knowledge. Empirical studies have proven that patients placed in an acuity-adaptable room have significant outcomes to patient safety, patient and family healing, staff stress and effectiveness, and improved overall health-care quality and cost. Significant clinical outcomes of the patient addressing length of stay, infection, medication errors, and reports of falls are strong evidence that this body of science needs to be pursued and examined. While it is difficult to conduct rigorous research on the impact of the acuity-adaptable patient room because the hospital system is so complex and it is difficult to isolate the impact of a single entity, several studies on acuity-adaptable care delivery model heralding effects of impact on patient outcomes make considerable progress in developing a knowledge base of evidence that this research area is relevant and it made a significant contribution to patient safety and quality of care.

This will be an excellent opportunity for a nurse researcher as well as fellow scientists to explore and add to the investigation of previous researches to strengthen the need of this kind of patient room in the future. Studies previously mentioned support the need to replicate the studies to gather more evidence that the acuity-adaptable patient room concept will be feasible, meaningful, and the most important priority for administrators or health-care designers to meet the challenges of the health-care trends that are coming to the industry with lightning-bolt speed.

ACKNOWLEDGMENTS

The authors thank Dr. Osama Gaber – Director of Transplantation, Ann Scanlon-McGinity, RN, PhD, Chief Nurse Executive, Katherine Walsh, DrPh, RN, Vice President of Nursing Operation, The Methodist Hospital, for executive support, Susan Xu, PhD – TMHRI Biostatitian, Data Collectors: Rhey Peralez, BSN, RN, MOTU Manager, Kristin Tran, BSN, RN, staff nurse and Jennifer Nguyen, BSN, RN, staff nurse and All the Multi-Organ Center Staff.

REFERENCES

AACN. (2003). Safeguarding the patient and the profession: the value of certification. *Am. J. Crit. Care.* 12(2):154-163.

Advanced Cardiac Life Support. (2006). Provider Manual. Dallas, TX: American Heart Association; 2006. ISBN0-87493-496-6.

American Nephrology Nurses Association. (2001). Core Curriculum for Nephrology Nursing. 4th ed. Pitman, NJ: American Nephrology Nurses Association.

Anonymous. (2004). The registered nurses population sample survey of registered nurses. Retrieved March 29, 2007 from http://bhpr.hrsa.gov/healthworkforce/reports/ rnpopulation/preliminaryfindings.htm

Barone CP, Martin-Watson AL, Barone GW. (2004). The postoperative care of the adult renal transplant recipient. *MedSurg. Nurs*.13(5):296-302.

Brown, K., and Gallant, D. (2006). Impacting patient outcomes through design. *Critical Care Nursing Quarterly*, 29(4), 326–341.

Brown, P., and Taquino, L. (2001). Design and delivering neonatal care in single rooms. *Journal of Perinatal Neonatology Nursing*, 15(1), 68–83.

Buerhaus, P., Steiger, D., and Auerback, D. (2000). Implication of an aging registered nurse workforce. *Journal of American Medical Association*, 283(22), 2948–2954.

Bush, C., Reisman, B., Anstine, L., Gallaher, C., and Davis, M. (2005). The Ohio State University Richard M. Ross Heart Hospital in the academic environment. *The American Heart Hospital Journal*, 3(2), 120–127.

Chang, V. and Nelson, K. (2000). The role of physical proximity in nosocomial diarrhea. *Clinical Infectious Diseases*, 3,717-722.

Chaudhury, H., Mahmood, A., and Valente, M. (2006). Nurses' perception of single-occupancy versus multioccupancy rooms in acute care environments: An exploratory comparative assessments. *Applied Nurse Research*, 19(3), 118–125.

Cho, S. H., Ketefian, S., Barkauskas, V. H., and Smith, D. G. (2003). The effects of nurse staffing on adverse events, morbidity, and medical cost. *Nursing Research*, 52(2), 71–79.

Clark, E., Roberts, C., and Traylor, K. (2004). Cardiovascular single-unit stay: A case study in change. *American Journal of Critical Care*, 13(3), 406–409.

Corazon Consulting (2004). National trends in cardiac universal bed utilization. (white paper). Pittsburgh, PA: Corazon consulting, Inc.

Douglas, C., Steele, A., Tood, S., and Douglas, M. (2002). Primary care trusts, a room with a view. *Source Health Service Journal*, 112(5827), 28–29.

Gallant, D. (2006). The transformational hospital: Patient room of the future, research on the acuity adaptable and universal room concepts. Paper presented at: Hill-Rom; 2006; Batesville, Indiana.

Gallant, D., and Lanning, K. (2001). Streamlining patient care processes through flexible room and equipment design. *Critical Care Nursing Quarterly*, 24(3), 59–76.

Gutch C, Stoner M, Corea A. (1999). Review of Hemodialysis for Nurses and Dialysis Personnel. 6th ed. St Louis, MO: Mosby.

Hendrich, A., Fay, J., and Sorrells, A. (2004). Effects of acuity-adaptable rooms on flow of patients and delivery of care. *American Journal of Critical Care*, 13(1), 35–45.

Hendrich, A., and Lee, N. (2005). Intra-unit patient transports: Time, motion, and cost impact on hospital efficiency. *Nursing Economics*, 23(4), 157–164.

Holechek M, Armstrong G. Kidney transplantation.(2008). In: Ohler L, Cupples S, eds. Core Curriculum for Transplant Nurses. Philadelphia, PA: Mosby Elsevier; 513-553.

Hill-Rom (2002). The patient room of the future. IN: Hill-Rom Publication. *JAMA* (2000). Vol.283, No.22, 2948-2954.

Janssen, P., Harris, S., Soolsma, J., Klein, M., and Seymour, L. (2001). Single room maternity care: The nursing response. *Birth*, 28(3), 173–179.

Janssen, P., Klein, M., Harris, S., Soolsma, J., and Seymour, L. (2000). Single room maternity care and client satisfaction. *Birth*, 27(4), 235–243.

Morgan B. (2006).Principles of continuous renal replacement therapy. http://www.ihsc.on.ca/criticare/icu/elearning/crrt/crrt.html. Accessed November 10, 2006.

Ohler L, Cupples S. (2008).Electrolyte imbalance in adults. In: Core Curriculum for Transplant Nurses. Philadelphia, PA: Mosby Elsevie:663-675.

PACEP. http://www.pacep.org/pages/start/ref.html? xin=sccm. Accessed February 12, 20106.

Passweg, JR., Rowling, PA., Atkinson, KA., Barret, AJ., Gale, RP., Gratwohl, A., Jacobsen, N., Klein, JP., Ljungman, P., Russell, JA., Schaefer, UW., Sobocinski, KA., Vossen, JM., Zhang, M-J, and Horowitz, MM. (1998). Influence of protective isolation on outcome of allogenic bone marrow transplantation for leukemia. *Bone Marrow Transplantation*, 21, 1231–1238.

Rashid, M. (2006). A decade of adult intensive care unit design: A study of the physical design features of the best-practice examples. *Critical Care Nurse Quarterly*, 29(4), 282–311.

Richter, L. (2001, May) Innovation in care delivery: The cardiovascular single unit stay", Poster session presented at the AACN-NTI Exposition, Anaheim, California.

Shactman, D., Altman, S., Eilat, E., Thorpe, K., and Doonan, M. (2003). The outlook for hospital spending. *Health Affairs*, 22(6), 12–26.

Shirani, K., McManus, G., Vaughan, W., McManus, B., Pruitt, B., and Mason, A. (1986). Effects of environment on infection in burn patients. *Archives of Surgery*, 121(1), 760–786.

Solucient. (2002). Demographics to take long-term toll on U.S. hospitals: expect hefty increase in demand for beds and services. Retrieved March 29, 2007 from http://www.solucient.com/news_press/news2002110502.shtml

The Advisory Board. (2001). The heart of the enterprise. (pp. 42–43).Washington, DC: The Advisory Board Company.

The Advisory Board. (2002). Impact of building a freestanding heart center. (pp. 3–4). Washington, DC: The Advisory Board Company.

Thompson, J., Meredith, W., and Molnar, J. (2002). The effect of burn nursing units on burn wound infections. *Journal of Burn Care and Rehabilitation*, 23(4), 281–286.

Ulrich, R., Quan, X., Zimring, C., Joseph, A., and Choudhary, R. (2004). The role of the physical environment in the hospital of the 21st century: A once-in-a-lifetime opportunity. Concord, CA: Center for Health Design.

U.S. Bureau of Labor Statistics. (2004). Occupational employment projections to 2012. Monthly Labor Review, February 2004, 80–105.

U.S. Census Bureau. (2000). Census 2000 brief: overview of race and Hispanic origin. Retrieved March 28, 2007 from http://www.census.gov/prod/2001pubs/cenbr01-1.pdf

Wallace M. (2003).What is new with renal transplantation? *AORN J.* 77(5):946-966.

Walsh, W. F., McCullough K. L., and White, R. D. (2006). Rooms for improvement: Nurses' perceptions of providing care in a single room newborn intensive care setting. *Advance Neonatal Care*, 6(5), 261–270.

Wysong P, Driver E. (2009). Patient's perception of nurse' skill. *Critical Care Nurse*. 29(4):24-37.

APPENDIX

Scholarly presentations regarding acuity-adaptable patient room and acuity-adaptable patient care delivery:

1. Oral Presenter – *"Daily Leadership Visibility: Mission Possible"* and a poster presenter – *"Acuity-Adaptable Care Delivery Improves Renal Transplantation Outcomes"* at the 21st International Nursing Research Congress, July 12-16, 2010, Orlando Florida.

2. Oral Presentation – *"Developing Bedside Leader: Transforming Care at the Bedside"* and *"Using Technology to support an Acuity-Adaptable Care Delivery in a Renal Transplantation: An Innovative Patient Care Delivery of the Future"* at the 20th Sigma Theta Tau International Annual Research Congress, July 13-17, 2009, Vancouver, Canada

3. Invited Speaker- *"Acuity-Adaptable: Patient Room of the Future"* at the 2nd Planning & Creating the Patient Room of the Future Conference held in Dallas, Texas, March 26-27, 2009.

4. Invited Speaker- *"Acuity- Adaptable: Patient Room of the Future"* at The Quality Celebration 2008 held at the Michael E. DeBakey VA Medical Center, Houston, Texas, October 21, 2008.

5. Invited Speaker- *"Acuity-Adaptable: Patient Room of the Future"*, at the Planning & Creating the Patient Room of the Future Conference held in Houston, Texas, September 26, 2008.

6. Poster Presentation- *"Acuity-Adaptable: Patient Room of the Future"* at the 17th Annual International Transplant Nurses Society Symposium in St. Louis, Missouri, September 25-27, 2008.

7. Oral presentation - *"Mentoring: A Win-Win Strategy to Engage Seasoned Nurses To Take Ownership in Professional Development"*, *"From Good to Best: An Education Strategy to Match an Acuity-Adaptable Care Delivery of the Renal Transplant Patients"* at the 19th International Nursing Research Congress Focusing on Evidence-Based Practice, Singapore, July 8, 2008.

8. *"A Kidney Transplant CORE Curriculum for Acuity-Adaptable Care Delivery"* - Abstract selected for the Inaugural ANCC Magnet ™ Practice Innovation at the Virginia Henderson International Nursing Library (VHINL), posted July 1, 2008.

9. Invited Speaker - *"Acuity-Adaptable: Patient Room of the Future"* speaker at the 13th Far Eastern University Alumni Association Grand Reunion held in Orlando, Florida, June 29, 2008.

10. Podium Speaker *"Using Technology to Blend Different Levels of Care: A Leadership Strategy to Create an Evidence Based Nursing Environment"*, at Rutgers 26th Annual International Computer and Technology at Las Vegas, June 4-7, 2008 and at the 19th International Nursing research Congress Focusing on Evidence-Based Practice, Singapore, July 8, 2008.

11. Oral presenter- *"Using Technology to Support Acuity-Adaptable Care Delivery of Renal Transplant Patients"* speaker at the Go for the Gold-Regional Learning Exchange held in Houston, December 7, 2007 at the Hilton Hotel.

12. Oral Presenter in the concurrent session -*"An Educational Strategy to Support an Acuity-Adaptable Care Delivery"*, at the 16th Annual International Transplant Nursing Society Symposium held at Denver, Colorado, October 3-6, 2007.

13. Speaker -*"Acuity-Adaptable Care Delivery Improves Renal Transplantation Outcomes"* speaker at The Methodist Hospital Research Institute Investigator Colloquium held in Houston, Texas, September 24, 2007 at The Trevisio.

14. Concurrent speaker -*"Acuity-Adaptable: Patient Room of the Future"*, *"Leading Change: Developing Bedside Leaders"*, *"The Making of a High-Acuity Unit"* and *" A Transdisciplinary Collaboration Using Performance Improvement Evidence-Based Practice"*, concurrent session speaker at the *18th International Nursing Research Congress Focusing on Evidence-Based Practice-Collaboration: A Transdisciplinary Roadmap to Discovery* held in Austria Center, Vienna, July 11-14, 2007.

15. Concurrent session speaker -*"Patient Room of the Future"* at the *National Indian American Conference* held in Houston, May 5, 2007.

In: Toward Healthcare Resource Stewardship   ISBN: 978-1-62100-182-9
Editors: J.S.Robinson, M.S.Walid and A.C.M.Barth   © 2012 Nova Science Publishers, Inc.

Chapter 13

OBESITY – THE AMERICAN EPIDEMIC: THE IMPACT OF OBESITY ON HOSPITAL COST IN OBSTETRICS AND GYNECOLOGY: A REVIEW

Courtney L. Barnes, Mistie P. Mills and Mira Aubuchon [*]
Department of Obstetrics, Gynecology and Women's Health,
School of Medicine, University of Missouri-Columbia, US

U.S. OBESITY TRENDS

Obesity is defined as a body mass index (BMI) of 30 or greater. BMI is calculated from a person's weight and height and provides a reasonable indicator of body fatness and weight categories that may lead to health problems.

During the past 20 years there has been a dramatic increase in obesity in the United States. In 2009, only Colorado and the District of Columbia had a prevalence of obesity less than 20%.

Thirty-three states had a prevalence equal to or greater than 25%; nine of these states (Alabama, Arkansas, Kentucky, Louisiana, Mississippi, Missouri, Oklahoma, Tennessee, and West Virginia) had a prevalence of obesity equal to or greater than 30%.

It is estimated that future mortality related to obesity is expected to exceed that of smoking-related conditions contributing in the United States to 112,000 preventable deaths per year [1, 2]. Numerous studies support the relationship between obesity and serious health consequences. Obese adults are more likely to experience hypertension, hyper-cholesterolemia, type 2 diabetes mellitus, coronary artery disease, stroke, gallbladder disease, osteoarthritis, sleep apnea, respiratory disorders, depression, blood clots, and cancer of the prostate and colon [3]. Adult obesity is also associated with a reduction in quality of life, possibly due to social stigmatization and discrimination [4]. Obese women additionally

---

[*] Corresponding Author: Mira Aubuchon, 500 N. Keene Street, Suite 203, Columbia, MO 65201. E-mail: aubuchonm@health.

experience higher rates of pregnancy complications, infertility, complications of gynecologic surgery, contraceptive failure, and uterine cancer [5-11].

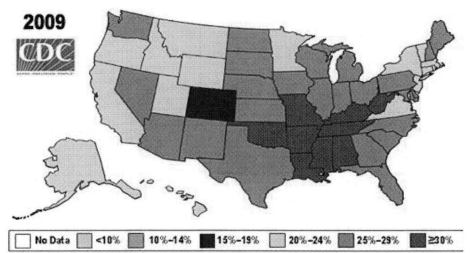

Quoted from Centers for Disease Control and Prevention (CDC) Website: http://www.cdc.gov/ obesity/data/trends.html.

Page accessed: June 5, 2011.

Content source: Division of Nutrition, Physical Activity and Obesity, National Center for Chronic Disease Prevention and Health Promotion.

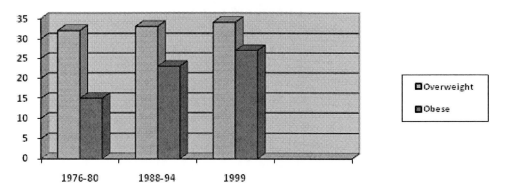

Figure 1. Prevalence of overweight and obese adults 1976 to 2000 – The National Health and Nutrition Examination Survey. Y-axis reflects percent of U.S. population.

For developed countries worldwide, the number of overfed people now rivals that of underfed people [1]. From 1995-2000, the number of obese adults increased by 50% to 300 million globally. The prevalence of adult obesity in the United States has increased by 2.4 million from 2007-2009 [1] (Figure 1). The majority of adults (61%) have a body mass index (BMI) ≥ 25 kg/m^2 with an estimated 72 million obese adults having a BMI $\geq$30 kg/m^2 [1]. Six percent of the adult population is extremely obese with BMI ≥ 40 kg/m^2 (4). Nearly one-third of the population is obese, with a disproportionately higher prevalence among non-Hispanic Blacks (36.8%), Hispanics (30.7%), persons ≥ 50 (62%) and those lacking high school diplomas (32.9%) [12].

The burden of obesity on our healthcare system is astonishing. Annual medical care costs for obese Americans are estimated to be $147 billion. Persons who are obese have medical costs that are $1,429 higher than lean patients [13]. From 1987 to 2001, 27 % of increased US healthcare costs were attributable to obesity-related diseases. For each obese patient, Medicare pays $95 more for an inpatient service, $693 more for a non-inpatient service, and $608 more for prescription coverage than with normal weight patients [13]. Likewise, Medicaid pays $213 more for an inpatient service, $175 more for a non-inpatient service, and $230 more for prescription drugs when comparing obese patients to normal weight patients [13]. The association of obesity to increased healthcare costs extends to private insurers as well, with $443 more spent for inpatient service, $398 more spent for non-inpatient services, and $284 more spent for prescription drugs for obese patients than normal weight patients [13].

OBESITY RELATED MEDICAL COMORBIDITIES IN PREGNANCY

In the United States, the incidence of obesity among pregnant women ranges from 18.5% to 38.3% [14]. Obese pregnant women experience higher rates of pregnancy complications, including hypertension, preeclampsia, late fetal death, and gestational diabetes [15].

Diabetes

It is estimated that there are > 14 million adult type 2 diabetes mellitus patients in the United States [1]. More than half of patients with type 2 diabetes are overweight, and approximately half are obese [16]. The risk of developing type 2 diabetes is 5 times greater with a BMI of 25 kg/m^2, 35 times greater with a BMI of 30 kg/m^2, and 93 times greater with a BMI of 35 kg/m^2 when compared to a base risk at a BMI of 21 kg/m^2 [17][18]. The physiologic changes of pregnancy further predispose to a diabetogenic state.

Gestational diabetes affects 3% of all pregnancies [19]. Even overweight patients have a 1.8-6.5 fold higher risk of developing gestational diabetes than lean gravidas, while obese women have up to a 20 fold increased risk [20, 21]. Women with untreated gestational diabetes experience nearly twice the risk of perinatal mortality (defined as death to the neonate during the first week of life) [19]. Therefore, increased prenatal surveillance for gestational diabetes in these populations is warranted [19].

Women with elevated serum glucose at the time of 1-hour glucose challenge testing undergo the 3-hour glucose tolerance test (GTT), whereby abnormal GTT glucose levels establish the diagnosis of gestational diabetes. After a diagnosis has been made, these patients receive extensive education about gestational diabetes, with a central focus on nutrition and exercise. These patients must also learn to use a glucometer, a machine that tests blood glucose levels, and must then check blood sugar four times per day. If hyperglycemia is not controlled with diet and exercise, the patient might require oral medications and sometimes even insulin injections during the prenatal period [19]. All of these represent significant costs in terms of staff time, hospital, and outpatient resources.

Table 1. Cost of Obesity-Related Complications and Care

Item	Cost
Operating room time	$1,670 - $2,750 per hour
Hospital days	$1,100 per day
ICU days	$2,100 per day
Bariatric surgical table	$10,000-$14,000
Special stirrups	$3,000
Readmission for postoperative infection	$16,600 - $17,900
DVT treatment	$2,394 - $17,168
Blood transfusion	$1,600 - $2,400 per unit
Neonatal intensive care stay for obesity-related complicated delivery	$5,000 per day
Hospitalization of pregnant mother with obesity-related complication	$975 per day
Cesarean Delivery	$7,500
Vaginal Delivery	$5,000
Antenatal Testing	$165 to $494
Meconium Aspiration Treatment	$16,000 to $67,000

Gestational diabetics also require antenatal testing to evaluate the well-being of a fetus in utero. This evaluation is routinely performed through an ultrasound-based biophysical profile or by doppler non-stress testing. At the University of Missouri Women's and Children's Hospital, women with diabetes in pregnancy receive a biophysical profile and a non-stress test weekly, which may begin 12 weeks before the estimated due date. The hundreds of dollars spent for antenatal quickly multiply with increased testing frequency [22] (Table 1). Ultrasound-based fetal surveys indicate that women whose fetuses were exposed to very high glucose levels during the first trimester are more likely to have infants with congenital anomalies. These include cardiac malformations such as neural tube defects [23].

Estimated fetal weights can be important for women with diabetes because glucose is a molecule that easily crosses the placenta. When a pregnant woman has hyperglycemia, or high glucose levels, the fetus responds to this state with an increased production of pancreatic insulin, thus stimulating fetal growth. Poorly controlled hyperglycemia can result in the growth of a very large infant, termed macrosomia. Macrosomic infants are more likely to experience neonatal respiratory distress syndrome, with subsequent neonatal intensive care unit (NICU) admission, and often require a cesarean section for delivery. When these large infants are born vaginally, there is a higher prevalence of shoulder dystocia [19]. Shoulder dystocia is an obstetric emergency that results when an infant's head is delivered and the shoulders are trapped behind the pubic bone [19]. Because physical exam to estimate fetal weight may be limited due to habitus, use of ultrasound for this purpose increases, further contributing to cost.

Shoulder dystocia places an infant at risk for hypoxia, brain injury, traumatic injury, neurological injury, and even death. Four to 40% of infants whose births were complicated by shoulder dystocia experience neurologic injury to the brachial plexus (a nerve bundle that is present in the neck), and 10% of those injuries are permanent [24]. Shoulder dystocia also increases maternal morbidity. In a study of 236 shoulder dystocia cases, 11% of women experienced postpartum hemorrhage and 3.8% had a severe (4th degree) laceration to the perineum [25]. Any of these complications can translate to prolonged maternal hospitalizations and NICU admissions. Lastly, shoulder dystocia is implicated in a significant portion of obstetric litigation cases. The cost of litigation can be substantial.

During labor, women with gestational diabetes require close monitoring of serum glucose levels and treatment of hyperglycemia with insulin therapy. Following delivery, infants born to women with a diagnosis of gestational diabetes are more likely to need treatment for hypoglycemia, respiratory distress, and jaundice [26]. In one series following women with gestational diabetes and preexisting type 2 diabetes in pregnancy, NICU admissions occurred in 29% of GDM pregnancies and in 40% of pregnancies affected by type 2 diabetes. Of the infants admitted to the NICU, 51% had hypoglycemia and 40% required support for respiratory distress [26]. Costs for critically ill children in the neonatal intensive care unit can be extremely high when inpatient days accrued and professional ancillary fees are taken into consideration [27] (Table 1).

Hypertension and Pre-Eclampsia

Women who are overweight or obese are more likely to have preexisting hypertension and are also more likely to develop high blood pressure in pregnancy. High blood pressure in pregnancy can be associated with preeclampsia, characterized by maternal hypertension, proteinuria, and renal and hepatic dysfunction [28]. Preeclampsia affects approximately 5% of pregnancies and is a leading cause of perinatal mortality, preterm birth, and maternal morbidity [29]. Obese women are 2.5 times more likely to develop preeclampsia than women who are of normal weight [30]. Maternal complications of severe preeclampsia include pulmonary edema, acute renal failure, liver hematoma, postpartum hemorrhage, clotting disorders, multiorgan failure, hypertensive encephalopathy, ischemia, edema, infarcts, and cardiorespiratory arrest [31]. Severe preeclampsia can result in prolonged maternal or neonatal hospitalization including ICU stays.

Post Dates Pregnancy

Pregnancies delivered post-dates, defined as a delivery greater than 2 weeks beyond the estimated due date, are more likely to have intrapartum and postpartum complications. A study evaluating the impact of body mass index on post dates pregnancy found that women with a BMI of 35 kg/m^2 or more were 50% less likely to experience a spontaneous onset of labor [32]. The risk of post-dates pregnancy is increased in women who had excessive weight gain between the first and third trimesters [32]. Babies that are delivered post-dates are more likely to be hospitalized during the first years of life and are at greater risk of developing epilepsy, neurodevelopmental problems, and Asperger's syndrome in later life [33-36].

Another complication associated with post dates is fetal meconium aspiration syndrome. As the placenta ages and the due date is passed, the placenta does not function as well and oxygen supply to the infant decreases. The infant responds by relaxing the anal sphincter muscles and passing stool into the amniotic fluid. When the fetus breathes this material into the lungs, meconium aspiration syndrome can occur. The average cost of managing an infant with meconium aspiration syndrome is costly [22] (Table 1).

Labor Induction

Women who are obese are 50% less likely to experience a spontaneous onset of labor and they often require an induction of labor [32]. Induced labors are associated with costly medical interventions, cesarean deliveries, and operative vaginal deliveries via a vacuum assistance device or forceps [32]. The cost of an induction was 10% to 30% more than the baseline cost of a vaginal delivery (Table 1). If the induction resulted in a cesarean delivery, there was an additional 5% to 20% in expenditures [22].

Intrapartum Anesthesia Difficulty

Obese women are more likely to require repeated epidural catheter placements in order to achieve successful regional anesthesia during labor and delivery [37]. Pregnant women as a whole are considered high-risk candidates for general anesthesia due to swelling of the throat during pregnancy and the increased risk of aspiration pneumonia. Obese gravidas are considered to be even higher risk candidates for intubation, and frequently have difficult intubations [37].

Cesarean Section

Obese women are also more likely to have cesarean sections. In one study, the cesarean section incidence for morbidly obese women increased by 250% when compared with matched control women weighting less than 126.4 kg [37]. Prolonged cesarean operative time > 2 hours and estimated blood loss > 1L were reported in 56% and 38% respectively of patients with weight ≥ 113.6 kg; these rates were more than double that of controls [38]. The mean cost of a cesarean section is 50% more costly than a vaginal delivery [39] (Table 1). However, overall maternal and infant expenses are more significantly impacted by NICU admissions than route of delivery, suggesting that there should be greater focus on maternal and child comorbidities that impact hospital costs rather than focusing only on decreasing cesarean section rates [27].

Postpartum Complications

Women who are obese are more likely to experience postpartum complications such as hemorrhage, wound infection, and endometritis [30]. Postpartum hemorrhage remains the leading cause of maternal mortality worldwide [23]. Treatment may involve intensive fluid resuscitation with additional intravenous access, blood products, multiple medications, surgical procedures, and ICU monitoring. Wound complications, further exacerbated by hyperglycemia, are more likely to occur among women who are obese [30]. Intensive wound care management may involve frequent visits to the clinic and home care visits. Lastly, women who are obese are more likely to have endometritis, a uterine infection, requiring antipyretics, antibiotics, and prolonged hospitalizations [30]. Left untreated, endometritis can progress to sepsis, pelvic abscesses, and long-term sequelae including infertility and chronic pelvic pain [23].

Quantifying Obesity-Specific Obstetric Costs

It is difficult to quantify the actual economic impact that obesity has on obstetric inpatient care. The primary method of assessment is reviewing diagnosis codes from inpatient admissions, but obesity is rarely coded as a diagnosis in pregnancy unless it was associated with a comorbidity or extreme obesity [5]. Despite this limitation, obesity was found to be associated with a $3,476 increase in charges and a $2,387 increase in costs, most likely due to 2.89 fold increased cesarean section rate and increased length of hospital stay [5]. This translated to a mean $1,805 increase in charges per patient. Applying these numbers to the percentage of obese women in 2005, it is estimated that obesity diagnosed in women hospitalized during pregnancy accounted for $106.8 million in economic costs [5].

It is important to note that these costs are maternal only and do not account for the increased costs of caring for children born of obese mothers. Furthermore it would be remiss not to recognize the non-hospital outpatient costs including medications dispensed from the outpatient pharmacy, telephone calls to the office, and increased number of prenatal visits [40]. This increased use of health care resources exacts a significant financial impact on the medical system.

Addressing the Problem

Johns Hopkins Healthcare created "Partners with Mom," to identify mothers who might generate high-dollar healthcare claims during their pregnancies from a NICU admission. The program identifies women who are high-risk and partners them with a social worker. One of the main focuses of the program is to identify women with diabetes and hypertension in pregnancy. The program participants were screened and met with their social worker to set realistic goals, perform regular assessments throughout the pregnancy, coordinating medical care, reporting any subtle changes that might affect health status, and evaluate outcomes for the participant [27]. Since the initiation of the program in 1999, the percentage of NICU births has decreased by 30% [27]. In addition to significantly decreasing NICU admissions, the program also noticed a 17% drop in inpatient hospital costs per day (due to a quicker transition of these NICU babies to a lower acuity hospital setting) [27]. This is certainly a positive step that begs replication in other locations.

Gynecologic Impact of Obesity

Obesity is directly linked to the development of gynecologic disease such as disordered menstruation, endometrial cancer, contraceptive failure and infertility. Furthermore, obese women often require more resources to diagnose disease and to provide surgical treatment.

Finally, staff injuries in caring for the obese gynecologic patient are an under-recognized factor in hospital cost.

Diagnostic Limitations of Obesity

Obesity can complicate the evaluation and physical exam of a female patient [41]. In a normal weight patient, abnormalities such as fibroids or ovarian cysts may be recognized on a simple pelvic exam. A gynecologic exam that is limited in the obese body habitus can result in the need for hospital-based radiologic studies such as computerized tomography (CT) scans and ultrasounds [41] costing hundreds or magnetic resonance imaging (MRI) costing thousands of dollars to determine uterine or ovarian pathology.

Routes of Gynecologic Surgery

Surgery, including hysterectomy, is a mainstay of treatment for fibroids and other gynecologic pathology and costs of this are increased with obesity. Morbidly obese women undergoing vaginal or abdominal hysterectomies require almost twice the length of hospital stay with twice the expense per day when compared to average weight patients (Table 1). Laparoscopic approaches decreased the length of stay but remained associated with increased cost per day for the obese patient [42] (Table 1). Postoperative complications include wound infection, delayed ambulation, and slow return of bowel function all of which contribute to a delay of hospital discharge and an increased hospital stay cost.

Common routes of surgery for gynecologic surgery include the abdominal approach with open laparotomy and the vaginal approach. Unfortunately, obesity increases complications regardless of route, although this is controversial for cancer-related gynecologic surgeries [43,44]. Abdominal surgeries, both obstetric and gynecologic, have been associated with significantly higher operative site infections [45-47] and wound complications in obese patients [6,7] that can lead to increased cost due to readmission (Table X). Obesity was directly linked to a longer operating time for hysterectomy in both abdominal and vaginal approaches for benign pathology, although the vaginal route was associated with fewer overall perioperative complications [48]. Rates of intraoperative injury to adjacent organs, most often the bladder, are also higher in obese patients [6,7][48, 49].

The well-documented association of surgical complications with obesity has led to an increase in the use of minimally invasive surgical techniques such as conventional and robotic-assisted laparoscopy. Obesity has been previously considered a relative contrain-dication to laparoscopy [50,51], but recent studies have demonstrated the safety of laparoscopy in this population [52,53]. Benefits from laparoscopic surgery include less pain, earlier ambulation and shorter hospital stays [54]. However, hospitals incur higher direct cost for equipment required to perform these types of procedures. Furthermore, the obese patient is 13 times more likely to require a conversion to laparotomy due to lack of visualization or bleeding [55].

Direct and Indirect Surgical Costs

Hospitals can experience several direct costs and indirect costs when treating surgical patients with obesity. Direct costs particularly arise from the need for special equipment in order to care for these patients, which include bariatric tables, stirrups, and bariatric surgical instrument trays [56] (Figure 2-4, Table 1). Anesthesia requirements may also be greater due to the need for more advanced intubation equipment (Table 1). Indirect costs include more staff requirements for lifting and transferring obese patients and movement and exchange of necessary equipment (Table 1).

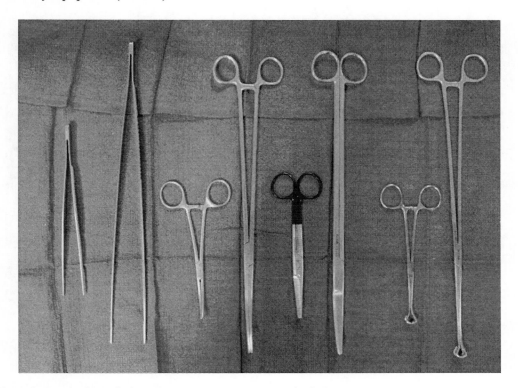

Figure 2. Standard Surgical Instruments versus Longer Bariatric Instruments.

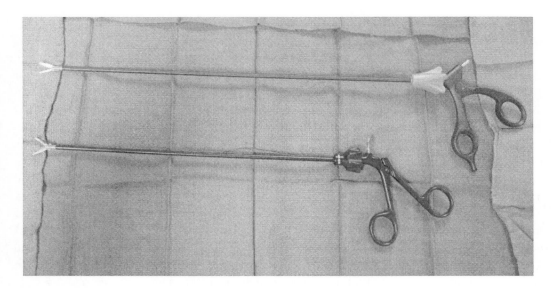

Figure 3. Standard Length Laparoscopy Instrument versus Bariatric Length.

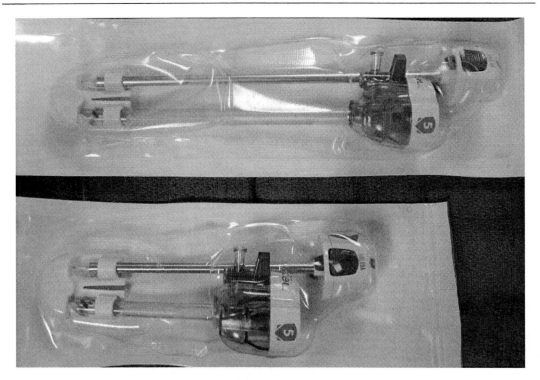

Figure 4. Standard Length Trocar versus Bariatric Length Trocar.

Unfortunately, obesity as a complication for surgical outcomes and hospital admissions has grossly been underestimated. Obesity is often a secondary or tertiary diagnosis which is often omitted during the reporting process. For that reason, it is difficult, and out of the scope of this review, to grasp the exact cost obesity plays in hospital admissions and surgical complications.

Operative Bleeding and Thromboembolic Disease

Obese patients are at higher risk of bleeding and requiring transfusions during the surgical and postsurgical period. Excessive bleeding requiring blood transfusion during or after surgery was reported in 6% of vaginal hysterectomies, with more blood loss noted in obese women than normal-weight patients [6,7]. A single unit of packed red blood cells has an acquisition cost of $200, but an actual cost that is up to 12 times higher [57] (Table 1).

One of the most common postoperative complications is thromboembolic disease such as pulmonary embolism or deep vein thrombosis. These are a major cause of mortality; at the time of autopsy, 24% of patients in acute-care hospitals, 22% in chronic-care hospitals and 5% of outpatients were noted to have pulmonary embolism [58]. Analysis of the database of the National Hospital Discharge Survey [59] strongly implicates obesity as a risk factor for initial and recurrent thromboembolic disorders [60]. Among hospitalized patients, rates of deep vein thrombosis and pulmonary embolism among the non-obese patient were 0.8% and 0.3% respectively, while these rates more than doubled in obese patients [61]. When comparing an obese patient with a non-obese patient under the age of 40, the obese female has a relative risk of 6.10 for deep vein thrombosis [60]. Hospitalized obese female patients are also at more risk than their male counterparts for pulmonary embolus and have nearly a 3 fold higher relative risk of developing deep vein thrombosis [60]. In 1999, the overall cost for treating a deep vein thrombosis ranged from $3,906 to $17,168 for inpatient care and $2,394 to $3,369 for outpatient care [62] (Table 1).

Endometrial Cancer

The United States has experienced a 0.3% increase in endometrial cancer over the last decade [63], with a 13 fold greater risk in obese women than the general population [9]. Increased endogenous estrogen produced by adipose and frequent chronic anovulation predispose obese women to endometrial cancer. The recent increase in survival rates [63] is fortunate, but correspondingly translates to higher overall costs given increased need for surgical and medical treatment with longer continued surveillance of survivors.

Infertility

Due to associated anovulation and other mechanisms, obese women have more difficulty conceiving and often have to resort to advanced fertility techniques [11]. While many infertility costs are directly borne by the patient for outpatient expenses, IVF increases risks of severe ovarian hyperstimulation syndrome and high-order multiple pregnancies [64], both of which directly increase hospital costs in terms of inpatient stay duration, neonatal and sometimes maternal intensive care.

Contraceptive Failures

In 2002, the direct medical cost of unintended pregnancy in the United States was $5 billion [65]. Contraceptive failure in the obese patient has been well-documented for oral contraceptives, particularly low-dose birth control pills. Oral contraceptive failure was noted to be 60% higher in patients weighing $\geq$ 70.5 kg [8]. Transdermal birth control methods were also noted to have similar findings, particularly in women with a mean weight of 74.5 kg compared to those 64.4 kg [66]. Gu et al also noted higher failure with contraceptive implants was 5 times more likely in those weighing 70 kg than those weighing 50 kg [66]. In fact, the prescribing information packet for a widely used implant describes potential decreased effectiveness in women 130% over ideal body weight [67]. As most pharmaceutical studies of birth control agents exclude patient populations with a BMI $\geq$ 35. There is limited information on contraceptive efficacy for obese women.

Obesity-Related Injuries to Hospital Staff

Hospitals often overlook direct and indirect costs associated with musculoskeletal injuries related to the care of the obese patient. In 2008, musculoskeletal injuries in the health care worker accounted for $7.4 billion per year [68]. Nurse's aides and orderlies suffered the highest prevalence at 18.8% [69]. Many more women staff the obstetric and gynecologic services than men, which likely contributes to the disproportionately high 269,000 annual cases of work-related back pain among females [69]. Although injuries can occur even with low to moderate weight patients, they are much more likely with the obese patient. In recognition of this issue, National Institute for Occupational Safety and Health is currently evaluating a project aimed at improving safety while lifting and moving bariatric patients [70].

Summary

Without a doubt, obesity is a factor in the development of several chronic diseases in pregnancy that result in increased prenatal monitoring and antenatal testing. Pregnant women with chronic disease are more likely to experience cesarean sections, complications from their deliveries, perinatal morbidity, and have infants admitted to the NICU. Obesity also significantly adversely impacts gynecologic care. Gynecologic patients have increased gynecologic conditions including endometrial cancer and infertility. The surgeries for obese patients are longer and these patients have increased postoperative complications. Each one of these factors has an implication on obstetric and gynecologic hospital costs. The global impact, while not clearly quantifiable, is assuredly significant.

REFERENCES

[1]   O'Brien PE, Dixon JB. The extent of the problem of obesity. *Am. J. Surg.* 2002;184:4S-8S.

[2]   Flegal KM, Graubard BI, Williamson DF *et al.* Excess deaths associated with underweight, overweight, and obesity. *Jama* 2005;293:1861-7.

[3]   Health NIo. Clinical guidelines on the identification, evaluation, and treatment of overweight and obesity in adults--the evidence report. *Obes. Res.* 1998;6:51S-209S.

[4]   U.S. Department of health and human services- office of the surgeon general. The surgeon general's vision for a healthy and fit nation. Http://www.Surgeongeneral.Gov. Accessed December 27, 2010 2010.

[5]   Trasande L, Lee M, Liu Y *et al.* Incremental charges, costs, and length of stay associated with obesity as a secondary diagnosis among pregnant women. *Med. Care* 2009;47:1046-52.

[6]   Moller C, Kehlet H, Utzon J *et al.* [hysterectomy in denmark. An analysis of postoperative hospitalization, morbidity and readmission]. Ugeskr Laeger 2002;164: 4539-45.

[7]   Harris WJ. Early complications of abdominal and vaginal hysterectomy. *Obstet. Gynecol. Surv.* 1995;50:795-805.

[8]   Holt VL, Scholes D, Wicklund KG *et al.* Body mass index, weight, and oral contraceptive failure risk. *Obstet. Gynecol.* 2005;105:46-52.

[9]   Kwon JS, Lu KH. Cost-effectiveness analysis of endometrial cancer prevention strategies for obese women. *Obstet. Gynecol.* 2008;112:56-63.

[10]   Ramsay JE, Greer I, Sattar N. Abc of obesity. Obesity and reproduction. *Bmj* 2006; 333:1159-62.

[11]   Dokras A, Baredziak L, Blaine J *et al.* Obstetric outcomes after in vitro fertilization in obese and morbidly obese women. *Obstet. Gynecol.* 2006;108:61-9.

[12]   . Vital signs: State-specific obesity prevalence among adults --- united states, 2009. *MMWR Morb. Mortal Wkly Rep.* 2010;59:951-5.

[13]   Finkelstein EA, Trogdon JG, Cohen JW *et al.* Annual medical spending attributable to obesity: Payer-and service-specific estimates. *Health Aff.* (Millwood) 2009;28:w822-31.

[14] Galtier-Dereure F, Boegner C, Bringer J. Obesity and pregnancy: Complications and cost. *Am. J. Clin. Nutr.* 2000;71:1242S-8S.

[15] Sebire NJ, Jolly M, Harris JP *et al.* Maternal obesity and pregnancy outcome: A study of 287,213 pregnancies in london. *Int. J. Obes. Relat. Metab. Disord.* 2001;25:1175-82.

[16] Leibson C, Milton LJ, 3rd, Palumbo PJ. Temporal trends in diabetes incidence and prevalence. *Diabetes Care* 1997;20:460-2.

[17] Colditz GA. Economic costs of obesity and inactivity. *Med. Sci. Sports Exerc.* 1999; 31:S663-7.

[18] Wolf AM, Colditz GA. Current estimates of the economic cost of obesity in the united states. *Obes. Res.* 1998;6:97-106.

[19] Coustan DR. Gestational diabetes. In: Queenan JT, Hobbins JC, Spong CY, eds. Protocols for high risk pregnancies: Blackwell Publishing, 2007:224-6.

[20] Abrams B, Parker J. Overweight and pregnancy complications. *Int. J. Obes.* 1988;12: 293-303.

[21] Perlow JH, Morgan MA, Montgomery D *et al.* Perinatal outcome in pregnancy complicated by massive obesity. *Am. J. Obstet. Gynecol.* 1992;167:958-62.

[22] Kaufman KE, Bailit JL, Grobman W. Elective induction: An analysis of economic and health consequences. *Am. J. Obstet. Gynecol.* 2002;187:858-63.

[23] Zlatnik FJ. Obesity. In: Queenan JT, Hobbins JC, Spong CY, eds. Protocols for high risk pregnancies: Blackwell Publishing, 2007:221-3.

[24] Acog practice bulletin clinical management guidelines for obstetrician-gynecologists. Number 40, november 2002. *Obstet. Gynecol.* 2002;100:1045-50.

[25] Gherman RB, Goodwin TM, Souter I *et al.* The mcroberts' maneuver for the alleviation of shoulder dystocia: How successful is it? *Am. J. Obstet. Gynecol.* 1997;176:656-61.

[26] Watson D, Rowan J, Neale L *et al.* Admissions to neonatal intensive care unit following pregnancies complicated by gestational or type 2 diabetes. *Aust. N. Z. J. Obstet. Gynaecol.* 2003;43:429-32.

[27] Diehl-Svrjcek BC, Richardson R. Decreasing nicu costs in the managed care arena: The positive impact of collaborative high-risk ob and nicu disease management programs. *Lippincotts Case Manag.* 2005;10:159-66.

[28] Foidart JM, Schaaps JP, Chantraine F *et al.* Dysregulation of anti-angiogenic agents (sflt-1, plgf, and sendoglin) in preeclampsia--a step forward but not the definitive answer. *Journal of Reproductive Immunology* 2009;82:106-11.

[29] Bodnar LM, Ness RB, Markovic N *et al.* The risk of preeclampsia rises with increasing prepregnancy body mass index. *Annals of Epidemiology* 2005;15:475-82.

[30] Magann EF, Doherty DA, Chauhan SP *et al.* Pregnancy, obesity, gestational weight gain, and parity as predictors of peripartum complications. *Arch. Gynecol. Obstet.* 2010.

[31] Sibai BM. Pre-eclampsia. In: Queenan JT, Hobbins JC, Spong CY, eds. Protocols for high risk pregnancies: Blackwell Publishing, 2007:441-9.

[32] Denison FC, Price J, Graham C *et al.* Maternal obesity, length of gestation, risk of postdates pregnancy and spontaneous onset of labour at term. Bjog 2008;115:720-5.

[33] Lovell KE. The effect of postmaturity on the developing child. *Med. J. Aust.* 1973;1:13-7.

[34] Ehrenstein V, Pedersen L, Holsteen V *et al.* Postterm delivery and risk for epilepsy in childhood. *Pediatrics* 2007;119:e554-61.

[35]   Lindstrom K, Fernell E, Westgren M. Developmental data in preschool children born after prolonged pregnancy. *Acta Paediatr.* 2005;94:1192-7.

[36]   Cederlund M, Gillberg C. One hundred males with asperger syndrome: A clinical study of background and associated factors. *Dev. Med. Child. Neurol.* 2004;46:652-60.

[37]   Hood DD, Dewan DM. Anesthetic and obstetric outcome in morbidly obese parturients. *Anesthesiology* 1993;79:1210-8.

[38]   Johnson SR, Kolberg BH, Varner MW *et al.* Maternal obesity and pregnancy. *Surg. Gynecol. Obstet.* 1987;164:431-7.

[39]   Kazandjian VA, Chaulk CP, Ogunbo S *et al.* Does a cesarean section delivery always cost more than a vaginal delivery? *J. Eval. Clin. Pract.* 2007;13:16-20.

[40]   Chu SY, Bachman DJ, Callaghan WM *et al.* Association between obesity during pregnancy and increased use of health care. *N. Engl. J. Med.* 2008;358:1444-53.

[41]   Silk AW, McTigue KM. Reexamining the physical examination for obese patients. *JAMA* 2011;305:193-4.

[42]   Becker ER. National trends and determinants of hospitalization costs and lengths-of-stay for uterine fibroids procedures. *J. Health Care Finance* 2007;33:1-16.

[43]   Chapman GW, Jr., Mailhes JB, Thompson HE. Morbidity in obese and nonobese patients following gynecologic surgery for cancer. *J. Natl. Med. Assoc.* 1988;80:417-20.

[44]   Soisson AP, Soper JT, Berchuck A *et al.* Radical hysterectomy in obese women. *Obstet. Gynecol.* 1992;80:940-3.

[45]   Dindo D, Muller MK, Weber M *et al.* Obesity in general elective surgery. *Lancet* 2003; 361:2032-5.

[46]   Pitkin RM. Abdominal hysterectomy in obese women. *Surg. Gynecol. Obstet.* 1976; 142:532-36.

[47]   Myles TD, Gooch J, Santolaya J. Obesity as an independent risk factor for infectious morbidity in patients who undergo cesarean delivery. *Obstet. Gynecol.* 2002;100:959-64.

[48]   Chen CC, Collins SA, Rodgers AK *et al.* Perioperative complications in obese women vs normal-weight women who undergo vaginal surgery. *Am. J. Obstet. Gynecol.* 2007; 197:98 e1-8.

[49]   Makinen J, Johansson J, Tomas C *et al.* Morbidity of 10 110 hysterectomies by type of approach. *Hum. Reprod.* 2001;16:1473-8.

[50]   Gadacz TR, Talamini MA, Lillemoe KD *et al.* Laparoscopic cholecystectomy. *Surg. Clin. North Am.* 1990;70:1249-62.

[51]   Miles RH, Carballo RE, Prinz RA *et al.* Laparoscopy: The preferred method of cholecystectomy in the morbidly obese. *Surgery* 1992;112:818-22; discussion 22-3.

[52]   Heinberg EM, Crawford BL, 3rd, Weitzen SH *et al.* Total laparoscopic hysterectomy in obese versus nonobese patients. *Obstet. Gynecol.* 2004;103:674-80.

[53]   Hsu S, Mitwally MF, Aly A *et al.* Laparoscopic management of tubal ectopic pregnancy in obese women. *Fertil. Steril.* 2004;81:198-202.

[54]   Safran D, Sgambati S, Orlando R, 3rd. Laparoscopy in high-risk cardiac patients. *Surg. Gynecol. Obstet.* 1993;176:548-54.

[55]   Thomas D, Ikeda M, Deepika K *et al.* Laparoscopic management of benign adnexal mass in obese women. *J. Minim. Invasive Gynecol.* 2006;13:311-4.

[56] Venture medical- skytron 6001 surgery table. Http://www.Venturemedical.Com/ products/surgical_tables/skytron_6001_surgery_table/. . In: Accessed December 27, 2010.

[57] Hannon T. The contemporary economics of transfusions. In: Perioperative transfusion medicine: Lippincott Williams and Wilkins, 2006.

[58] Nordstrom M, Lindblad B. Autopsy-verified venous thromboembolism within a defined urban population--the city of malmo, sweden. *Apmis* 1998;106:378-84.

[59] . Us deparment of health and human services, public health service, national center for health statistics national hospital discharge survey 1979-1999 multi-year public-use data file documentation. Http://www.Cdc.Gov/nchs/about/major/hdasd/nhds.Htm. . In: Accessed January 12, 2010.

[60] Stein PD, Beemath A, Olson RE. Obesity as a risk factor in venous thromboembolism. *Am. J. Med.* 2005;118:978-80.

[61] Stein PD, Goldman J. Obesity and thromboembolic disease. *Clin. Chest Med.* 2009;30: 489-93, viii.

[62] O'Brien JA, Caro JJ. Direct medical cost of managing deep vein thrombosis according to the occurrence of complications. *Pharmacoeconomics* 2002;20:603-15.

[63] . National cancer institute surveillance epidemiology and end results. Http://seer. Cancer.Gov/statfacts/html/corp.Html In: Accessed December 27, 2010.

[64] Fauser BC, Devroey P, Macklon NS. Multiple birth resulting from ovarian stimulation for subfertility treatment. *Lancet* 2005;365:1807-16.

[65] Trussell J. The cost of unintended pregnancy in the united states. *Contraception* 2007; 75:168-70.

[66] Gu S, Sivin I, Du M *et al.* Effectiveness of norplant implants through seven years: A large-scale study in china. *Contraception* 1995;52:99-103.

[67] . Implanon full prescribing information. Http://www.Spfiles.Com/piimplanon.Pd.Pdf. . In: Accessed December 27, 2010.

[68] Waehrer G, Leigh JP, Miller TR. Costs of occupational injury and illness within the health services sector. *Int. J. Health Serv.* 2005;35:343-59.

[69] Guo HR, Tanaka S, Cameron LL *et al.* Back pain among workers in the united states: National estimates and workers at high risk. *Am. J. Ind. Med.* 1995;28:591-602.

[70] Collins JW. U.S. Department of health and human services. Safe patient handling and lifting standards for a safer american workforce. Http://www.Hhs.Gov/asl/testify/ 2010/05/t20100511a.Html. Accessed December 27, 2010 2010.

In: Toward Healthcare Resource Stewardship ISBN: 978-1-62100-182-9
Editors: J.S.Robinson, M.S.Walid and A.C.M.Barth © 2012 Nova Science Publishers, Inc.

Chapter 14

PERSPECTIVES ON PSYCHIATRIC COMORBIDITIES OF LATE LIFE AND THEIR COST IMPLICATIONS FOR MEDICAL CARE

Lee A. Hyer,[1,2,] Ciera V. Scott[1] and Catherine A. Yeager[3]*
[1]Georgia Neurosurgical Institute, Macon, GA, US
[2]Mercer University School of Medicine, Macon, GA, US
[3]Eisenhower Army Medical Center, Ft Gordon GA,US

Although prevalence estimates for specific psychiatric syndromes are lower among older adults as compared to other age groups, older individuals in need of care are three times less likely than their younger peers to receive treatment (Karlin, 2007). Recently, attempts have been made to improve mental healthcare access and treatment for older individuals, but this group continues to receive such care at very low rates. This is unfortunate as poor mental health is associated with higher disease burden, causes increased problems in overall medical care, adds to cost of care, and results in a lower quality of life. There is also evidence to show that when older adults receive mental healthcare, they often receive an insufficient amount of treatment (including both pharmacotherapy and psychotherapy), which is below recommended guidelines (Harman, 2005; J. Unutzer, Katon, W., Sullivan, M., and Miranda, J., 1999).

In this chapter we discuss the importance of mental health in the context of older adults and the gaps of this treatment experienced by older adults. First, we provide some perspective on the plight of older adults from an economic perspective. As a group, they are both in need of and over-utilize healthcare services. The extent to which psychiatric conditions influence this, we believe, is considerable. Next, we discuss the ideal of person-centered care and control of healthcare utilization (i.e., personal responsibility and participation). We then provide 10 suggestions aimed at improving care quality and care efficiency for older adults. We consider cost of care throughout this chapter.

---

[*] Corresponding Author: Lee A. Hyer, Georgia Neurosurgical Institute, 840 Pine Street, Suite 880, Macon, GA 31201. E-mail: leehyer@ganeurosurg.org.

HEALTH PERSPECTIVE

Where age is concerned, America has experienced an extraordinary cultural shift. In 1959, older people had the highest poverty rate (35%), followed by that of children (27%); by 2007, the proportion of older adults in poverty was only 10%. In fact, in 2007 older people in the middle income group made up the largest share of elders by category (33%), with those in the high income group (31%) coming in second (*Older Americans 2010: Key Indicators of Well-Being*). Health self-ratings also have improved: in 2008, 75% of people 65 years and older rated their health as good, very good, or excellent. For those 85 years and older, these ratings were still respectable at 66%. But, as life expectancy has increased, so too has a growing burden of chronic diseases (Hurwicz, 2011).

For this growth in life expectancy, there is a cost. More than 1/5 of hospital patients in 2008 were born in 1933 or earlier. Twenty-two percent of all admissions to U.S. hospitals in 2008 were for patients born the year that Franklin D. Roosevelt was first inaugurated President of the United States or earlier. Those who ranged in age from 75 to 84 years accounted for almost 14% of the 40 million admissions to U.S. hospitals that year, while patients age 85 and over made up another 8%. Together, these most senior of America's elders accounted for 8.7 million hospital admissions in 2008 compared to the 5.3 million admissions of relatively younger seniors – that is, those between 65 and 74 years of age (Agency for Healthcare Research and Quality, 2008). (Quality, 2008)

Percentages of lifestyle problems are also noteworthy. For starters, if you are a male in the US and 65 years old, you can now expect to live an average 18.5 years more than your predecessors; if you are 85, you can expect 6.8 more years of life. Life expectancy has actually increased by a year just in this past decade; the time spent seriously ill, however, is now 1.5 years and the time spent disabled has increased by 2 years. For people 65 years or over, heart disease, followed by malignant neoplasms, and then stroke lead the way toward death. Older men and women have hypertension and arthritis at rates of over 50%. In 2008, 32% of people 65 years or older were obese (BMIs of $\geq$ 30) and 11% smoked. Notably, 25% of older Americans spent time at leisure, but watching TV occupied most of their free time (>50%) (*Older Americans 2010: Key Indicators of Well-Being*).

Utilization of healthcare services increased only slightly from 336/1,000 in 2007 from 306/1,000 in 1992, but skilled nursing care went from 28/1000 to 81/1000 in 2007. Also, the number of physician visits and consultations increased to just over 13 per year; but the number of home health visits decreased from 8.4 in 1996 to 3.4 in 2007. This decrease occurred during a time when home health was viewed as beneficial. Not unimportant, average health care costs per year were directly related to income: those living in poverty cost $21,033 compared with those with more means at $12,440. Of these monies, inpatient healthcare was 25% (down from 32% in 1994) and prescription costs were 16% (up from 8% in 1997). Older adults paid 60% of prescription costs out-of-pocket, compared with public programs at 35% and private insurers at 38%. Finally, virtually every older person was paying some out-of-pocket expenses (95%). From 1977 to 2006 the percentage of household income that people aged 65 years and older allocated to out-of-pocket spending for healthcare services increased from 12% to 28%. Today, over 50% of monies are going toward medication (*Older Americans 2010: Key Indicators of Well-Being*).

Compared to other age groups, older adults have the highest numbers of doctor visits, hospital stays, and prescription medication usage (Bureau). In 2004 the average annual cost per older person ≥ 65 years) was $3899 (Statistics). Left unchecked, healthcare expenditures will likely rise from the current level of ~15% to 29% of gross domestic product (GDP) in 2040. AS intimated, medication use is of course high among the elderly. As much as 30% of the prescriptions and 40% of over-the-counter drugs can be attributed to use among this group. Adverse drug reactions account for a substantial amount of emergency room use, hospital admissions, and other healthcare expenditures. Only 50% of medication is taken properly, and there are 1.9 million drug-related injuries (Cogbill, 2010). Taking just blood pressure medication as an example, only 25% of older patients remain in treatment and consistently take their medications in sufficient amounts for blood pressure control (Cogbill, 2010). Several barriers have been attributed to poor medication use. These include physical illness, medication side effects, cognitive dysfunction, psychiatric conditions (mood disorders), functional loss, social loss, and inability to afford the medication at full dosing (Cogbill, 2010).

These data dovetail with the reality of the functional limitations of older age. In the 2000 US census, the most prevalent type of limitation or disability among Americans over 65 years was physical (28.6%), followed by limitations that affect leaving the house (20.8%), then sensory limitations (14.2%), followed by cognitive (10.6%) and self care limits (Freedman, 2004). The overall prevalence of disability among older adults was 41.9%, and even higher for elders living in poverty (Hurwicz, 2011). As people age, activities of daily living (ADLs) decline dramatically between 65 and 74 years - a fourfold change in ADLs and three fold change in independent activities of daily living (IADLs). Looking more closely at functional decline, adults older than 75 years account for 59% of fall-related deaths, but make up only 5% of the population ((D. Haber, Logan, W., and Schumacher, S., 2011)). Also, a sedentary lifestyle leaves older adults at risk for just about everything. Both obesity and malnutrition increase with age; currently, about 1/3 are obese and 1/5 are malnourished (D. Haber, 2010; , "Medicare screenings, vaccines underused", 2002). Fortunately, smoking and alcohol use are lower (15%) than that of younger groups, but it still is a concern. Finally, while only 5% of those over 65 years reside in a nursing home, between 10% and 15% of community dwelling elders require considerable support and assistance to remain in their own homes.

MENTAL HEALTH PROBLEMS FOR OLDER ADULTS

Medical care is directly related to mental health. When older adults do seek help for mental health problems, they go to their family physicians or attend primary care clinics. It is estimated that over 70% of medical problems, especially unexplained ones, are attributed to mental health issues (REF). Modal problems for older adults in the areas of cognitive decline, depressive symptoms, anxiety issues, or unexplained somatic concerns are well over 50%. Patients with depression and significant comorbidities are especially costly to the healthcare system. The acronym MUPS has been applied to Medically Unexplained Symptoms. Depressed patients with diabetes, for example, have more trouble adhering to their diets and checking blood glucose levels, plus they exercise less, smoke more, and die at about twice the rate as those without depression. Clearly, it is more costly *not* to treat the depression.

Older adults have historically utilized mental health services at substantially low rates. Unfortunately, although recent policy developments portend an increase in service use, there has been scant empirical attention devoted to the current or recent utilization of mental health interventions by the elderly, and almost nothing is known about the correlates of mental health service need and service use among older adults. Karlin (2007) examined patterns of serious mental illness, specific mental health syndromes, and service use among older (65+) and younger (18-64) adults throughout the United States, and the extent to which various factors predicted mental health need and use, and magnitude of actual treatment. In addition, Karlin's study examined factors related to unmet need, as well as age-group differences in perceived benefit from treatment. Findings revealed that older adults are three times less likely than their younger counterparts to receive any outpatient mental health treatment. Additionally, only 2.5% of older individuals utilized any outpatient mental health service in the preceding year, as compared to 7% of younger adults. These results suggest that the low rate of utilization by older adults may be partly a function of limited subjective mental health need. Importantly then, mental health problems appear to be significantly undertreated in older age groups.

The pathways leading to comorbidity of mental and medical disorders are complex and bidirectional (Katon, 2003). Medical disorders may lead to mental health conditions, mental health conditions may place a person at risk for medical disorders, and mental health and medical disorders may share common risk factors. We should expect that comorbidity between medical and mental health conditions is the rule rather than the exception. In the 2001–2003 National Comorbidity Survey Replication (NCS-R), a nationally representative epidemiological survey, more than 68% of adults with a mental health condition (diagnosed via structured clinical interview) reported having at least one general medical disorder, and 29% of those with a medical disorder had a comorbid mental health condition (Alegria, 2003; R. C. Kessler, Berglund, P., Chiu, W. T., Demler, O., Heeringa, S., Hiripi, E., Jin, R., Pennell, B. E., Walters, E. E., Zaslavsky, A., Zheng, H., 2004). In addition to the high prevalence of these conditions, there also is evidence that having each type of disorder is a risk factor for developing the other. For example, among respondents to the 1999 National Health Interview Survey (REF), a nationally representative epidemiologic survey, the likelihood of having major depression diagnosed via a screening instrument increased with each additional reported comorbid chronic medical disorder.

Medical conditions are most often grouped into "triads" (i.e., common co-occurrences of three diseases together). Notably, psychiatric disorders were among seven of the top ten most frequent diagnostic comorbidity triads. This category of disorders resulted in the most expensive 5% of Medicaid beneficiaries with disabilities. The commonest triad was 1) a psychiatric condition, 2) cardiovascular disease, and 3) central nervous system disorders. This triad was present in 9.5% of all beneficiaries and 24% of the most expensive group of beneficiaries. Indeed, at least in the US, one of the most important drivers of the high numbers of individuals with comorbid mental and medical conditions is the combination of a psychiatric condition and a chronic disease (Foundation, 2011). As noted above, the 2001–2003 National Comorbidity Survey Replication found that approximately 25% of American adults meet criteria for at least one diagnosable mental disorder in any given year (C. Kessler, W. T., Demler, O., and Walters, E. E., 2005), and more than half report one or more chronic medical conditions (Hoffman, 1996).

When mental and medical conditions co-occur, this combination is associated with elevated symptom burden, functional impairment, decreased longevity and quality of life, and increased cost (Dickerson, 2008; Egede, 2007); (Katon, 2003); (Stein, 2006). The impact of having comorbid mental and medical conditions is at least additive and at times may be synergistic, with the cumulative burden greater than the sum of the individual conditions. Comorbid mental and medical conditions are associated with substantial individual and societal costs as well (Druss, 2002); (R. C. Kessler, Heeringa, S., Lakoma, M. D., Petukhova, M., Rupp, A. E., Schoenbaum, M., Wang, P. S., Zaslavsky, A. M., 2008)). Melek and Norris analyzed the expenditures for comorbid medical conditions and mental disorders using the 2005 Medstat Market Scan national claims database (Melek, 2008). They looked at the medical expenditures, mental health expenditures, and total expenditures of individuals with one of ten common chronic conditions with and without comorbid depression or anxiety. They found that the presence of comorbid depression or anxiety significantly increased medical and mental health care expenditures, with over 80% of the increase occurring in medical expenditures. For example, the average total monthly expenditure for a person with a chronic disease and depression is $560 dollars more than for a person without depression; the cost difference for people with comorbid anxiety is $710.

In publicly insured populations, the proportion of clients receiving treatment for one or more chronic conditions is extraordinarily high; data from the 2001 Medical Expenditure Panel Survey indicate that more than 80% of Medicare recipients report being treated for one or more chronic illnesses (Anderson, 2005); and national claims-based data from 2002 indicated that 79% of disabled and 56% of nondisabled adult Medicaid enrollees nationwide had one or more chronic conditions (Adelmann, 2003; Kronick, 2009). It is also important to mention that socioeconomic status (SES) factors, such as low income and poor educational attainment, are associated with comorbid mental disorders and medical conditions. A consistent inverse association exists between SES and a variety of health indicators, health behaviors and mortality (Harper, 2007; Lantz, 1998; Lorant, 2003). For example, a recent meta-analysis showed that people of low SES are 1.8 times more likely to report being depressed than people who have a higher status (Lorant, 2003). SES may both contribute to the onset of mental disorders and be a consequence of the "downward drift" associated with a history of psychiatric disorders (Eaton, 1999).

There is one other element we need to respect: the combined effects of age and low SES. Crimmins, Kim and Seeman (2009) examined poverty and biological risk, and their findings provide some plausible explanations for why age and mortality are not linearly related in clinical settings. Their data were collected from two National Health and Nutrition Examination Survey (NHANES) samples, which they then linked to the National Death Index. The NHANES data revealed that poor people in each decade of life (20s through 70s) had higher levels of biological risk than people of similar age who are not poor, thus supporting the notion of premature aging in those who endure poverty. The graph below reflects this problem. Decline in mean cognition scores as we age is ineluctable, but it is biased against those with a psychiatric history or with a disadvantaged childhood, or both. While there are certainly independent moderating effects at later life, it is clear that this trend bodes poorly for older adults, especially with psychiatric histories or current problems, or with built-in socioeconomic disadvantages.

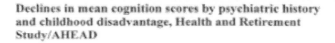

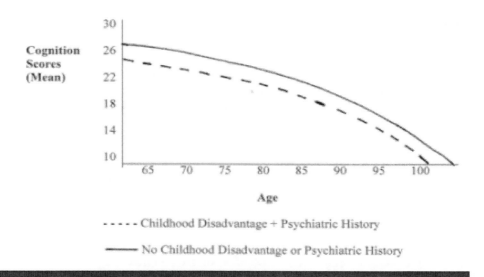

Declines in mean cognition scores by psychiatric history and childhood disadvantage, Health and Retirement Study/AHEAD

- - - - - Childhood Disadvantage + Psychiatric History

———— No Childhood Disadvantage or Psychiatric History

QUIXOTIC THINKING

Of course, the goal for older adults is better self-care and prevention. Many chronic medical conditions require patients to maintain a self-care regimen in order to manage symptoms and prevent disease progression, both of which may be hampered by comorbid mental health conditions. Self-care behaviors include taking medication as prescribed and adhering to lifestyle modifications, which may include exercise, diet and stress relief (Lorig, 2003). Depression may decrease the motivation and energy needed to perform self-management behaviors and may also adversely impact interpersonal relationships, including collaboration with caregivers, physicians and other healthcare providers (Katon, 2003). A meta-analysis indicated that the odds of noncompliance with medical treatment regimens are three times greater for depressed patients in comparison to that of nondepressed patients (DiMatteo, 2000).

The issue for providers, healthcare administrators, and policy makers is to balance the essential tension between good care and cost. This is not easy as it requires a thoughtful program of preventative self-care and reasoned medical service utilization based on patient-centered input by the older adult and his/her caregiver/family. In the Institute of Medicine report, *Retooling for an Aging America* (2008), a vision of health in America is laid out. First, the healthcare needs of the older population will be best served by a patient-centered, preference-sensitive approach. Patient-centeredness includes taking into account the increasing socio-demographic and cultural diversity of older Americans. Second, services will need to be efficient so that wasteful and ineffective care is reduced. Third, interdisciplinary teams will provide comprehensive, seamless care across various delivery sites, and be supported by easily accessible health information systems fitted to emerging care needs and delivery modalities. Last, older adults will be active partners in their own care until they no longer have the capacity for competent decision making. Ideally, there will be a partnership between provider and patient that includes: 1) clear information; 2) adoption of healthy lifestyles; 3) informed self-management of chronic conditions; and 4) increased participation in one's own care.

Patient-centeredness and control of one's health, then, are primary aims of a transformed high quality healthcare system. Under this model, the health care provider fosters the integration of care and education, focusing on both disease management and health promotion. With older adults, a shift needs to occur from a provider-driven focus on specific interventions for set symptoms to a person-centered focus on treatment response, problem remission/recovery, wellness, resilience, and maintaining community integration and social support. Implied here is the interplay between data and the person as is exemplified by evidence-based practices (EBPs). This is conceived as a road map, not necessarily sequentially, but logically and strategically. The ultimate demonstration of the evidence is the quality of fit between the individual at a particular point in time as judged by the participation and response of that person. To date, there are little data articulating the road map of using EBPs with older individuals, despite their appeal.

The empirical basis for personalizing treatment principally consists of post hoc analyses of unitary treatments (e.g., a course of an antidepressant or psychotherapy). While this knowledge is necessary, it is not sufficient for two reasons. First, depressed elderly persons face a bewildering constellation of health threats and social constraints and thus have many different contributors to poor treatment outcomes. Second, the professional skills available in various treatment settings and sectors can promote or inhibit treatment success. Therefore, to benefit depressed elderly patients in the community, personalization of care must employ comprehensive care algorithms targeting both modifiable predictors of poor outcomes and organizational and community barriers to care. Accordingly, the model of geriatric depression needs to integrate the current biological concepts of depression with older patients' unique reactions to adverse experiences and with their unmet social and healthcare needs. The care algorithms based on this model should: 1) target clinical/biological predictors of adverse outcomes of depression; 2) address unmet needs through linkages to appropriate social services; 3) enhance the competencies of elderly persons so that they make good use of their resources; and 4) attend to patient psychoeducation needs (Andreescu, 2008). This is done best with an interdisciplinary team with knowledgeable care managers in a primary care setting, where there are likely to be built-in efficiencies and sensitivities to cost. Often, this model of care can be implemented by utilizing the home, so that there are fewer office visits and more telephone-based monitoring and consults.

Finally, we highlight a caution in regard to the evidence driving change in healthcare delivery. The measures used to monitor treatment effectiveness are frequently confusing because 'outcomes' are nebulous. Concepts of morbidity have clouded discussion on and research about health trends. Studies have shown that, during a single time period, there are different trends for different components of health in the elderly population and that the correlations between different components also change. For example, going back to statements made at the beginning of this chapter about increasing life expectancy in the face of increasing morbidity among older adults, data show that prevalence of symptoms, disease, and functional limitations is expanding at the same time that disability is being compressed, or at least postponed. Researchers must clarify the implications of these different trends. Symptoms and disease imply need and demand for medical services. Functional limitations imply rehabilitative and compensatory activities, whereas disability among elderly people often entails need for social services and/or long-term care (Parker andThorslund, 2007).

Obviously, the nature and direction of health trends are highly contingent upon the indicator used (Gudex, 2000). As pointed out by Crimmins (1996), health indicators reflect different health dimensions, and there are logical reasons why trends in different components of health show disparity. Looking at results for different kinds of health indicators reveal a general pattern that prevails in spite of differences in methodology: there are clear increases in health problems as measured by specific items such as diseases and symptoms, and as measured by medical records and tests of physical function. Measures of significant disability (e.g., ADLs), however, show improvement or little change. Studies that use only disability measures provide optimistically misleading results in regard to total resource need (e.g., from specialized medical care to long-term-care facilities to simple but essential home services) in the future for aging adults. Therefore, if the study of health trends is going to be of any use in planning resource allocation in the future, investigators must examine the different components of health separately, using a variety of measures as indicators (Parker and Thorslund, 2007).

NEW TREATMENT MODELS FOR OLDER ADULTS AND COST

In this section, we identify 10 treatment issues for older adults. Presented are what we believe are the best targets for treatment and methods, taking cost and reality into consideration. Throughout, depression is used as the marker syndrome for examining EBPs for elders with medical and psychiatric comorbidities.

1. Care Managers and Primary Care Teams

Multi-disciplinary care is common with older adults whether it is recognized as such or not. Older adults are typically treated by multiple practitioners, and rarely is any of that care coordinated (i.e., interdisciplinary). This is now good evidence showing that interdisciplinary geriatric teams result in better clinical outcomes, especially when those teams exhibit positive, supportive, and frequent communication among their members (Lemieux-Charles, 2006; Sheehan, 2007; Sheehan D., 2007) . Central to the interdisciplinary team model is the care manager, usually a nurse or medical social worker, who stays in touch with the patient, monitors the patient's health markers, and coordinates general medical and mental healthcare among team members and specialists.

Older primary care patients with major depression who have access to care managers are more likely to have their depression treated appropriately and to have reduced suicidal ideation and increased remission rates over two years compared with a similar population who receive usual care, according to the Prevention of Suicide in Primary Care Elderly: Collaborative Trial (PROSPECT) (Bruce, 2004) . This study included 599 patients, 60 years and up with depression, at 20 primary-care practices in urban, suburban, and rural settings. In the intervention group, patients had access to specially trained care managers, including social workers, nurses, or psychologists, who helped physicians, monitor depressive symptoms, medication adverse events, treatment adherence, as well as offer treatment for depression with an antidepressant medication and/or a brief course of interpersonal psychotherapy (IPT).

Care-management systems such as the one in PROSPECT are increasingly needed, as today's primary-care physicians do not have the time or resources to provide the chronic care required by depressed older patients. Doctors are under pressure to see as many patients as possible just to pay their expenses, so the typical patient receives only about 10 minutes of their doctor's time – hardly enough time for a physician to recognize depressive symptoms much less address the problem. Indeed, PROSPECT showed that only 50% - 60% of depressed older patients in the study's usual-care group got treated. It appears likely that health maintenance organizations (HMOs) will adopt this care-management approach in the coming years because they recognize that it is "financially feasible" for them to do so. However, HMOs represent only a small part of healthcare delivery in the United States.

One other model is also worth noting, the *Improving Mood-Promoting Access to Collaborabitve Treatment* (IMPACT) model. This model extends findings from PROSPECT (J. Unutzer, Katon, W. J., Callahan, C. M., Williams, J. W., Hunkeler, E., Harpole, L., Hoffing, M., Della Penna, R. D., Noel, P. H., Lin, E. H. B., Arean, P. A., Hegel, M. T., Tang, L., Belin, T. R., Oishi, S., and Langston, C. , 2002) by demonstrating the benefits of a team approach and collaboration among care delivery systems to chronic care management. It shows that improving quality of care and frequency of contacts for elders with chronic disease and depression not only helps over the first 12 months but also that these patients are likely to stay better over the ensuing 12 months (see model description below).

While these models seem effective and cost sensitive, mental health care is usually more complicated than medical care. The interactive care of older adults by psychiatry and primary care is not without its problems. At base, primary care providers are reluctant to prescribe psychiatric medications; psychiatric clinics are reticent to deal with physical maladies. We believe that, except for patients with serious and chronic mental illness or those with complex psychiatric pictures (e.g., severe depression, OCD, complex PTSD, and eating disorders), psychiatry clinics are fast becoming anachronistic. For example, currently such clinics have little to offer older adults with garden variety dementia or Mild Cognitive Impairment (MCI). In psychiatry the treatment of choice for dementia, for example, is primarily cognitive enhancing medications with no adjunctive psychosocial intervention. The effect sizes are low for these drugs and the time period for any effective medication assistance is limited (18 months at best). The NIH Alzheimer's and Cognitive Decline Conference (2010) indicated the limits of medicine and suggested prevention comes mostly in the form of lifestyle interventions – exercise, active leisure activity, and cognitive activity, as well as caregiver support.

In effect, treatment for older adults' mental health problems is stock and not particularly effective. Clearly as physical care relates to mental health, attention to chronic medical care, especially toward cerebral and vascular risk factors, is important. But, older adults are not really carefully treated psychiatrically with empirical support. Those prescribed psychiatric medications tend to continue with these regardless of etiology. Wright et al (2009), for example, assessed 2737 healthy older adults with no baseline indicators of cognitive impairment. The CNS meds taken at Years 1, 3, and 5 were then monitored. A cognitive measure (3MS) was also administered. Results showed that in Year 5, 7.7% had cognitive impairment and 25.5% had cognitive decline; CNS med use was 13.9%, 15.2%, 17.1% over the 5 years. This trend to prescribe psychiatric drugs, therefore, increased over time and was associated with cognitive decline (>5 point decrease). Longer treatment durations and increased dosing, potentially leading to adverse effects on cognition, also were problems.

Importantly, collaborative care approaches have been found to be highly cost-effective from a societal perspective (Katon et al, 2005; (Gawande, 2011; Schoenbaum, 2001);Gawande, 2011). Cost-effectiveness indicates a good value for society, but does not necessarily mean that cost-effective programs will save money or result in a "cost-offset" (Von Korff, 1998). However, more recent clinical trials have suggested that cost savings may be achievable over the long term, particularly among the costliest and most complex patients, such as those older adults with comorbid diabetes and depression (Katon et al, 2008; Unutzer et al, 2008). There are challenges, however, in moving from cost-effectiveness findings to policy change, given the realities of healthcare financing in the United States (see Gawande, 2011). For instance, if a program reduces emergency room visits or hospital admissions, funding for that program typically does not reap any financial benefits from these savings (Mauskopf, 2007). Cost-effectiveness analyses need to be supplemented with budget impact analyses that seek to understand these costs from the perspective of cost offsets as well as the organizations that implement these programs (Leatherman, 2003; Mauskopf, 2007; Neumann, 2007).

Noted above, the most widely disseminated model is IMPACT (2002) (see www.impact-uw.org). Care managers, either nurses or psychologists trained to provide education and apply a brief psychotherapy intervention for depression, were embedded in the primary care clinic. They collaborated with the PCP to optimize treatment (including antidepressant medication and/or short-term problem-solving therapy) acutely and they followed up with patients regularly for 12 months. An examination of cost over 4 years revealed that IMPACT patients incurred lower average costs for all of their medical care (approximately $3300 less) as compared to those patients receiving usual care (J. Unutzer, Katon, W. J., Fan, M. Y., Schoenbaum, M. C., Lin, E. H., Della Penna, R. D., and Powers, D., 2008)Unitzer et al., 2008).

Similarly, more than 90 clinics have participated in an initiative known as DIAMOND (Depression Improvement Across Minnesota, Offering a New Direction), which uses the IMPACT model of collaborative care delivery in Minnesota. DIAMOND components include: a care manager, consulting psychiatrist, a patient registry for long term health monitoring, stepped care that includes EBP-based pharmacotherapy and brief psychotherapy, and relapse prevention. Of 151 depressed patients enrolled in the program who had been contacted after being in the program for 6 months 42% were in remission, and an additional 12% had seen at least a 50% improvement in their depressive symptoms (Jaeckles, 2009). To finance this care model, the DIAMOND project applies the concept of a case rate payment (as opposed to fee-for-service) for depression care. Minnesota health plans are paying a monthly per person case rate to participating clinics for a bundle of services, including a care manager and consulting psychiatrist, under a single billing code. Because the payments are being made from the health care side of the system, there is an opportunity for any cost savings to accrue directly to the health plans paying for the program.

In the Community Care of North Carolina (CCNC) project, Medicaid enrollees receive health care and care management through local networks made up of physicians, hospitals, social service agencies and county health departments. Preliminary evidence suggests that this project may help improve quality of care for chronic medical illnesses and save money (Steiner, 2008). The CCNC project is a primary care case management model that could serve as a prototype for accountable care organizations, providing care management, outcome measurement, and quality infrastructure needed by small practices. In the last several years four CCNC networks have worked with state and regional mental health authorities to pilot a model for integrating mental health and primary care (Wilhide, 2006). To date, these networks have reported considerable cost savings.

Primary care, then, is where the action is, but here, too, there are problems. These involve the competency to handle psychiatric problems and use psychiatric medications appropriately. A review of 30 years of health services research on depression outcomes concluded that patients with major depression had poor outcomes in primary care, especially for older adults (Callahan, 2001). In a meta-analysis of 50,000 across the world Mitchell et al. (2009) found that for every 20 true cases, 10 were diagnosed correctly, 10 were missed, and 15 non-depressed patients were seen as depressed. This same trend was seen by Berardi et al. (2005): A depression diagnosis had 80% "hits" with 40% of patients actually prescribed antidepressants, but 45% were false positives (Berardi, et al., 2005). Anxiety conditions fare no better: Medication utilization increases with the number of anxiety diagnoses (Kroenke, 2007). Furthermore, we have found anecdotally that, if a patient reports to their PCP that the presenting problem is somatic, the PCP is very likely to miss the psychiatric overlay. For collaborative medical and mental health care to work, then, the "gatekeeper" must be well educated about the many faces of depression, including clinical presentations influenced by developmental stage and/or culture.

2. Taxonomy Crisis for Normal and Clinical Aging

Any clear demarcation between normal aging and clinical aging is at present unclear. Most medical conditions that have a slow onset can be viewed as a chronic condition. This implies two fundamental needs for health care providers: (1) the need for ever-increasing specificity of syndromes and familiarity with these syndromes as they evolve; and (2) the need for good normative data across multiple health domains and health assessment tools. A strategy for effective assessment and treatment of chronic conditions is to identify changes early in the syndrome and intervene. With older individuals, pathological changes are hypothesized to begin during what would be classified as normal aging and as such go undetected. In studying pathways toward disability, Fried, Bandeen-Roche, Chaves, and Johnson (2000) posited that changes in the ability to complete tasks of daily living are preceded by changes in physical functioning, suggesting that the concept of pre-disability or subclinical disability status, a stage that lies before 'dependence' on the disability spectrum, should be attended to by providers. Pre-disability and mild cognitive impairment provide clinical-like categories for those elders whose symptoms do not yet meet the criteria for a geriatric syndrome.

The question of norms therefore becomes important: What, for instance, is the normal range of scores for older adults in domains such as sleep, pain, gait speed, and flexibility? How much daily variability can one expect in scores on assessments of depression, cognition, and pain, for example? Normative data are commonly influenced by age, education, and historical and/or ethnocultural factors, so that we must be careful when applying what norms we have to our patients.

In medicine, Oslerian teachings hold to "Ocam's razor," an idea that fosters the distillation of a disease presentation into a single diagnosis. With older adults in particular, we are arguing that such simplification leads to a poor outcome, especially among a modal older adult patient where chronic, multi-morbid conditions and deficits in both health and well-being are present. Often these are lumped into one ICD or DSM diagnosis. Any given older patient might have a combination of hypertension, Type 2 diabetes, new onset shortness of breath, allergies, cognitive impairment, depression, and pain, as well as social isolation, impaired IADLs, and limited family support. But the interplay of chronic disease and external factors may create a very different clinical picture from patient to patient. In fact, just minimal increases in allostatic load correlate greatly with frailty over a three year period (Gruenewald, 2009).

Looking at cognitive decline specifically, the issue of whether a dimensional or categorical model best represents the neuropsycyhiatric construct of "dementia" crystallizes this problem. Dementia is prevalent (5% of adults and growing). As it is currently defined in the DSM-IV, dementia is too categorical, exclusive, and arbitrary for ascertaining and addressing cognitive impairment. There unfortunately is no objective taxonomic boundary separating those who do and those who do not meet criteria for dementia. By creating a dichotomy between dementia and nondementia, we don't do justice to the spectrum of cognitive problems seen at older ages. For instance, over 22% of people older than 70 years have memory impairment. This often departs from the plaques and tangles we associate with "Alzheimer's Disease." Although we commonly use cut scores to connote dementia, they do not represent the taxon boundary between health and pathology. Converting what is observed in the way of soft signs and symptoms into hard categories fails to capture the complexity of the common co-existence (and probable interaction) of cerebrovascular disease and Alzheimer disease, as well as other contaminants, for example. Jack et al. (2010) noted how the value of biomarkers changes in AD over time. The focus, rather, should be on identifying signs, symptoms, and behaviors that place a person on the continuum of cognitive decline, not whether s/he qualifies to be in a particular diagnostic group. It is time to shift the focus from thresholds of dementia/no dementia to a continuum of cognitive impairment, from the late to the early stages, and from effects to causes.

Other psychiatric constructs (e.g., depression, anxiety) also are best thought of as dimensional. The idea that one can be depressed and be like other depressives with 5/9 signs and symptoms is not realistic. The idea too that "subsyndromal" problems are different from syndromes is also fallacious. With older adults, the mix of psychiatric problem states with medical conditions as well as with situational stressors requires a broad view and one that respects common sense, empirically based interventions, as well as cost. Treatment of such a complex person requires a team, requires vision, and requires a cost-offset mindset.

3. Point of Care and the Long View

A related third concept is point-of-care as defined by the American Colleges of Medicine and the Association of American Colleges of Nursing (2010), which points to issues and procedures associated with face-to-face patient care. According to the recent report by the

Association of American Medical Colleges and American Association of Colleges of Nursing (2010), *point-of-care learning* is defined as learning that occurs at the time and place of a health provider - patient encounter. Point-of-care learning is most often distinguished by its context, i.e., the active encounter between the clinician and the patient at the healthcare site, home, or elsewhere. It is during this process that information needs are identified and the opportunity for clinician and patient education, clinical decisions, and patient management all intersect. The provider - patient encounter traditionally has occurred face-to-face in a clinical setting; however, in this age of growing information and communication technologies and new approaches to healthcare delivery, patient encounters may also include telephone calls, email communications, and video conferencing. The most basic of provider skills in the point-of-care environment is knowledge management, including the ability to identify learning needs, know and understand what resources to use, how to access and critically appraise information, and how to apply it. A second basic skill is the ability to self-assess, that is, to accurately assess one's own learning needs, impact on patient outcomes, and need for performance change.

Related is the fact that patients' psychiatric problems wax and wane over time, but do not extinguish easily. The mood or behaviors that influence illness presentation may be malleable but not substantially alterable in any easy way. Adults experience repeated depression at levels as high as 80%, depending on the number of earlier incidents of depression. Barlow (2004) notes: "Advances in knowledge in the psychopathology of mood disorders seem to make it clear that the wrong target has been addressed. That is, it is now known that the major depressive episodes will respond to most reasonable treatments in the short term or will remit on their own, but they will almost always recur. To be truly effective, treatments, whether psychological or pharmacological, must prevent recurrence of future depressive episodes" (p.873). (Barlow, 2004)

In short, the provider needs to keep the long view in mind and focus on mitigating the impact of psychiatric vulnerabilities on medical conditions. So the busy health care provider is really tasked at the point-of-care to maximize the intervention for the current incident while keeping the long-view of care in mind. This requires developing a care mentality that is not short sited, cost limiting, or validation-poor. After all, a solitary, acute response to developing medical issues would be very short sighted. Several models noted above have suggested as much. And, as described above, the primary care movement in the last decade also reaches deep and seeks interdisciplinary collaborative care, home-based care, social care, and the integration of psychiatric care.

4. Aging Is Complex and Variable Clinically

Aging is indeed complex. We do not know what causes aging and how can we prevent the harmful aspects of old age (LeCouteur, 2010). Older age itself is associated with progressive impairment of mitochondrial function, increased oxidative stress, and immune activation. It is best characterized by the decline of anatomical integrity and function across multiple organ systems and a related ability to respond to stress. This decline is associated with increasing pathology, disease, and a progressively higher risk of death. We do not know well what cell senescence is or what causes the allostatic load to not be processed well. Both genetics and environment are responsible for this (resulting in aging phenotype). Aging is then a part of a modulation of gene/environment interaction.

Indeed, variability is itself not an optimal sign at older ages, because it is thought to reflect a breakdown in 'system' integrity. Intra-individual variability (IIV) is associated with developing cognitive deficits, especially in working memory (WM), brain volumetric decline, demyelination, reduced blood flow, vascular injury, and many other neurological conditions. The more variability in the system, the more medical probems that are likely to arise.

As challenges, we can say that even small changes in core capacities can lead to large changes in complex behavior (Salthouse, 2001). Presumably the true savings in 'number of years added' for most of our treatment efforts will be important and known. In time we may know also the "real" upper limit of cure for most disorders, given the best care, is somewhere less than 50%. Just the idea of an 85 year old individual who is optimally healthy, coming for care, is problematic. Within five years 80% of the healthy oldest old will still develop considerable medical issues (Beckman, 2005).

Clinically, common problems when working with elders run the gamut from basic safety issues to reasonable prevention, as well as issues related to the specific disease(s) itself. Clinical areas of focus include polypharmacy, adverse drug events, medication compliance, falls prevention, continence care, and caregiver management of problem behaviors. These issues can significantly impact the quality of everyday life of older adults and therefore need to be addressed aggressively. Common concerns are:

Conditions go undiagnosed and untreated: Too much of the time, common and treatable conditions, such as cognitive impairment, nutrition problems, sleep disorders, fall risk, overactive bladder and incontinence, mobility disorders, and depression, are undiagnosed.

Health and care needs of the oldest old: Included in this vulnerable group are many very old minority and rural elders. Individuals 85 years and up are the fastest growing group in the older population and these individuals place the greatest demands on the healthcare system.

Minority/disadvantaged elders: African American and Hispanic elders, especially, are at high risk for chronic health problems such as Type 2 diabetes, obesity, and high blood pressure, and they typically receive less treatment, and less quality treatment, for their conditions.

Health literacy: The Institute of Medicine has indicated that 90 million people have difficulty understanding and acting upon health information. The prevalence of limited health literacy is highest among older adults, minority populations, those who are poor, and the medically underserved. Training of healthcare professionals to improve their ability to communicate with older patients is critical.

5. Prevention Works

This has been a fact of public life for over 100 years. The frequent medical care utilizers or the "indicated group" are especially ripe for preventive measures (Smits, 2008). While the recent NIH Alzheimer's and Cognitive Decline Prevention Conference (2010) noted that there is very little that can be recommended strongly for the care of AD or cognitive decline, there should be a focus on prevention. This includes exercise, leisure, cognitive activity, as well as a therapeutic emphasis on cerebral vascular risk factors. It is also noteworthy that enriched environments assist in the delay of cognitive decline as synaptic connectivity is increased. This even applies to diabetes, as schooling, for example, mediates the relationship of glucose hypometabolism and impaired ADL performance. Cognitive retraining also has an impact on all older adults, including MCI.

Targeting exercise, for example, Herring ,O'Connor, and Dishman (2010) reviewed 40 English-language articles published from January 1995 to December 2008 in scholarly journals involving sedentary adults with chronic illness. They independently calculated the Hedges *d* effect size from studies of 2914 patients and extracted information regarding potential moderating variables. Compared with no treatment conditions, exercise training significantly reduced anxiety symptoms by a mean Delta effect of 0.29 with a 95% confidence interval between 0.23 and 0.36. Largest anxiety improvements resulted from exercise programs lasting no more than 12 weeks, using session durations of at least 30 minutes and an anxiety report timeframe greater than the past week. The authors concluded that exercise training reduces mental health symptoms among sedentary patients who have a chronic illness.

Good nutrition, social interaction, low levels of stress, and personal meaning-making are co-incident with exercise in the application of good health habits and better quality of life. Again, the physician/health care provider is challenged to examine the cost/benefit of these kinds of care ideals given the case mix and reality of the older adult. Many of the features of quality care including the recruitment and training of a competent behavioral health workforce, the development of service delivery models, bridging science and service and facilitating the dynamic, an iterative learning process resulting from their interplay, the fostering of intervention designs, the development of basic and applied research, the development of decisional algorithms for referral to specialty services, and the implementation of outcome-driven, culturally-informed, evidence-based intervention strategies.

6. Home Care and Caregiver Input

As with health homes (or "medical homes"), prevention is emphasized. Early identification and intervention, chronic disease management, person-centered approaches, and implies adoption of EBP. As noted, there are now several compelling examples of high value integrated care interventions targeting mental health and substance-use in elderly adults that include psychological interventions/supervision. We have already discussed IMPACT, DIAMOND, and PROSPRECT.

A core issue is home care, especially home care with a caregiver focus. Hicken and Plowhead (2010) outlined the effective use of home care for depression, anxiety, and many health-related conditions like Type 2 diabetes and heart disease, as well as traumatic brain injury. In 2007, the Veterans Health Administration (VA) Office of Mental Health Services began offering home-based psychological services. The typical home care patient in this system has eight or more chronic medical conditions and 47% have reached *dependent* status on two or more ADLs. Depression and/or anxiety are typically part of the picture. The issues that require special attention in this setting were provided: confidentiality, environmental distractions, role confusion and boundaries, time management, safety, and provider competence.

The PATH (Home Delivered Problem Adaptation Therapy for Depressed, Cognitively Impaired, Disabled Elders; (Kiosses, 2010)) model also has been applied. This model focuses on the patient's ecosystem – patient, caregiver, and home. Problem solving therapy is applied. Environmental adaptation tools and caregiver participation are required. Environmental tools are designed to bypass any behavioral and functional limitations identified in the patient. The PATH tools include calendars, checklists, pictures, notebooks, notepads, alarms, signs, colored tags, diaries, timers, timed prerecorded messages, voice alarms, customized audio tapes, and a step-by-step division of tasks. This intervention is done in the home in 12 sessions with the caregiver's participation. A trial comparing PATH with standard treatment revealed that the PATH care model was more efficacious than standard treatment in reducing depression and disability in these especially vulnerable patients. At this time, cost data that compares PATH to usual catre points in the direction of savings in terms of utilization and quality of life.

As in PATH, other studies have shown that the role of the caregiver is critical in the treatment of dementia. Caregiving is far from a simple task, however (Schulz and Martire, 2004)(Schulz, 2004). In general, data show that caregiver involvement is an important aspect of a comprehensive, multifaceted approach to cognitive rehabilitation (Berger, 2004; Koltai, 2001; Moniz-Cook, 1998; M. P. Quayhagen, and Quayhagen, M., 1989; M. P. Quayhagen, Quayhagen, M., Corbeil, R. R., Roth, P. A., and Rodgers, J. A., 1995; Zarit, 2004). When caregivers are distressed, the patient almost invariably does poorly, so adjunctive care for the caregiver is beneficial to both. Several caregiver treatment models (e.g., (Hepburn, 2003) and adjunctive methods (e.g., Resources for Enhancing Alzheimer's Health (REACH project)) have been applied to aging in general and dementia in particular. These models have addressed the caregiver directly and the problem solving process in caregiving, either preventively or via treatment. Again, the data point in the direction of a cost savings.

As noted, most older adults with dementia will be cared for by primary care physicians, but the primary care practice setting presents numerous challenges to providing quality care for these individuals. Callahan et al. (2007) conducted a clinical trial of 153 older adults with Alzheimer's disease and their caregivers, with the dyad randomized by physician to receive collaborative care management (n=84) or augmented usual care (n=69) at primary care practices within two US university-affiliated health care systems. Intervention patients received 1 year of care management by an interdisciplinary team led by an advanced practice nurse working with the patient's caregiver. The team used standard protocols to initiate treatment and identify, monitor, and treat behavioral and psychological symptoms of dementia, stressing nonpharmacological management. The Neuropsychiatric Inventory (NPI) was administered at baseline and at 6, 12, and 18 months. Secondary outcomes included the Cornell Scale for Depression in Dementia (CSDD), cognition, activities of daily living, resource use, and caregiver's depression severity.

Initiated by caregivers' reports, 89% of intervention patients triggered at least one protocol for behavioral and psychological symptoms of dementia with a mean of four protocols per patient from a total of 8 possible protocols. Intervention patients were more likely to receive cholinesterase inhibitors (79.8% vs 55.1%; p=.002) and antidepressants (45.2% vs 27.5%; p=.03) than patients receiving usual care. Intervention patients had significantly fewer behavioral and psychological symptoms of dementia. Intervention caregivers also reported significant improvements in distress. Collaborative care for the treatment of Alzheimer's disease therefore resulted in substantial improvement in the quality of care and in behavioral and psychological symptoms of dementia among primary care patients and their caregivers. These improvements were achieved without significantly increasing the use of antipsychotics or sedative-hypnotics. Cost was also a benefit.

7. Assist the Brain

Last year, Americans spent $265 million on "brain fitness" software and web-based programs that claim to boost brainpower. But can playing Word Scramble or Rock, Paper, Scissors on a computer really fend off dementia? These exercises may or may not work. A recently published study with over 11,000 volunteers ages 18 to 60 years found that computer-based brain training did not significantly improve mental fitness (Katsnelson, 2010). Other studies, including a 2006 investigation led by Pennsylvania State University psychologist Sherry Willis have suggested that brain training can improve cognitive function in elderly patients and those in the early stages of Alzheimer's disease (Willis, 2006).

Overall Ideas

- Big Idea: Aging compromises the basic operating characteristics of biological hardware; training and experience can assist with the software of the cognitive system (Mayr, 2008)
- Constantly adapting CNS is receptive to training – plasticity, symmorphosis, brain reserve, enriched environments
- Training can assist in Attention and Working Memory (WM). Targeted training of Executive Functions – set shifting, inhibition, and updating – are especially helpful (Dahlin, 2008)
- More "holistic" training can provide benefits that extend beyond Attention and WM if applied to complex, goal-directed activities (Basak, 2008; Stine-Morrow, 2008)
- Environmental enrichment makes a difference: having occupation or avocation, active leisure, complexity in life, mental training
- Health: enhanced cardio-vascular health and neurocognitive function (Herzog et al., 2009, as well as exercise (Erickson, 2009) make a difference

Memory Training Applied to Cognitively Healthy People

- Mnemonic strategies are beneficial
- Improvement in memory can be seen, but less so compared with younger groups
- Can maintain skilled memory performance for 6 months

Memory Training Applied to Cognitively Less Healthy People

- Training shows little transfer to other skills Affect, attitude, effort, and ambient stress matter
- Several studies show promise (Lowenstein, et al, 2004; (Belleville, 2006; Unverzagt, 2007);Yesavage et al., 2009)
- Caregivers really can help with compensatory strategies (Hyer, et al., 2007)
- Multi-method packages for patient/caregiver dyads are available (Hyer et al., in press)

What does work and is it worth it? The hard line is that researchers still don't know. We noted above that the NIH concluded that there is no clear evidence to support most interventions (NIH Alzheimer's and Cognitive Decline Prevention, 2010). The softer line is that there is considerable promise in memory clinics and memory training for at least healthy older adults. In the box below we present the overall picture of memory training, as well as where the better patient training and better results occur. In the real world, consideration of the problems related to cognition is time well spent in developing cost of care models as this variable is highly related to just about all outcomes. Cognition influences adjustment, functionality, and quality of life across the board of settings - from home to nursing home.

In our clinic (Hyer et al, 2011) we have been able to show changes in both older patients with MCI using a computer-based program (Cogmed) and older patients with varied memory complaints using a 6-session holistic model emphasizing concentration techniques. Satisfaction was high, function was improved, and quality of life was positive. These cognitive retraining methods allow for several curative factors that are more general but important -- coping, practice, consistent application, and improved affect. In sum, cognitive retraining resulted in many positive outcomes.

8. Assessment of the Patient over Time

Assessments of domains of interest over time are informative for cost-saving treatment adjustments, and are best accomplished by incorporating self-report of abilities, a performance-based test of abilities, a collateral report of abilities, and an analysis of the consistency or discrepancy between the reports. For behavioral health treatments, i.e., alcohol, pain, nutrition, treatment adherence, the assessment process is often intertwined with a brief educational component, assessment of patient beliefs, and even a brief motivational interviewing intervention. Of note, psychosocial and functional assessments are at least as valid as most medical tests and are less expensive than many (Meyer, 2001).

Moreover, as a prelude to and follow-up after psychotherapy, psychological assessment can enhance the therapeutic process in several ways: 1) a clearer delineation of clinical symptomatology; 2) hypothesis testing and decision-making regarding differential diagnoses; 3) assisting in case formulation; 4) predicting a client's ability to participate as well as the degree of participation in psychotherapy; 5) predicting healthcare utilization; 6) hypothesis testing for therapy impasses or looming therapy failure; 7) monitoring treatment effects over time; 8) the confirmation (or disconfirmation) of perceived psychotherapy outcomes (as in improving prediction of relapse); and 10) enabling the health care provider to respond to managed care and other external pressures (Anthony, 2002).

At late life comorbid depression and generalized anxiety have special meaning and must be assessed thoroughly. This is most common problem at late life. Problems with frontal lobe functioning are prevalent, either subtly as in working memory or working memory dysfunction, or more globally as in an under-active prefrontal cortex and disinhibited amygdale (Beaudreau, 2008). For example, cross sectional investigations generally support the hypothesis that the presence and severity of anxiety in an older adult is associated with lower cognitive performance. An older adult who is anxious has a reasonable probability of having cognitive problems as well, especially in processing speed and/or executive functioning. Longitudinal studies that took into account baseline performance levels have shown that clinically significant anxiety predicted accelerated cognitive decline (Sinoff, 2003). As such, a thorough pre-therapy assessment of the elder who presents with depression and/or anxiety is vital for understanding the full complement of issues that may be playing a role in the chief complaint.

9. Enter Mental Health and Reasonable Psychological Profiles

The role of the behavioral health provider will only become more essential. Mental health and substance-use problems are the leading cause of combined disability and death of women and second highest in men in the United States. Currently, only 7% of health care expenditures go to mental health treatment. This, despite the fact that over 70% of people dually eligible for Medicare and Medicaid have mental illness. We know too that 67% of adults and more than 92% of people with serious mental illness do not receive effective mental health and substance-use treatment. This is due to multiple variables that affect success and acceptability of care. The estimated cost by Institute of Medicine (IOM) that excessive costs stemming from waste and inefficiency within the nation's health care system currently total between $750-$785 *billion* annually. Much of this is due to ignoring mental health.

One model that assists in this process is the transdiagnostic model. Brown and Barlow (2005) held that all emotional disorders that lie on the depression and anxiety continuums have a similar underlying structure and that there is a unified approach to treating them. This model holds that a single negative affective (NA) vulnerability influences the development of an anxiety disorder and/or depressive disorder. Individuals high in NA show an increase the likelihood of negative life events, have high levels of physical and mental health problems, are prone to multiple psychiatric diagnoses, and have multiple poor lifestyle habits (Lahey, 2009). Individuals with NA undergo multiple learning experiences over the life span that promotes fears and depression, which eventuate in medical and psychiatric comorbidities. Day to day, these individuals are excessively irritable, sad, anxious, self-consciousness, and vulnerable that is out of proportion to their circumstances. A good intervention protocol would take a multimodal approach and treat a profile of problems, some are syndromal and sone subsdromal, including: psychoeducation, cognitive restructuring, breathing training, exposure techniques to address feared objects/activities, and self-monitoring.

Procedurally, a case driven formulation under the umbrella of the transdiagnostic model is given to patients using parallel care strategies (not serial) and a holistic understanding of the person. Treating, for example, depressive symptoms in isolation of the patient's cognitive and physical limitations risks slower or less effective reduction in depressive symptoms. However, simultaneously targeting a profile of depression, cognitive impairment, and physical disability, provides a multi-pronged approach to helping patients cope with their problems, which in turn increases the likelihood of a successful outcome for depression treatment. Although evidence for such multi-faceted approaches to treatment is nascent, large-scale studies and further intervention development are currently underway. Given the high prevalence of depression in older adults, establishing more effective treatments is vital to improving geriatric mental health and quality of life for patients and their families. Better cost estimates will inevitably follow.

10. Too Many Best Care Practices

In a JAMA a few years ago, Boyd et al. (2005) presented the case of a 79 y/o female with the usual medical problems at later life (see box below). When her situation was carefully assessed, problems related to her care became obvious. She was receiving 13 medications daily (pills were taken multiple times a day) and she was subjected to 18 non-pharmacological interventions. This woman represents the other side of the coin, excessive care that is not coordinated.

---

79 y/o Female: Osteoporosis, Type 2 Diabetes, Arthritis, Hypertension, COPD, and Depression.

- 13 medications, dosed for 21 times/day
- Medications costs were greater than $400.00/month
- 18 non-pharmacological activities, such as dieting, self-monitoring
- 6 medications had a 100% chance of drug/drug interactions and 100% for non-pharmacological intervention interactions
- Best Practice Guidelines did not comment on the time or burden of self-management, or raise the issue of likely poor compliance due to burden

---

This case is not meant to cause providers to shelve diagnostic best practices but to be prudent about them, to develop a coordinating team process, and to monitor progress. The typical older adult has greater than four medical conditions, has sensory problems, has subsyndromal mental health symptoms, has limited means, is isolated, and has a high requirement to develop and maintain good lifestyle habits (socialization, cognitive retraining, exercise, health, etc.). This person is likely to have health literacy issues and may be unable to afford medications or comply with suggestions/prescriptions. Obviously cost will suffer here also.

This medicalization into life has been excessive. Consumerism and the medical/industrial complex have made us a bundle of risk factors to be plucked upon. In effect, there is little effective transformation of health care to disease care. With the increase of chronic diseases, with the effective treatment we currently have for these, and with the way we can prevent illnesses, health care has become tertiary, even reductive. This rise in expectations causes problems because we have less self responsibility and more demands on the system; health care is not only a right but where more is better. The results are not good as we rank lower in health care, average age and disease numbers than most industrial countries. Health in this sense has become an end in itself, not a means to an end.

CONCLUSION

The case just described cries out for more innovative and less costly models of care for older adults. This means placing emphasis on prevention, personal participation, and case-managed interdisciplinary care. Mental health must not be forgotten because neglected mental health problems ultimately increase the cost of care. Single specialty clinics are not the answer as they are no more effective and of course costly. In fact, we provided 10 suggestions to consider in the holistic care of older adults.

In a review of long term care and the value of psychiatric medication, Reichman and Conn (2010) noted that the evidence in support of various models of psychogeriatric services (in nursing homes) concluded that liaison-style services that employed educational approaches, treatment guidelines, and ongoing involvement of mental health staff are more effective than the purely case-based consultation model. This latter model almost exclusively involves the application of medication only. In a recent position statement on the role of geriatric psychiatry in long-term care, Reichman and Conn (2010) note:

> "We continue to rely nearly exclusively on medication management in our clinical nursing home practices, even though our confidence in the efficacy and safety of the historically most treasured psychotropic agents has been seriously eroded.... We must acknowledge that the newer generation medication therapies have not delivered substantial enough gains over their predecessors...it is time to shed our overreliance on biological determinants and the disease models of mental illness. It is time for a reappraisal." (p.1050-1052)

We have argued that a new look at the care of older adults is in order, one that addresses the co-incident mental health and physical health of older adults. These issues infect physical problems (as well as mental problem) and lead to increased cost and problems. As we noted, a reasonable design for the treatment of medical and mental health comorbidities is based on the public health target "indicated," where prevention is sought for high risk individuals before they become patients. As a common disorder with devastating outcomes, mental geriatric problems are major health hazards. Identification of predictors of treatment response and personalization of treatment (that is, matching the treatment to the patient) has long been contemplated as a strategy to increase efficacy, to prevent relapses, and to preempt disability, and to obviate a worsening of medical morbidity and cognitive decline. While we are not yet there, it is prudent to have a "problem watch" for at risk patients and to carefully monitor interventions for the need for timely treatment changes, discontinuations, or implementation of different interventions. In this way, we believe that the costs of medical care at late life can be more effectively reined in.

From the 30,000 foot level, the additive effect of both genetic and environmental risk factors likely provides the best accounting of the data. In fact, a balance of positive and negative genetic and good-living factors affects the brain throughout life to influence the degree of cognitive agility or impairment at late life. These factors increase or decrease oxidative stress, inflammation, insulin signaling components, size and frequency of infarcts, and concentration of growth factors, cortisol, and other hormones. In effect, an older individual's "fate" unfolds as we would expect it, based on reasonable personal actions and integrated preventative care. This occurs for mental as well as physical problems and represents a process of fiscally cost savings and effective outcomes.

REFERENCES

Adelmann, P. K. (2003). Mental and substance use disorders among Medicaid recipients: Prevalence estimates from two national surveys. *Administration and Policy in Mental Health*, 31(2).

Alegria, M., Jackson, J. S., Kessler, R. C., and Takeuchi, D. (2003). National Comorbidity Survey Replication (NCS-R), 2001-2003. Paper presented at the Inter-university Consortium for Political and Social Research, Ann Arbor.

Anderson, G. F. (2005). Medicare and chronic conditions. *New England Journal of Medicine*, 353(3).

Andreescu, C., Mulsant, B. H., Houck, P. R., Whyte, E. M., Mazumdar, S., Dombrovski, A. Y., Pollock, B. G., and Reynolds, C. F. III. (2008). Empirically derived decision trees for the treatment of late-life depression. *American Journal of Psychiatry*, 165(7), 855-862.

Anthony, M. M., and Barlow, D. H. (2002). Handbook of assessment and treatment planning for psychological disorders. New York: Guilford Press.

Barlow, D. H. (2004). Anxiety and Its Disorders: The Nature and Treatment of Anxiety and Panic (2nd ed.). New York: Guilford Press.

Basak, C., Boot, W. R., Voss, M. W., and Kramer, A. F. (2008). Can training in a real-time strategy video game attenuate cognitive decline in older adults? *Psychology and Aging*, 23(4), 765-777.

Beaudreau, S. A., and O'Hara, R. (2008). Late-life anxiety and cognitive impairment: A review. *American Journal of Geriatric Psychiatry*, 16(10), 790-803.

Belleville, S., Gilbert, B., Fontaine, F., Gagnon, L., Menard, E., and Gauthier, S. (2006). Improvement of episodic memory in persons with mild cognitive impairment and healthy older adults: Evidence from a cognitive intervention program. *Dementia and Geriatric Cognitive Disorders*, 22(5-6), 486-499.

Berger, G., Bernhardt, T., Schramm, U., Muller, R., Landsiedel-Anders, S., Peters, J., Kratzsch, T., and Frolich, L. (2004). No effects of a combination of caregivers support group and memory training/music therapy in dementia patients from a memory clinic population. *International Journal of Geriatric Psychiatry*, 19(3), 223-231.

Bruce, M. L., Ten Have, T. R., Reynolds, C. F., Katz, I. I., Schulberg, H. C., Mulsant, B. H., Brown, G. K., McAvay, G. J., Pearson, J. L., and Alexopoulos, G. S. (2004). Reducing suicidal ideation and depressive symptoms in depressed older primary care patients: A randomized controlled trial. *Journal of the American Medical Association*, 291(9), 1081-1091.

Bureau, U. C. Health status, health insurance, and health services utilization, 2001: household economic studies, 2006. 2009, from http://www.census.gov/prod/2006pubs/p70-106.pdf

Callahan, C. M. (2001). Quality Improvement Research on Late Life Depression in Primary Care. *Medical Care* 39(8), 772-784.

Cogbill, E., Dinson, K., and Duthie, E. . (2010). Considerations in Prescribing Medication to the Elderly. In V. Hirth, D. Wieland, and M. Dever-Bumba. (Ed.), Case-based geriatrics: A global approach. New York: McGraw-Hill.

Dahlin, E., Neely, A. S., Larsson, A., Backman, L., and Nyberg, L. (2008). Transfer of learning after updating training mediated by the striatum. *Science*, 320(5882), 1510-1512.

Dickerson, F., Brown, C. H., Fang, L., Goldberg, R. W., Kreyenbuhl, J., Wohlheiter, K., and Dixon, L. (2008). Quality of life in individuals with serious mental illness and type 2 Diabetes. *Psychosomatics*, 49(2).

DiMatteo, M. R., Lepper, H. S., and Croghan, T. W. . (2000). Depression is a risk factor for noncompliance with medical treatment: Meta-analysis of the effects of anxiety and depression on patient adherence. *Archives of Internal Medicine*, 160(14).

Druss, B. G., Marcus, S. C., Olfson, M., and Pincus, H. A. (2002). The most expensive medical conditions in America. *Health Affairs* (Millwood), 21(4).

Eaton, W. W., and Muntaner, C. (1999). Socioeconomic stratification and mental disorder. In A. V. Horowitz, and Scheid, T. L. (Ed.), A handbook for the study of mental health: Social contexts, theories, and systems (pp. 259-283). Cambridge: Cambridge University Press.

Egede, L. E. (2007). Major depression in individuals with chronic medical disorders: Prevalence, correlates and association with health resource utilization, lost productivity and functional disability. *General Hospital Psychiatry*, 29(5).

Erickson, K. I., and Kramer, A. F. (2009). Aerobic exercise effects on cognitive and neural plasticity in older adults. *British Journal of Sports Medicine*, 43, 22-24.

Foundation, R. W. J. (2011). Mental disorders and medical comorbidity: Emory University.

Freedman, V. A., Martin, L. G., and Schoeni, R. F. (2004). Disability in America. *Population Bulletin*, 59, 1-32.

Gawande, A. (2011). Medical report: The hot spotters-Can we lower medical costs by giving the neediest patients better care? [Electronic Version]. New Yorker. Retrieved January 24, 2011.

Gruenewald, T. L., Seeman, T. E., Karlamangla, A. S., and Sarkisian, C. A. (2009). Allostatic load and frailty in older adults. *Journal of American Geriatric Society*, 57(1525-1531).

Gudex, C., and Lafortune, G. (2000). An inventory of health and disability-related surveys in OECD countries. OECD Labour Market and Social Policy Occasional Papers No. 44.

Haber, D. (2010). Health promotion and aging: Practical applications for health professional. (5th ed.). New York: Springer.

Haber, D., Logan, W., and Schumacher, S. (2011). Health promotion and disease prevention. In V. Hirth, D. Wieland, and M. Dever-Bumba. (Ed.), Case-based geriatrics: A global approach. New York: McGraw-Hill.

Harman, J. S., Edlund, M. J., Fortney, J. C., and Kallas, H. (2005). The influence of comorbid chronic medical conditions on the adequacy of depression care for older Americans. *Journal of the American Geriatrics Society*, 53(12), 2178-2183.

Harper, S., and Lynch, J. (2007). Trends in socioeconomic inequalities in adult health behaviors among U. S. sates, 1990-2004. *Public Health Reports*, 112(2).

Hepburn, K. W., Lewis, M., Sherman, C. W., and Tornatore, J. . (2003). The Savvy Caregiver Program: Developing and testing a transportable dementia family caregiver training program. *The Gerontologist*, 43(6), 908-915.

Hoffman, C., Rice, D., and Sung, H. Y. (1996). Persons with chronic conditions: Their prevalence and costs. *Journal of the American Medical Association*, 276(18).

Hurwicz, M. L., and Tumosa, N. (2011). Cultural competence in geriatric care. In V. Hirth, D. Wieland, and M. Dever-Bumba. (Ed.), Case-based geriatrics: A global approach. New York: McGraw-Hill.

Hyer, L., Dhabliwala, J., and Salvatierra, J. (2011). CogMed for Older Adults: Update on Program. Paper presented at the The 22nd Annual Southeastern Regional Student Mentoring Conference in Gerontology and Geriatrics, Tybee Island, GA.

Hyer, L., Scott, C., and Islom, F. (2011). Effects of a Holistic Memory Clinic for Older Adults. Paper presented at the The 22nd Annual Southeastern Regional Student Mentoring Conference in Gerontology and Geriatrics, Tybee Island, GA.

Jaeckles, N. (2009). Early DIAMOND adopters offer insights. *Minnesota Physician*.

Katon, W. J. (2003). Clinical and health services relationships between major depression, depressive symptoms, and general medical illness. *Biological Psychiatry*, 54(3).

Katsnelson, A. (2010). No gain from brain training. *Nature*, 464(22), 1111.

Kessler, C., W. T., Demler, O., and Walters, E. E. (2005). Prevalence, severity, and comorbidity of 12-month DSM-IV disorders in the national comorbidity survey replication. *Archives of General Psychiatry*, 62(6).

Kessler, R. C., Berglund, P., Chiu, W. T., Demler, O., Heeringa, S., Hiripi, E., Jin, R., Pennell, B. E., Walters, E. E., Zaslavsky, A., Zheng, H. (2004). The US National Comorbidity Survey Replication (NCS-R): Design and field procedures. *International Journal of Methods in Psychiatric Research,* 13(2).

Kessler, R. C., Heeringa, S., Lakoma, M. D., Petukhova, M., Rupp, A. E., Schoenbaum, M., Wang, P. S., Zaslavsky, A. M. (2008). Individual and societal effects of mental disorders on earnings in the United States: Results from the National Comorbidity Survey Replication. *American Journal of Psychiatry*, 165(6).

Kiosses, D. N., Teri, L., Velligan, D. I., and Alexopoulos, G. S. (2010). A home-delivered intervention for depressed, cognitively impaired, disabled elders. *International Journal of Geriatric Psychiatry*, 26(3), 256-262.

Koltai, D. C., Welsh-Bohmer, K. A., and Schmechel, D. E. (2001). Influence of anosognosia on treatment outcome among dementia patients. *Neuropsychological Rehabilitation: An International Journal*, 11(3 and 4), 455-475.

Kroenke, K., Spitzer, R. L., Williams, J. B. W., Monahan, P. O., and Lowe, B. (2007). Anxiety disorders in primary care: Prevalence, impairment, comorbidity, and detection. *Annals of Internal Medicine*, 146(5), 317-325.

Kronick, R. G., Bella, M., Gilmer, T. P. (2009). The faces of Medicaid III: Refining the portrait of people with multiple chronic conditions: Center for Health Care Strategies, Inc.

Lahey, B. B. (2009). Public health significance of neuroticism. *American Psychologist*, 64(4), 241-256.

Lantz, P. M., House, J. S., Lepkowski, J. M., Williams, D. R., Mero, R. P., Chen, J. M. (1998). Socioeconomic factors, health behaviors, and mortality: Results from a nationally representative study of US adults. *Journal of the American Medical Association*, 279(21).

Leatherman, S., Berwick, D., Iles, D., Lewin, L. S., Davidoff, F., Nolan, T., and Bisognano, M. (2003). The business case for quality: Case studies and an analysis. *Health Affairs*, 22(2).

LeCouteur, D. G., and Sinclair, D. A. (2010). A blueprint for developing therapeutic approaches that increase healthspan and delay death. *The Journals of Gerontology Series A: Biological Sciences and Medical Sciences,* 65A(7), 693-694.

Lemieux-Charles, L., and McGuire, W. . (2006). What do we know about health care team effectiveness: A review of literature. *Medical Care Research and Review*, 63(3), 1-38.

Lorant, V., Deliege, D., Eaton, W., Robert, A., Philippot, P., Ansseau, M. (2003). Socioeconomic inequalities in depression: A meta-analysis. *American Journal of Epidemiology*, 157(2).

Lorig, K. R., and Holman, H. (2003). Self-management education: History, definition, outcomes, and mechanisms. *Annals of Behavioral Medicine*, 26(1).

Mauskopf, J. A., Sullivan, S. D., Annemans, L., Caro, J., Mullins, C. D., Nujiten, M., Orlewska, E., Watkins, J., and Trueman, P. (2007). Principles of good practice for budget impact analysis: Report of the ISPOR task force on good research practices--Budget impact analysis. Value in Health, 10(5).

Mayr, U. (2008). Introduction to the special section on cognitive plasticity in the aging mind. *Psychology and Aging*, 23(4), 681-683.

Medicare screenings, vaccines underused. (2002). American Medical News, 7.

Melek, S., and Norris, D. (2008). Chronic conditions and comorbid psychological disorders. Seattle: Milliman.

Meyer, G. J., Finn, S. E., Eyde, L. D., Kay, G. G., Moreland, K. L., Dies, R. R., Eisman, E. J., Kubiszyn, T. W., and Read, G. M. (2001). Psychological testing and psychological assessment: A review of evidence and issues. *American Psychologist*, 56(2), 128-165.

Moniz-Cook, E., Agar, S., Gibson, G., Win, T., and Wang, M. (1998). A preliminary study of the effects of early intervention with people with dementia and their families in a memory clinic. *Aging and Mental Health*, 2(3), 199-211.

Neumann, P. J. (2007). Budget impact analyses get some respect. *Value in Health*, 10(5).

Quality, A. f. H. R. a. (2008). National healthcare quality report (No. 09-0001). Rockville, MD.

Quayhagen, M. P., and Quayhagen, M. (1989). Differential effects of family-based strategies on Alzheimer's Disease. *The Gerontologist*, 29(2), 150-155.

Quayhagen, M. P., Quayhagen, M., Corbeil, R. R., Roth, P. A., and Rodgers, J. A. (1995). A dyadic remediation program for care recipients with dementia. *Nursing Research*, 44(3).

Salthouse, T. A. (2001). Structural models of the relations between age and measures of cognitive functioning. *Intelligence*, 29(93-115).

Schoenbaum, M., Unutzer, J., Sherbourne, C., Duan, N., Rubenstein, L. V., Miranda, J., Meredith, L. S., Carney, M. F., and Wells, K. (2001). Cost-effectiveness of practice-initiated quality improvement for depression: Results of a randomized controlled trial. *Journal of the American Medical Association*, 286(11).

Schulz, R., and Martire, L. M. (2004). Family caregiving of persons with dementia: Prevalence, health effects, and support strategies. *American Journal of Geriatric Psychiatry,* 12(3), 240-249.

Sheehan, D., Robertson, L., and Ormond, T. . (2007). Comparison of Language Used and Patterns of Communication in Interprofessional and Multidisciplinary Teams. *Journal of Interprofessional Care*, 21(1), 17-30.

Sheehan D., R. L., and Ormond T. . (2007). Comparison of Language Used and Patterns of Communication in Interprofessional and Multidisciplinary Teams. *Journal of Interprofessional Care*, 21(1), 17-30.

Sinoff, G., and Werner, P. (2003). Anxiety disorder and accompanying subjective memory loss in the elderly as a predictor of future cognitive decline. *International Journal of Geriatric Psychiatry*, 18(10), 951-959.

Smits, F., Smits, N., Schoevers, R., Deeg, D., Beekman, A., and Cuijpers, P. (2008). An epidemiological approach to depression prevention in old age. *American Journal of Geriatric Psychiatry*, 16(6), 444-453.

Statistics, B. o. L. Age of reference person: Average annual expenditures and characteristics. Consumer Expenditure Survery, 2004., 2009, from http://www.bls.gov/cex/2004/Standard/age.pdf

Stein, M. B., Cox, B. J., Afifi, T. O., Belik, S. L., and Sareen, J. (2006). Does co-morbid depressive illness magnify the impact of chronic physical illness? A population-based perspective. *Psychological Medicine*, 36(5).

Steiner, B. D., Denham, A. C., Ashkin, E., Newton, W. P., Wroth, W. P., and Dobson, L. A. (2008). Community care of North Carolina: Improving care through community health networks. *Annals of Family Medicine*, 6(4).

Stine-Morrow, E. A. L., Parisi, J. M.*, Morrow, D. G., and Park, D. C. . (2008). The effects of an engaged lifestyle on cognitive vitality: A field experiment. . *Psychology and Aging*, 23, 778-786.

Unutzer, J., Katon, W. J., Callahan, C. M., Williams, J. W., Hunkeler, E., Harpole, L., Hoffing, M., Della Penna, R. D., Noel, P. H., Lin, E. H. B., Arean, P. A., Hegel, M. T., Tang, L., Belin, T. R., Oishi, S., and Langston, C. . (2002). Collaborative care management of late-life depression in the primary care setting: A randomized controlled trial. *Journal of the American Medical Association*, 288, 2836-2845.

Unutzer, J., Katon, W. J., Fan, M. Y., Schoenbaum, M. C., Lin, E. H., Della Penna, R. D., and Powers, D. (2008). Long-term effects of a collaborative care for late-life depression. *American Journal of Managed Care*, 14(2).

Unutzer, J., Katon, W., Sullivan, M., and Miranda, J. (1999). Treating depressed older adults in primary care: Narrowing the gap between efficacy and effectiveness. *Milbank Quarterly*, 77(2), 225-256.

Unverzagt, F. W., Kasten, L., Johnson, K. E., Rebok, G. W., Marsiske, M., Koepke, K. M., Elias, J. W., Morris, J. N., Willis, S. L., Ball, K., Rexroth, D. F., Smith, D. M., Wolinsky, F. D., and Tennstedt, S. L. (2007). Effect of memory impairment on training outcomes in ACTIVE. *Journal of the International Neuropsychological Society*, 13(6), 953-960.

Von Korff, M., Katon, W., Bush, T., Lin, E. H. B., Simon, G. E., Saunders, K., Ludman, E., Walker, E., and Unutzer, J. (1998). Treatment costs, cost offset, and cost-effectiveness of collaborative management of depression. *Psychosomatic Medicine*, 60(2).

Wilhide, S., and Henderson, T. (2006). Coomunity care of North Carolina: A provider-led strategy for delivering cost-effective primary care to Medicaid beneficiaries. Washington: American Academy of Family Physicians.

Willis, S. L., Tennstedt, S. L., Marsiske, M., Ball, K., Elias, J., Koepke, K. M., Morris, J. N., Rebok, G. W., Unverzagt, F. W., Stoddard, A. M., and Wright, E. (2006). Long-term effects of cognitive training on everyday functional outcomes in older adults. *Journal of the American Medical Association*, 296(23), 2805-2814.

Zarit, S. H., Femia, E. E., Watson, J., Rice-Oeschger, L., and Kakos, B. (2004). Memory club: A group intervention for people with early-stage dementia and their care partners. *The Gerontologist*, 44(2), 262-269.

In: Toward Healthcare Resource Stewardship   ISBN: 978-1-62100-182-9
Editors: J.S.Robinson, M.S.Walid and A.C.M.Barth   © 2012 Nova Science Publishers, Inc.

Chapter 15

HOSPITAL COSTS AND THE EMERGENCY DEPARTMENT

Ulf Martin Schilling[1,2,*]

[1]Department of accidents and emergencies,
Linköpings University Hospital and IKE, Linköping, Sweden
[2]Department of Clinical and Experimental Medicine,
Faculty of Health Sciences, Linköping University, Linköping, Sweden

ABSTRACT

All over the world, hospital costs are increasing. In many hospitals, the emergency department is one of the major cost-factors due to the high number of patients attended and the volume of investigations and the required staffing. In our hospital, it is the department accounting for the highest laboratory and radiology costs but even serves the highest number of patients.

This chapter gives an overview over cost distribution at the emergency department and different approaches to reduce expenditures for emergency work-flow and procedures from a Swedish perspective. The impact of the introduction of specialized emergency physicians, point-of-care analysis, revised working time models and several studies of physician's knowledge and behaviour as well as the impact of hospital flow and bottlenecks are presented and discussed in the chapter.

INTRODUCTION

All over the world, hospital costs are increasing. The actual part of the gross domestic product spent on health has risen to 15.7% in the US (2007) and is still rising [1].

At the same time the availability of health care is highly dependent upon local economic factors and reflects directly in mortality and morbidity rates even in privileged regions as urban environments of the developed world. Rapid urbanization with insufficient

---

* E-mail: mschillingdeu@netscape.net.

infrastructure, poverty and overcrowding of slum-alike environments result in poor health and an increased risk for the transmission of contagious disease. At the same time, health problems are a major direct cause of poverty [2, 3]. Poverty and disease are found in countries under ongoing industrialization and urbanization as well as in industrialized countries, but in the latter there is the advantage of a generally better availability of basic infrastructure and emergency health care.

In emergency care, one must be careful to directly compare emergency departments between different countries or even within the same district. Emergency care can be defined by the provider as found in the medical dictionaries, or by the attending patient. As stated in Wikipedia: "Emergency medical services (abbreviated to the initialism "EMS" in some countries) are type of emergency service dedicated to providing out-of-hospital acute medical care and/or transport to definitive care, to patients with illnesses and injuries which the patient, or the medical practitioner, believes constitutes a medical emergency." As a result, all patients can define themselves as suffering an emergency, even if not considered so by the medical provider.

Not only will this fact result in conflicts regarding emergency investigation and therapy between providers and non-emergent patients, but depending on local jurisdiction and the extend of personal liability medically doubtful or unnecessary investigation will be performed due to safety reasons and to avoid malpractice-claims. Alternatively, patients will be unnecessarily admitted to the hospital for security reasons if beds are available.

In many medical systems even non-emergent patients cannot be rejected by the emergency department due to legal issues. Furthermore, the distinction between emergent and non-emergent problem often cannot be made but after emergent conditions have been ruled out on a clinical basis or by relying on further diagnostic modalities as the patients' symptoms can be similar for emergent life-threatening and non-emergent disease.

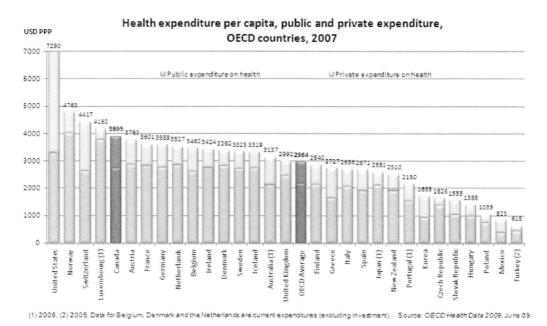

Figure 1. Health expenditure per capita, OECD countries, 2007 (OECD Health Data 2009).

Basic health care is seen as a gate-keeper in many health care systems, mainly taking care of non-emergent problems and referring emergencies and special problems to the emergency department or respective specialties. However, basic health care will reflect local economy even if founded by the government. As a result of poor local economy and a resulting reduced availability of basic health care, emergency health care is sought as an alternate way into the health care system. Depending on local circumstances, this results in a high percentage of total hospital expenditures spent on emergency care for even non-emergent problems. This invariably results in a major use of resources by the emergency department for the diagnosis and treatment of medically non-emergent conditions on cost of higher specialized services in the hospitals budget.

This results in the paradox that hospitals in economic poor districts usually find themselves with a low funding but a high medical demand and a chronically overcrowded emergency department (ED) draining the economic resources for more specialized departments, whilst well-funded hospitals in rich districts have a good funding and a moderate demand of emergency service, but well equipped specialized departments and research facilities. As a direct result, emergency care in poor districts will be able to provide limited service only to the individual patient.

COST DISTRIBUTION AT THE EMERGENCY DEPARTMENT

Emergency care is defined by demand and acuity. The demand of emergency care is heavily dependent on local circumstances, but in general it can be defined as unlimited due to the constant need of emergent assessment of both "real" medical emergencies and patients presenting with "emergent" symptoms. On the other hand, all emergency departments are attended by numbers of acutely ill patients in critical conditions, which are in need of urgent medical help which sometimes requires a high standard of knowledge, but most of all staff-intensive care. Due to this fact, emergency departments need a high amount of staffing all times of the day. Even if adopting working times to the patient's flow for improved use of personnel resources there must be staff available for immediate surges due to minor accidents with increased numbers of casualties or mass-casualty incidents.

As the number of patients attending the emergency department is high, numbers of laboratory and radiological investigations will be performed. A huge amount of basic care material is required for emergency patients, and emergency departments require a lot of space to permit an adequate work-flow, protection of the patient's integrity and protection against contagious disease. Decontamination units are often connected to the emergency department, and cleansing and disinfection must be conducted regularly and often to prevent nosocomial infection. Security must be provided all times of the day. Used by a high number of patients with a fast turnover, material at the emergency department will wear out rapidly both in the waiting area and in the emergency rooms, resulting in elevated material costs compared to the "ordinary" medical ward.

At our emergency department, approximately 40.000 patients are cared for every year. The total budget for our ED is 25.200.000 US$. 133 employees are involved in taking care of these. 33 physicians, 40 nurses, 20 nurse-aides, 30 secretaries and 10 administrative staff are currently employed at our ED. Statistically, each employee takes care of 300.75 patients per year on 200 legal working days, i.e. 1.5 patients per day. Statistics however does not show reality as each patient is treated by at least one physician, one nurse and often a nurse-aid, whilst secretaries and administrative staff are occupied with administrative services mainly. Cost for staffing thus can be split into administrative costs and costs for medical personal. Recalculating by occupation workload is 1.212 patients per physician, 1.000 per nurse, 2.000 per nurse-aid per year. Wages, taxes and social security for each physician is approximately 160.000 US$, for each nurse approximately 80.000 US$, each nurse-aid approximately 67.500 US$, each secretary 67.500 US$ and each administrative personal 80.000 US$, resulting in a total of 12.655.000 US$ total staffing costs divided into 2.825.000 US$ administration and 9.830.000 US$ medical service (22.3% administration and 77.7% medical staff). Calculated on each single patient, this results in a staffing cost of 316,375 US$ on each visit.

Reimbursement in the Swedish emergency department is heavily regulated. Essentially, the health care system is governmental, and delegated from the central government to the county council Landsting. The county council provides the fixed budget for general medical service, a budget which in turn is split between the parts of the county and on the sublevel in the several institutions, which in turn split the remaining budget between the different departments and health-care providers. A minority of the budget is provided by the central government indirectly through the participation in the centrally funded university education for medical staff. Private funding is negligible in our health care system.

Patients pay for the majority of health costs by taxes, but have to pay a 16.67 US$ on each visit with a maximum of 150 US$/year without further costs on diagnostic procedures but they are charged for medication bought at the pharmacy up to 500 US$/year. Health care for children is free of charge. All patient fees are redistributed to the county council, so that the department cannot calculate with possible revenues from patient-fees.

The reimbursement for the different departments is decided by the institution depending on the departments specialty, number of beds, number of patients, availability and procedures performed and partly by the DRG as by ICD10, resulting in a complex calculation for the distribution of the fixed budget. In summary, each department has to rely on the budget provided to maintain its production, with very limited possibilities to increase its revenues.

As costs are increasing due to inflation, increases in wages and the technical progress in medicine (including the introduction of new, more efficient drugs and the application of new international guidelines), the different departments at the hospital are forced to reduce costs as they can. One very common way to try to reduce costs is to reduce hospital and departmental capacity, by reducing several hospital beds within the same department at a single time. This way, complete teams of physicians, nurses and nurse-aides can be laid off, and as fewer patients can be taken care of actual costs do decline. Unfortunately, as demand by emergency patients is increasing due to the aging population this strategy inevitably results in a reduction of accessibility for non-emergent patients, resulting in long time waiting for non-urgent procedures and an increased rate of complications due to the delay. In the Swedish system, patients submitted to such a delay can demand to be treated elsewhere, mostly in the limited Swedish private sector on the respective departments' costs - and cannot be refused to do so. This way, costs effectively do increase instead as the department has to pay for the emergent patient, the non-urgent patient treated elsewhere and yet is expected to take care of eventual complications resulting from the therapy performed external.

Another method to reduce costs without getting charged for negligence is by "outsourcing" investigations and patients to other departments, so that only the "right" patients with a confirmed diagnosis and mandatory treatment are accepted to the specialized ward. In essence, both strategies result in an increased number of patients attending the ED for non-emergent problems to reduce the waiting time, to treat any occurring complication due to delayed therapy or to treat complications arising from therapy performed elsewhere. Furthermore, the latter strategy mandates that patients are nearby completely evaluated and investigated at the ED and in primary care before being accepted for further treatment. In this context it is essential to know that the ED is the only department of the hospital that legally is not allowed to refuse a patient. As a result, physicians at the ED are forced to perform investigations not essentially mandatory for ED therapy or decision, to be able to help the patient to get further care. This in turn results in an increased waiting time at the ED and increased ED overcrowding.

When the surgical department at our hospital tried to implement the strategy of accepting patients after the majority of diagnostic procedures was performed at the ED to find the "right" patients, admission rate to the surgical department fell from 34.75% to 30.66% with a constant number of patients attending for surgical problems. Laboratory and radiological costs, however, increased by 16.04 and 23.84%, totalling an increase of 18.99% in costs per patient at the emergency department, and an increase of 11% in the number of radiological investigations (analysed 1931 patients june-juli 2007 compared to 1892 patients june-july 2008). In total figures, direct costs increased by 47 US$/patient at the ED (totaling +88924 US$), whilst 91 patients less were admitted to the surgical ward (977,18US$ in costs for the ED per admission avoided to the surgical department). This strategy might seem to be cost neutral for the total of the hospital (a day at the surgical ward costing approximately 850-950 US$ depending on the patients needs), but not for each single department involved.

OVERCROWDING

Overcrowding at the ED is a common problem. However, the term overcrowding still is discussed in the scientific community and definitions of overcrowding vary. Some common definitions of overcrowding at the ED include an increase in waiting and processing time, a lack of ED bed/room-capacity during prolonged periods of the day, a general perception of being rushed by physicians and nursing staff and diversion of ambulances as well as an increased numbers of patients leaving the ED without being seen by a doctor [4]. Essentially, it might be defined as an extreme volume of patients in ED treatment areas, forcing the ED to operate beyond its capacity. [5] Factors contributing to overcrowding are increased demand due to reduced availability in primary care (increased inflow), high number of complex patients (processing shortage), lack of nursing staff (processing shortage) and lack of hospital beds or hospital capacity (outflow obstruction). As overcrowding is difficult defined with a multitude of local definitions existing, the cost of overcrowding is difficult to determine.

Krochmal et al analysed the cost of overcrowding as soon as 1994 showing that patients remaining at the ED due to outflow obstruction had a 12% increased time of hospitalisation later on, resulting in concomitant increase in the total cost of care. [6]

As 25% of all admitted patients were subjected to a delay of more than 24 hours, it can be calculated on an overall admission rate of 30% that the costs at the ED will increase by at least 2160 US$/patient (1.5 US$/minute), and that on 100 patients/day the cost for the ED will increase by 16.200 US$ (7.5x2160 US$) due to waiting time alone – not counting the increased costs for further therapy at the ED and at the hospital ward. The indirect costs due to reduced quality of care, increased risk for malpractice, resulting liability issues and loss of highly educated staff (i.e. human resources) at the ED are difficult to calculate, especially as there are extremely few scientific studies regarding this issue.

Furthermore, overcrowding impacts on surge-capacity, the capacity needed to deal immediately with increased ED-demand in cases of major incidents with multiple patients arriving within a short period of time. This is a major problem in the US as well as in the rest of the world, notably in Sweden, the country with the lowest number of hospital beds per inhabitant in the industrialised world. [7, 8]

In the struggle to reduce overcrowding, several strategies have been investigated. Ambulance and patient diversion was shown not to be cost-efficient due to the loss in revenue, the loss of time due to connected administration and general patient dissatisfaction. Repeated public education revealed to be beneficial to avoid non-emergent patients at the ED as shown in Singapore. In the same setting, the introduction of fees for ED-attendance showed to reduce the number in non-emergent patients when the fees exceeded the fees for primary care visits. [9, 10]

Fast-track admission is under current investigation in several settings and has yet to show its cost-effciency. Specialised nurses might be an option as shown in a study from the Netherlands, in which the diagnosis and therapy of ankle-strains was compared between specialised nurses and house officers, showing no significant difference in costs between both groups but a reduced total waiting time and an increased patient satisfaction in patients treated by the specialised nurse. [11, 12]

EMERGENCY PHYSICIANS

The training of subspecialiced emergency physicians was started in Sweden in 2006 and the subspecialty was acknowledged as late as 2008 by the Swedish Board of health. At the current date, only a minority of Swedish ED's are staffed by emergency physicians [13]

Theoretically, emergency physicians are cheaper compared to subspecialised physicians as the latter is highly competent in taking care of a subset of patients, but often limited in other patients. A general surgeon, for example, is certainly qualified to care about any surgical patient attending the ED, but might have limitations when patients with stroke or acute myocardial infarction, atrial fibrillation or diabetic complications have to be attended. As the final diagnoses and problems patients are attending for can vary highly, ED's have to staff multiple specialties at all times, which generates costs. Furthermore, as patients symptoms can be caused by different pathologies which might be medical, surgical or other, cross-referral at the ED will invariably happen and result in increased waiting time, overcrowding, an increase in diagnostic procedures and finally in increased costs. Elderly patients with diffuse symptoms, patients with epigastric pain without evident or multiple minor injuries after falls are prone to be referred between different specialties when attending a hospital.

With the introduction of emergency physicians competent of taking care of the majority of patients non-regarding the final diagnosis and distribution as medical/surgical/other, and the flexibility to "swab" between patients of different specialties, this obstacle might be reduced resulting in a possible reduction in staffing and reduced time a patient attends at the ED.

However, the introduction of new specialties and subspecialties tends to be regarded with caution, as it has to be assured that the quality of care provided by the physicians is at least comparable to the quality provided at the actual level. To find out if our emergency physicians did provide the appropriate level of care, we conducted a cohort study. The introduction of the specialty was assumed to result in improved diagnostic security, improved quality of care and a reduction in ED costs. At the current date, studies still are going on to show if these aims could be fulfilled. It has been shown that the introduction of attending emergency physicians reduces the number of liability claims to the ED, and that the number of reimbursements declined significantly when ED-physicians were introduced in the US-setting [13]. In a single-center study at our university hospital, we compared the performance of emergency physicians in compparison with internal medicine physicians.

Background

Detecting the emergency of non-fulminant pulmonary embolism (PE) still is one of the major problems presenting to the emergency physician. Signs and symptoms of PE most often are discrete and non-specific. Non-invasive investigation and laboratory parameters can be misleading, and the final diagnosis often is stated by radiologic investigation. To help physicians to suspect PE several scoring systems have been developed. In Sweden, the use of the Wells score is emphasized by the national board of health.

Emergency medicine in Sweden still is a developing field of medicine and was recognized as late as 2008 as a subspecialty. Thus, most of the emergency physicians working at the emergency department still are residents under continuous education and the guards are shared by emergency physicians and physicians otherwise working at the different wards.

Objective

Due to their specialisation in the field of emergency medicine, it could be suspected that emergency physicians might be better in detecting the otherwise discrete findings of pulmonary embolism in emergency patients. To confirm this hypothesis, a single centre retrospective cohort-study was performed.

Methods

During the three-month periods (march till may) 2007 and 2008 the findings in all patients undergoing pulmonary CT-angiography at the emergency department of our university hospital were reviewed. The investigations were attributed to emergency physician (EP) or internal medicine physician (IP). Both negative and positive findings were evaluated, and the number of medical patients treated by the respective group were calculated according to the computerized triage system as each emergency physician signs for the patient he is treating. Statistical analysis was performed by the Students-T-test, and probability levels of 5% were accepted as significant.

Results

During march till may 2007, a total of 2847 patients attended for medical problems, 576 of which were treated by EP (20.23%). The rest of the patients (79.77%) were treated by IP. In march till may 2008, 2408 patients searched for medical problems and 625 (25.95%) were attended by EP. During this period, EP ordered a total of 34 pulmonary CT in 2007 and 35 in 2008. 17.64% (2007) and 22.86% (2008) of these resulted in confirmation of the diagnosis of pulmonary embolism. IP ordered a 77 (2007) and 64 (2008) pulmonary CT during this period, resulting in 12.98% (2007) and 10.93% (2008) of positive findings, respectively. Calculating these numbers on the total of patients attended by the different groups, EP ordered pulmonary CT for 5.9% (2007) resp. 5.6% (2008) of their patients, whilst IP performed CT-scans in 3.39% (2007) resp. 3.59% (2008) of their patients (p=0.0108). This means, that EP have a higher index of suspicion for the diagnosis of PE in the context of the emergency department (1.74 (2007) resp 1.56 (2008) vs 1.0 for the IP).

For the total of patients attended at the emergency department, this resulted in positive findings for pulmonary CT in 1.04% (2007) and 1.28% (2008) for the EP, and in 0.43% (2007) and 0.39% (2008) for the IP (p<0.01). This means that EP are more accurate in detecting PE in the context of the emergency department.

Thus, the odds-ratio to have a positive finding on a pulmonary CT by an EP compared to an IP was 2.43 (2007) resp 3.26 (2008).

The total percentage of positive findings for the hospital including the emergency department was 14.29% (2007) and 14.15% (2008) on a total of 259 resp 212 CT-scans, and excluding the emergency department 14.19% (2007) and 13.27% (2008) on 148 resp 113 CT-scans. No significant difference could be found between the positive findings for all the hospital compared to the EP (p=0.38) or IP (p=0.27).

Conclusion

Emergency physicians seem to have a higher index of suspicion for PE than internal medicine physicians and are more accurate in detecting PE at the emergency department. Compared with the total of our university hospital, emergency physicians are at least comparable in diagnosing PE.

However, does this mean that emergency physicians are more cost-efficient at the ED than other specialised physicians? Even if they might be better in detecting subtle signs of PE, they do warrant a higher amount of investigations and thus higher actual costs with a rising total. On the other hand, the use of emergency physicians might be beneficial as a lower number of physicians might be needed. In our ED we were able to reduce the number of physicians from 4 to 3 at night shift hours (i.e. a decrease of 25%) when emergency physicians are on duty keeping patient flow unimpaired.

POINT OF CARE ANALYSIS

Point of care analysis (POCA) has been integrated at ED workflow during recent years. POCA refers to analysis which is fast, easy and bedside. Both blod-sample and other specimens as well as apparative diagnosis can be regarded as POCA. Under this point of view, the stethoscope, the thermometer and the ECG must be regarded to rank among the eldest POCA systems. Currently, the most interesting POCA at the ED are laboratory analysis including breath analysis and ultrasound imaging.

POCA can be cost efficient, even if the costs for single blood tests might be higher than analysis at the central laboratory. Three aspects are of major concern when questioning the cost efficiency of POCA: Can the faster test-result enhance caretaking both in quality and speed? Is the test result reliable? Which are the overall costs of testing for POCA compared to central analysis?

In the US, it is warranted that the test result for emergency laboratory investigation should be available within 30 minutes. If this can be achieved, the need for further even faster investigation is limited from the clinical point of view. In this case, only in urgent emergencies as for example major trauma or bleeding, acute myocardial infarction or stroke the need for POCA is evident as therapy might be influenced by the test results and as speed is mandatory. In other countries as Sweden, there is no such governmental regulation. Thus, time for test results may vary significantly. We conducted a study comparing the actual time from the taking of a blood sample until the available result between the POCA iStat™ (Abbot) and the local central laboratory for the tests of arterial blood gas (CG4+), extended electrolyte status (Chem8+) and troponin TnI in 40 patients. The study revealed that in our setting a potential 48.5 minutes per patient could be saved by using the available POCA when all tests were conducted (48.5±28.7). On a total of 40.000 patients this would be 32333 hours per year. Even if the potential saving in time could be achieved in as much as 10% only, a reduction of 3233 working hours/year would result in substantial economic saving.

In direct comparison, the different tests modalities performed with a good correlation.

This led us to the question: Beside the potential indirect impact on costs, how would a direct impact of the use of POCA be on the local budget? To answer this question, we directly compared the offer from the manufacturer for all necessary equipment based on the calculation of 25000 tests per year with the actual prices as offered by our central laboratory for the same analysis. Our results revealed the potential of a saving of approximately 70 US$/patient in direct laboratory costs by POCA. However, it must be considered that local circumstances, prices and need of testing might result in completely different figures in your clinical setting.

If calculating the costs for staffing from another point of view each minute of staffing the ED will costs 24.08 US$ if assuming that staffing is distributed evenly over the year. 40.000 patients per year means that statistically, every 13.14 minutes a new patient will arrive at the ED. With an average stay of 3.5 hours (210 minutes) there will be constantly 16 patients at the emergency department, at a staffing cost of 1.5 US$/patient/minute, i.e. . By reducing the waiting time, more patients could be attended decreasing relative staffing costs, alternatively staffing could be reduced. In the study above, we could show a potential reduction of up to 32333 hours/year (1939980 minutes), which would translate into 2.909.700 US$ in indirect savings beside the potential 2.800.000 US$ savings due to analysis by POCA on 40.000 patients.

RADIOLOGY

A high number of patients at the ED will undergo radiologic diagnosis, in our setting as many as 65.24% of all attending patients (study sample 4996 unselected patients june/july 2008). Depending on local circumstances, radiology can be performed in the emergency room directly on the patients' bed, or in the radiology department. In our ED, investigations are performed at the radiology department. Thus, each patient investigated has to be transferred to radiology from the ED. Due to the high number of procedures, waiting time for these patients will invariably increase as the overcrowding at the ED results in overcrowding at the radiology department. Calculating that each minute of waiting time costs 1.5 US$/patient/minute, and that there is a 26.097 radiologic investigations will be performed on 40.000 patients, a median 15 minutes delay in radiology costs 587.174,34 US$ per year. Even here, POCA might prove beneficial if further radiology investigation can be avoided. The available POCA beside integrated X-ray systems is ultrasound, a bedside diagnostic system increasingly used in the ED. A selection of with ultrasound detectable pathology is listed in table 1. [14-20]

All these pathologies can be detected by experienced physicians at the ED within a few minutes (the transcranial protocol, one of the longest emergency ultrasound protocols, takes 15 minutes in total) with a reasonable level of security and a high sensitivity and specificity. By rendering further radiological investigation unnecessary, ultrasound as been proven to be cost-efficient. Beside the direct savings due to avoidance of further redundant investigation and by focusing further diagnostic procedures, indirect savings occur due to decreased waiting time and reduced overcrowding at the ED.

SCHEDULES

Staffing at the ED always is difficult, as workload is unplanned. However, local statistics will tell when the normal patient-flow is as highest and as lowest, and calculations can be based on that. Still, there has to be a certain level of overstaffing for immediate response to major incidents or catastrophes.

Historically, our ED was staffed with 6 physicians daytime (8-20) and 4 physicians nighttime (20-08). Three of these physicians were responsible for several wards during nighttime beside the actual ED. Patient inflow, however, had its peak around lunch and was constant until approximately 11pm, to gradually decline on the majority of days. As a result of inequal patient inflow and thus delays in processing the patients, waiting times started to rise around 1 pm to increase until 11pm, before gradually declining. A peak in waiting time could be seen around 4pm when physicians changed shifts. After the introduction of emergency physicians bound to the ED (before run by physicians from different departments put on the shift in a rotation system), approaches were started to decrease waiting time by staffing accordingly to patient inflow.

Table 1. Pathologies detectable by emergency ultrasound [14-20]

Cardiac arrest	Deep vein thrombosis
Asystole	Lokal infection
Tamponade	Abscess
Hypovolemia	Foreign body
Pulmonary embolism	Asthma/COPD
Pneumothorax	Pleural effusion
Pneumonia	Stroke
Pulmonary oedema	Carotid dissection
Major trauma	Testicular trauma
– Assessment of the Basic Haemodynamic State	Pregnancy viability assessment
	Foreign body detection
– Review response to haemodynamic interventions	Assessment for raised intracranial pressure
Focussed Assessment with Sonography for Trauma (FAST)	Vascular injury
– Haemoperitoneum	– Pseudoaneurysm
– Haemopericardium	– Arteriovenous fistula
Extended FAST (EFAST)	– Perivascular haematoma
– Pneumothorax	– Thrombosis
– Haemothorax	– Dissection
Intravascular filling status	
– Inferior vena cava size and respiratory variation	Procedural guidance
	– Intubation confirmation and endotracheal tube placement
Regional trauma	– Nerve blocks for analgesia
Cardiac and Thoracic aortic injury (trans-thoracic and trans-oesophageal echocardiography)	– Intercostal/paravertebral blocks for rib fractures
– Blunt myocardial injury	– Limbs blocks for limb trauma
– Penetrating cardiac injury	– Guide for compartment pressure monitors
– Traumatic aortic injury	– Vascular access
Fractures	– Central and peripheral venous
– Sternal fractures	– Arterial
– Rib fractures	– Foreign body removal
– Other fractures and dislocations	– Paracentesis/Intercostal
Soft-tissue injury	
– Muscle and tendon injuries	
Ocular trauma	
– Intra-ocular foreign bodies	
– Posterior ocular assessment in the presence of hyphaema or major periorbital haematoma	

As a first step, staffing was increased during the period between 10 am and 6 pm to meet the increased demand during this time of the day by shifting working hours for one of the physicians. In a next step, another sift was introduced between 6 pm and 2 am to increase the patient flow, so that the ED should not be overcrowded at 2 am. To keep these positions economically balanced, staffing was reduced between 2 am and 8 am. (Physicians local union tariffs include a 100% bonus during these hours, i.e. working time is paid as 200% of the ordinary wage). With ED-physicians covering all shifts, further savings might be possible.

SAVING COSTS

Introduction

Generally, cost awareness defined as the knowledge of costs for investigations and treatments is prioritized different among physicians in different health systems. During medical education in Germany, Spain, France and Sweden the author was confronted mostly to the medical aspects and not to the costs of diagnosis and therapy. In direct conference with colleagues our emergency department it seemed that a majority of the doctors was poorly informed about costs.

To get a general opinion about the awareness of Swedish physicians regarding the costs for a single examination we asked the doctors on call in internal medicine at the emergency department of our university hospital to anonymously estimate the cost of several investigations used in the diagnostic strategies to exclude pulmonary embolism (PE). We assumed that the awareness of costs for apparative investigations would correlate with the level of experience due to extended responsibilities among registrars and consultants.

Methods

30 doctors "on call" in internal medicine at emergency department of the university hospital of Linköping were enrolled by an anonymized questionnaire. Rank and experience of the physician and the estimated cost of the most common investigations in PE were recollected. The data were evaluated in relation to the physicians' experience divided into the groups less than 5 years (junior grade <5, JG5, n=11), 5 till 9 years (junior grade 5-9, JG9, n=10) and more than 9 years (senior grade, SG, n=9). Statistical analysis was performed by using the Student's T-Test, Kruskal-Wallis test and Pearsons correlations quotient as applicable. An correlation/probability of $p \leq 0,05$ was accepted as significant.

Estimated prices were compared to the costs 2007 as provided by the laboratory, radiology and department of clinical physiology of Linköpings university hospital accepting a 25% difference between estimated and real cost as described elsewhere [21, 22]. To allow a standardized approach the mean of the different charges for any investigation was accepted as the overall prize.

Results

Mean experience was 7.7 years varying between 2 months and 27 years of practice for the total of physicians, 2,15±1,4 years for the JG5, 6,9±1,6 years for the JG9 and 14,6±5,6 years for the SG. The difference in years of experience between each group was significant (p<0,01).

Mean accuracy was 27% for the JG5, 25% for the JG9 and 33% for the SG without any significant difference between the groups. No correlation could be shown between the knowledge about the cost of the items asked and the physicians' experience in years. (figure 2)

Mean deviation was ranged an average of 52% for the total of modalities. A general tendency to underestimation (53% vs. 16% overestimation) was observed. Junior doctors tended to underestimate costs, whilst senior doctors estimated more balanced. (JG5 60%, JG9 63%, SG 33%, p≤0,01). One physician estimated costs within the accepted margins for 5 of 6 items whilst 6 physicians did not estimate the cost of any item correctly.

Discussion

An average 28% of the estimations ranked within ±25% of the real costs for the total of investigations. This can be compared to the results published by Ryan et al [21, 22]. No statistical difference between the groups of junior and senior physicians could be shown. These results are similar to the international studies performed in the England, Scotland, Italy, Spain and Canada [21, 22, 23, 24, 25, 26, 27]. The cost-awareness had to be considered as generally low.

Younger doctors seem to underestimate the costs of investigation, which is in line with the results of a Canadian study [24]. Underestimation of prices has been connected to increased ordering of apparative and laboratory investigation [28].

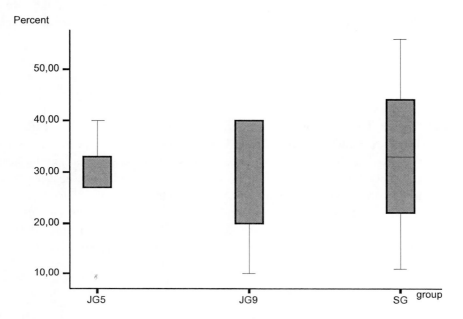

Figure 2. Percentage of deviation from the real costs in the group of physicians with less than 5 years experience (JG5), 5 to 9 years experience (JG9) and more than 10 years of experience (SG). No significant difference between the groups could be detected.

It has been shown that younger doctors are prone to order higher numbers of avoidable laboratory and radiological investigations than more experienced physicians [29]. Multiple reasons as missing experience, liability issues and diagnostic insecurity, as well as missing cost- awareness might contribute to the more expensive practice of junior physicians. In the stressful environment of the emergency department it might be more comfortable to confirm or exclude a diagnosis by radiology or laboratory analysis instead of asking for second opinion by senior physician, especially if the senior physicians are physically elsewhere at the hospital.

To cut costs, cost-awareness of health care providers is crucial as resources are limited. Cost awareness of all the staff involved has been shown to result in increasing economic efficiency in the clinical context [30]. The availability of price-lists for example has been featured as a helpful visual tool in improving the cost-awareness in the clinical milieu by Snyder-Ramos et al [30].

Conclusion

The results of our study showed that there is a generally low cost-awareness among the doctors working in the Swedish emergency department. No differences regarding knowledge of costs could be detected between inexperienced and experienced doctors. Further education of the doctors to increase their knowledge about the costs of the tests performed might be necessary. [31]

In the study above it was shown that physicians working at the Swedish emergency department often are unaware of the real costs for analyses and investigations performed. In a following study, the possible impact of price-lists as visual instruments on the overall laboratory and radiology costs at the emergency department of Linköpings university hospital (LUH) was evaluated [32]

Introduction

In the study above it was shown that physicians working at the Swedish emergency department (ED) often are unaware of the real costs for analyses and investigations performed [31]. With exploding costs in healthcare, programs to increase cost-awareness among health care personal are incited. Several approaches have been tested to increase cost-awareness among medical health care providers and to reduce costs, including the introduction of strict protocols, daily information about the costs of some of the most common tests and the use of price lists both experimentally and as a practical approach [30, 33-35]. In this study, the impact of price-lists on the overall laboratory and radiology costs at the internal medicine part of the ED of Linköpings university hospital (LUH) was evaluated.

Methods

Price lists including the 91 most common laboratory analyses and the 39 most common radiological investigations performed at the emergency department of LUH were created. The lists were distributed by the medical head of the ED to all physicians performing on-call duty in internal medicine through the hospitals internal email-provider in april 2008 and continuously exposed at the medical working stations at the ED. The study was performed among medical doctors at the ED blinded towards the follow-up of the intervention. The orthopaedic colleagues were considered as control group and were not informed about the price lists nor had direct access to them.

The mean costs for laboratory and radiologic investigations for all patients considered to be medical and orthopaedic during the months of june and july 2007 (control period) and 2008 (test period) were calculated. Neither clinical nor admission procedures were changed during this period. No further intervention aiming to reduce costs was performed at the same time. No pressure was exerted on the medical staff regarding the use of the lists or the reduction of costs. Statistical analysis was performed using the Student's T-test.

Results

A total of 1442 orthopaedic and 1585 medical patients were attended to during june and july 2007. In june and july 2008, 1467 orthopaedic and 1637 medical patients required emergency service (an increase of 1,7% of orthopaedic and 3,3% of medical patients).

No significant difference between the number of patients in 2007 and in 2008 could be detected.

The mean costs per patient were 163 US$ for orthopaedic and 180.16 US$ for medical patients in 2007, and in 2008 166.5 US$ (+1,95%, p+0,45) and 146.16 US$ (-18,8%, p=0,07) respectively.

In orthopaedic patients, laboratory costs decreased by 9% (p=0,2) whilst the costs for radiological examination increased by 5,4% (p=0,4). In medical patients, the costs for laboratory analysis decreased by 21,4% (p=0,12) and for radiological examination by 20,59% (p=0,04).

The total number of radiological investigations decreased by 4,6% in orthopaedic (p=0,29) and by 6,8% in medical patients (p=0,17).

Discussion

Increasing costs and limited budgets are major issues in public health. Cost-awareness and cost-effectiveness are demanded by insurance companies and hospital administrations. During medical education, these aspects of the physicians often are neglected. [31]

Several approaches to increase cost-awareness among medical staff have been studied. Concise information about prices by repeated direct information or commonly accessible price lists showed to be valuable tools in increasing cost awareness among physicians and in reducing costs for the single patient. [30, 33, 34]

Price lists are relatively easy to create, cheap and reliable. Widespread distribution can be performed by the use of information systems such as the email-provider applied in this study Total material costs in our study were less than 16 US$. A continuous exposure of the price lists at the working stations was easily achieved.

By this single intervention, the costs for medical patients could be significantly reduced in our setting. Costs for the control group remained stable during the same period.

For the ED's economy, 46.150,50 US$ (16.15%) could be saved on medical patients within a two months period even during a 3,3% increase in total patient numbers, with an 8.265,50 US$ (3.5%) increase in costs for orthopaedic patients.

In a 12-months-period a 266.000 US$ could be saved on testing for internal medical patients by this method, with remaining potential for savings on orthopaedic or surgical patients.

Conclusion

Price lists are an effectiv tool to increase cost awareness at the emergency department. The use of price-lists resulted in a significant decrease in investigation costs. Further work has to be done to guarantee that the possible savings are not made on cost of the medical quality for the patient's therapy.

However, even as the introduction of price lists seemed to influence the costs at the emergency department positively, the acceptance at the emergency department was uncertain. To find out how the lists were regarded by our physicians, we performed another study. [36]

Background

In a recent study, it was shown that cost-awareness among physicians working at the Swedish emergency is very low non-regarding the level of experience of the physicians. [31] In another study, it could be shown that price lists provided at the emergency department effectively can reduce the number and costs of both laboratory and radiological investigations ordered. [32]

However, cost-cutting projects can result in irritation among physicians feeling themselves to be forced to implement cost-cutting in their daily work and might be considered to be both annoying and unnecessary. To get further understanding of physicians view towards price-lists in their daily work and as a general cost-cutting tool we performed an study at among physicians involved in taking care of patients attending the emergency department of a university hospital were asked about their views towards the available price-lists as a tool for their daily work and in cost-cutting.

Methods

An anonymized questionnaire was distributed among the physicians working in internal medicine in a Swedish university hospital. All physicians were invited to participate. The data asked for were the level of qualification of the physician (consultant, specialist, senior house officer/registrar (SHO) and junior house officer (JHO)), if the physicians regarded price lists as a usable tool in their daily work (positive/negative) and if they assumed that knowledge about the costs for investigations would have an impact on the total expenses for investigations performed at the clinic. The questionnaires were recollected by the hospitals internal mail. Statistical analysis was performed using the unpaired Student's T-test, accepting p-levels <0.05 as significant.

Results

A total of 27 questionnaires were recollected by our method. Four consultants, 3 specialists, 16 SHOs and 4 JHOs chose to participate in the study.

4 of 4 consultants (100%), 2 of 3 specialists (66.67%), 12 of 16 SHO (75%) and 4 of 4 JHO (100%) considered price-lists to have an impact on the costs for clinical investigations (p<0.01). 3 of 4 consultants (75%), 2 of 3 specialists (66.67%), 11 of 16 SHO (68.75%) and 4 of 4 JHO (100%) regarded price lists as a useful tool in their daily work (p=0.051).

Conclusion

Medical doctors at our hospital involved in the caretaking of emergency patients regard price-lists as a possibly useful tool in their daily work, and do consider readily available price-lists to have a major impact on cost-cutting. Interestingly, no difference could be seen between the most junior and the most senior doctors participating in this study regarding their positive attitude towards such lists.

With the knowledge of doctors being positively inclined towards price lists, which in turn resulted in major cost-cutting, the next step was to see how long the impact of a single intervention would last to give us the opportunity to repeat the intervention in optimal intervals. [37]

Background

Having shown that readily available price lists do have a positive impact on the cost-development at the emergency department, it was of further interest to reveal how long the effect of a single intervention might last. Earlier studies showed that the effect of price lists might decline during the following periode, however, no clear schedule for this process could be shown. Other studies showed that continuous education about costs might be beneficial for the cost-development in ward units.

In this study, we evaluated the declining performance of price lists distributed at a single time point in the context of the emergency department to find the optimum schedule for recurrent intervention.

Methods

Price lists including the 91 most common laboratory analyses and the 39 most common radiological investigations performed at the emergency department of LUH were created by using the information provided by the radiology department and the clinical chemistry department of the hospital. Different modalities (capillary vs. venous blood samples) were listed separately. The lists were distributed to all physicians on-call in internal medicin by the internal email-provider in april 2008. Further lists were exposed above the working stations at the ED continually until September 2008. The mean costs for radiologic investigations for all medical and orthopaedic patients during the months of june and july 2007 as a baseline and on a monthly base from june 2008 till mars 2009, the percentage of radiological investigations on the total of patients for the respective line and the percentage of admission of patients were calculated. Neither clinical nor admission procedures were changed during the period investigated. The physicians were blinded towards the study. Statistical analysis was performed on a bimonthly base using the Student's T-test. Probability levels <0.01 were accepted as significant.

Results

A total of 1442 orthopaedic and 1585 medical patients were attended to during june and july 2007. Between june 2008 and mars 2009, 7987 orthopaedic and 9302 medical patients were attended at our emergency department. The costs for medical patients for radiological examination started to climb in December 2008, (8 months after the intervention, +16%) resulting in a significant increase in february 2009 (10 months after the intervention, +48%, $p<0.001$), whilst the radiological costs for orthopaedic patients slightly increased in December (+13%, $p=0,1$) to stabilize afterwards. Admission rates for medical patients did not differ significantly during the period investigated, whilst a decrease in admission rates for orthopaedic patients could be observed ($p<0,01$). No significant difference in the rate of radiological investigations could be found for each line even if a 10% increase in both lines could be observed.

Conclusion

Price lists are an effective tool to reduce costs at the context of the emergency department. The effect of single interventions declined after 8 months, which is concordant with the existing literature. A repetition of interventions by price lists after a period of 6 to 8 months might be appropriate to conserve the cost-reducing effect of price-lists.

After conducting these studies, we introduced a new system of triage in our emergency department in which a routine pattern of blood samples was taken directly on arrival at the ED. We evaluated the effect of this intervention by following the cost development for laboratory analysis. [38]

Background

The triage system METTS has been shown to be a triage-system reducing mortality at the emergency department. It was stated that point-of-care-analysis of standardized laboratory samples in triage systems could reduce the costs for single patients. In this single centre study, we controlled if the costs for single patients at the emergency department could be reduced by standardized sampling according to METTS without point-of-care analysis.

Methods

The system was introduced as the triage system at our university hospital. The triage followed a standardized system following a user's guide, and standardized laboratory sample packages were created and taken accordingly. In contrast to the original concept using point-of-care-analysis, the samples were sent to the hospitals central laboratory.

The total costs for laboratory analysis during a three months period after the introduction of METTS at our emergency department were compared to their historical controls. The number of patients attended and the total costs for laboratory analysis were calculated according to the hospitals computerized attendance and accounting systems. Statistical analysis was performed using the unpaired two-tailed Student's T-test.

Results

A total of 9000 patients were attended from December 2008 to februari 2009 (period 1) and 8553 patients from December 2009 to februari 2010 (period 2, p = 0.39). Total costs for laboratory analysis was 439.3 ± 53 TSKR in period 1 and 670 ± 21.6 TSKR in period 2 (p = 0.0089). Mean laboratory costs per patient were 145.67 ± 7 SKR in period 1 and 235.33 ± 5 SKR (p < 0.001) in period 2, i.e. +61.55%.

Conclusion

The introduction of standardized laboratory analysis using the hospitals central laboratory instead of point-of-care-systems results in significant increase of costs. Economically, the use of standardized sampling coupled to primary triage without point-of-care-analysis should be discouraged.

CHANGING APPROACHES

A part of patients visiting the emergency department will do so due to general malaise, failing social systems and problems within the organisation of primary care, i.e. institutional and administrative reasons. Most of these patients will be geriatric patients which are at risk to stay a significantly longer time at the ED compared to younger counterparts, increase overcrowding and undergo highly expensive investigation.. Due to major cuts in the geriatric department, with concurrent impact on the flow of geriatric patients, a specialised geriatric team was introduced in the ED. In this team, a geriatric physician, geriatric nurses, paramedics (physiotherapists) with tight contact to primary care, advanced mobile care and community services work together. The team cares about elderly and multimorbide patients attending the ED, with special focus on recurrent attendees and patients attending for unspecified problems or general malaise and general weakness. The team is available 8 hours/day during working days, i.e. 40 hours a week. During the period from November 2009 until januari 2011 the team attended 754 patients with a median age of 85 years, of which 279 (37%) were admitted to the hospital. In a comparable university hospital (Lund, Sweden) admission rate for similar patients is around 90%. Internationally, patients at this age stay between 7 and 15 days at the hospital. [39, 40, 41]

Thus, the team could avoid 400 admissions (53%) which would have given between 2800 and 6000 days of hospitalisation. At a cost of 400 US$/day of geriatric hospitalisation the team could save between 1.120.000 and 2.400.000 US$ or 1485.41 US$ - 3183.03 US$/patient.

CONCLUSION

In conclusion, the emergency department usually is one of the biggest cost factors in hospitals. High patient turnover, unplannable patterns of demand and the need of surge-capacity challenge the ED to keep a high level of staffing. Wages, radiology and laboratory costs consume the majority of the ED's resources. Patient flow is subjected to several bottlenecks as radiology, laboratory and administrative processes, mainly lack of beds and capacity. External factors including hospital politics influence the patients flow and thus te costs at the ED. By introducing cost-saving programs, flow-orientated schedules, specialised emergency physicians and by the consequent use of the possibilities offered by bedside analysis both as laboratory point of care analysis as radiological modalities as for example ultrasound expensive waiting time and concurrent overcrowding can be reduced.

REFERENCES

[1]   World health statistics 2010 p136.
[2]   Haan M, Kaplan GA, Camacho T: "Poverty and health prospective evidence from the alameda county study." *Am. J. Epidemiol.* (1987) 125 (6): 989-998).
[3]   Diez Roux AV,Luisa N Borrell LN, Haan M, Jackson SA, Schultz R: "Neighbourhood environments and mortality in an elderly cohort: results from the cardiovascular health study." *J. Epidemiol. Community Health* 2004;58:917-923 doi:10.1136/jech.2003. 019596.
[4]   Hwang U: "Care in the emergency department: How crowded is overcrowded?" *Acad. Emerg. Med.* 2004;11:1097-1101.
[5]   Cowan RM, Trzeciak S: "Clinical review: Emergency department overcrowding and the potential impact on the critically ill." *Crit. Care.* 2005; 9(3): 291–295.
[6]   Krochmal P, Riley TA. "Increased health care costs associated with ED overcrowding." *Am. J. Emerg. Med.* 1994 May;12(3):265-6.
[7]   Harris A, Sharma A. "Access block and overcrowding in emergency departments: an empirical analysis." *Emerg. Med. J.* 2010 Jul;27(7):508-11.

[8]   Cherry RA, Trainer M: "The Current Crisis in Emergency Care and the Impact on Disaster Preparedness". *BMC Emergency Medicine* 2008, 8:7 doi:10.1186/1471-227X-8-7.

[9]   Falvo T, Grove L, Stachura R, Zirkin W. „The financial impact of ambulance diversions and patient elopements." *Acad. Emerg. Med.* 2007 Jan;14(1):58-62.

[10] Anantharaman V: "Impact of health care system interventions on emergency department utilization and overcrowding in Singapore." *Int. J. Emerg. Med.* (2008) 1:11–20 DOI 10.1007/s12245-008-0004-8.

[11] Derksen RJ, Coupé VMH, van Tulder MW,Veenings B, Bakker FC: "Cost-effectiveness of the SEN-concept: Specialized Emergency Nurses (SEN) treating ankle/foot injuries." *BMC Musculoskeletal Disorders* 2007, 8:99 doi:10.1186/1471-2474-8-99.

[12] Carter AJ, Chochinov AH. "A systematic review of the impact of nurse practitioners on cost, quality of care, satisfaction and wait times in the emergency department." *CJEM.* 2007 Jul;9(4):286-95.

[13] Press S, Russell SA, Cantor JC, Jerez E. Attending physician coverage in a teaching hospital's emergency department: effect on malpractice. *J. Emerg. Med.* 1994 Jan-Feb;12(1):89-93.)

[14] James C.R. Rippey, Alistair G. Royse: "Ultrasound in trauma. Best Practice and Research." *Clinical Anaesthesiology* 23 (2009) 343–362

[15] Stengal D, Bauwens K, Sehouli J and Rademacher G. "Emergency Ultrasound-based algorithms for diagnosing blunt abdominal trauma." Cochrane Database of Systematic Reviews (Online) 2009; (1).

[16] Melniker LA, Leibner E, McKenney MG et al. "Randomized controlled clinical trial of point-of-care, limited ultrasonography for trauma in the emergency department: the first sonography outcomes assessment program trial." *Annals of Emergency Medicine* 2006 Sep; 48(3): 227–235.

[17] Beck-Razi N, Fischer D, Michaelson M et al. „The utility of focused assessment with sonography for trauma as a triage tool in multiple-casualty incidents during the second Lebanon war." *Journal of Ultrasound in Medicine* 2007 Sep; 26(9): 1149–1156

[18] Raoul Breitkreutz, Felix Walcher, Florian H. Seeger: "Focused echocardiographic evaluation in resuscitation management: Concept of an advanced life support–conformed algorithm." *Crit. Care Med.* 2007; 35[Suppl.]:S150–S161

[19] Korner M, Krotz MM, Degenhart C et al. „Current role of emergency US in patients with major trauma." *Radiographics* 2008 Jan–Feb; 28(1): 225–242.

[20] Daniel A. Lichtenstein, Gilbert A. Meziere: "Relevance of Lung Ultrasound in the Diagnosis of Acute Respiratory Failure* The BLUE Protocol." *CHEST* 2008; 134:117–125.

[21] Ryan M, Yule B, Bond C, Taylor RJ. "Knowledge of drug costs: a comparison of general practitioners in Scotland and England." *Br. J. Gen. Pract.* 1992;42: 6-9.

[22] Ryan M, Yule B, Bond C, Taylor RJ. "Scottish general practitioners' attitudes and knowledge in respect of prescribing costs. " *Br. Med. J.* 1990;300:1316-8.

[23] Robertson WO. "Costs of diagnostic tests: estimates by health professionals." *Med. Care,* 1981;18:556-9.

[24] Innes G, Grafstein E, McGrogan J. "Do emergency physicians know the costs of medical care?" *CJEM.* 2000;2(2):95-102.

[25] Conti G, Dell'Utri D, Pelaia P, Rosa G, Cogliati AA, Gasparetto A. "Do we know the costs of what we prescribe? A study on awareness of the cost of drugs and devices among ICU staff." *Intensive Care Med.* 1998;24(11):1194-8.

[26] Muñoz-Ramón JM, Espla AF. "Level of information on prices in an anesthesia department." *Rev. Esp. Anestesiol. Reanim.* 1995;42(3):103-6.

[27] Fowkes FG. "Doctors' knowledge of the costs of medical care." *Med. Educ.* 1985;19(2): 113-7.

[28] Long MJ, Cummings KM, Frisof KB. "The role of perceived price in physicians' demand for diagnostic tests." *Med. Care* 1983;21:243-50.

[29] Miyakis S, Karamanof G, Liontos M, Mountokalakis TD. "Factors contributing to inappropriate ordering of tests in an academic medical department and the effect of an educational feedback strategy." *Postgrad. Med. J.* 2006;82(974):823-9.

[30] Snyder-Ramos SA, Bauer M, Martin E, Motsch J, Bottiger BW. "Accessible price lists at the anaesthesiologist's workplace enhance cost consciousness as a part of process and cost optimization." *Anaesthesist.* 2003;52(2):154-61.

[31] Schilling UM:" Cost awareness among Swedish physicians working at the emergency department." *Eur. J. Emerg. Med.* 2009 Jun;16(3):131-4.

[32] Schilling UM."Cutting costs: the impact of price lists on the cost development at the emergency department."*Eur. J. Emerg. Med.* 2010 Dec;17(6):337-9.).

[33] Roberts DE, Bell DD, Ostryzniuk T, Dobson K, Oppenheimer L, Martens D, Honcharik N, Cramp H, Loewen E, Bodnar S, et al.: "Eliminating needless testing in intensive care--an information-based team management approach." *Crit. Care Med.* 1993 Oct;21(10):1452-8.

[34] Seguin P, Bleichner JP, Grolier J, Guillou YM, Mallédant Y: „Effects of price information on test ordering in an intensive care unit." *Intensive Care Med.* 2002 Mar; 28(3):332-5. Epub 2002 Feb 9.

[35] Cummings KM, Frisof KB, Long MJ, Hrynkiewich G.: "The effects of price information on physicians' test-ordering behavior. Ordering of diagnostic tests." *Med. Care.* 1982 Mar;20(3):293-301.

[36] Schilling UM: " The acceptance of price lists at the emergency department: how do doctors think about it?" *Scandinavian Journal of Trauma, Resuscitation and Emergency Medicine* 2010, 18(Suppl 1):P32.

[37] Schilling UM: "The duration of cost-cutting effects of price-lists" *Scand. J. Trauma Resusc. Emerg. Med.* 2010; 18(Suppl 1): P35 Published online 2010 September 17. doi: 10.1186/1757-7241-18-S1-P35.

[38] Schilling UM, Rönnersten A: "Laboratory sampling according to triage – how much does it cost?" *Scandinavian Journal of Trauma, Resuscitation and Emergency Medicine* 2010, 18(Suppl 1):P19.

[39] K. Vijaya, E. Ravi Kiran: "Profile of Geriatric in-Patient Admissions. *Journal of the Academy of Hospital Administration* Vol. 16, No. 2 (2004-07 - 2004-12).

[40] Van Staden AM, Weich DJV: "Profile of the geriatric patient hospitalised at Universitas Hospital, South Africa." *SA Fam. Pract.* 2007;49(2):14.

[41] Wong CH, Wang TL, Chang H, Lee YK: "Age-related emergency department utilization: A clue of patient demography in disaster medicine." *Ann. Disaster Med.* 2003;1:56-69).

In: Toward Healthcare Resource Stewardship   ISBN: 978-1-62100-182-9
Editors: J.S.Robinson, M.S.Walid and A.C.M.Barth   © 2012 Nova Science Publishers, Inc.

Chapter 16

LONG –TERM ECONOMIC ANALYSIS OF OUTPATIENT FOLLOW-UP

Fernando Alfageme Roldan[1,]* and *Almudena Bermejo Hernando[2]*

[1]Department of Dermatology,
Hospital Universitario Puerta de Hierro - Majadahonda, Madrid, Spain
[2]Applied Economy Department,
Universidad Autónoma de Madrid, Madrid, Spain

ABSTRACT

Background: In recent economic evaluation studies of long-term follow up of medical or surgical conditions, estimations are excessively simplified or mathematically inaccurate.

Objectives: To establish practical cost evaluation guidelines in the long term, clearly specifying type costs and to bring them from future to present in order to compare them with other interventions or studies.

Methods: Direct and indirect costs are independently analysed, accurately depicting the clinical protocol in each clinical scenario of follow-up or intervention .

Direct costs include clinical visit to department with differentiation between first and successive visits and if the patient is a child or an adult. This cost is mainly dependant on human resources in the department (doctors, nurses, assistants…) and should also include overhead costs shared with other departments.

Indirect costs, mainly including loss of productivity for the employer and salary for the worker and transport cost for the patient if adult or parents if the patient is a child must be specified. Retirement age should be also be taken into account.

Present estimation of future costs is a function of the increase of life cost (inflation-deflation) and life expectancy of the patients and affected by a discount rate that is conventionally determined.

---

* Correspondending Author: Dr. Fernando Alfageme Roldan. Dermatologia, Hospital Universitario Puerta de Hierro – Majadahonda, Manuel de Falla, 1. 28222 Majadahonda (Madrid), Spain. E-mail: feralfarol@yahoo.es.

Results: A simplified but accurate method of cost evaluation is possible in long term outpatients follow-up programmes

Conclusion: Use of this method can help in the homogenisation of cost evaluation studies of health programmes

1. Introduction - Theoretical Aspects in Economic Analysis

a. Necessity of Economic Analysis in Healthcare

In the last 20 years the interest in economic analysis of health programs has increased. Three apparent axiomatic paradoxes can be the reason of increased necessity of health analysis in developed countries. First, resources are scarce but healthcare requirements of the population are unlimited and increases with time and economic development. This dissonance generates the concept of cost/opportunity: Some necessities cannot be fulfilled on behalf of other necessities that population or their political representatives consider more important. Second, healthier population demands a higher number of health services. The reason of this contradiction may be that necessity does not usually correspond to demand in individual and population. Third, as technical refinement in healthcare delivery progresses, prices of these marginal refinements increase not proportionally to the differential advantage added.

Economic analysis aims to rationally help in the assignment of economical resources to health programs that usually are designed by health administrative professionals. Therefore it is a necessity of health professionals to understand the principles of economic analysis to communicate in a clear and common language with administrative staff assigning budgets.

b. Necessity of Long Term Follow-Up in Medicine

Follow-up in medicine can be considered as an expression of preventive medicine stemming from the idea that "to prevent is better than to cure" and in economic terms "to prevent is cheaper than to cure".

One aspect of preventive medicine is screening for disease in very early stages (secondary prevention) or for premorbid conditions depending on known risk factors (primary prevention). Tertiary prevention has to deal with established illness and how disability can be prevented. These forms of preventive medicine serve as tools in clinical follow-up.

Some aspects of follow-up are dependent on the risk of the disease as risk is distributed along the patient's life. If risk is continuous, uniform follow-up intervals should be taken into account (i.e. melanocytic nevi follow-up and melanoma). If the risk is increased in certain stages of life, or due to gender differences or family history (i.e. breast cancer), these situations should be screened more carefully (with more complementary tests) and more frequently.

The clinical scenario (hospital, primary care center) and the health personnel needed for each follow-up (nurse, primary care physician, and specialist) are different depending on the pathology and have different costs. These variables (time, age, sex, risk factors) make follow-up possible and is an obligation for the clinician or epidemiologist to establish clear risk profiles which will be the target population of a follow-up program and which intervals should be optimal from a clinical and economical point of view (efficiency).

In many occasions complementary tests are needed. Medical visits are not usually much time-consuming for most follow-up programs. However, costs are numerous and not always evident to the patient, health professional, manager, supervisor or politician. Therefore, preventive programs may be taken closer to the population at risk for easier accessibility (mammogram, buses; school, vaccination).

As follow-up programs are time- and money-consuming, not every possible follow-up program is materially possible and assignment of budgets for one or another program depends on how the clinical, epidemiologist or program responsible person must convince those making decisions though clear clinical and economical reasoning.

The economical principle behind preventive medicine and follow-up is investing money in health to avoid consequences (illness) that would have an economic impact on the patient and the whole society (indirect costs). As the productivity of this person is reduced it also has an impact on society productivity; and solidarity with this person is also a cost assumed by the whole community.

Although this idea is evident, health professionals and managers usually lose sight of it. From an economic point of view costs incurred by these programs should be less than the consequences of not following these patients. In costs, not only economic cost of productivity should be taken into account. Disease has an impact on suffering of the individual, his/her family, and the community in general. The moral consequences of disease, disability, and live years lost have a value that is difficult to calculate. "Difficult to calculate" does not mean "void of value".

Costs may be difficult to estimate. Costs of visits are "piled up" and costs change as money value changes with time.

c. Economic Analysis Types in Health Sciences

As previously stated economic analysis is a decision tool in the assignment of resources. If a decision is based in the cost or results of a treatment the decision would be a *partial analysis*. This is the most basic analysis type and should be avoided unless necessary. If a decision is based on the costs and results (efficiency) of *several alternatives* to control and minimize expenses to reach maximal health results then analysis is considered complete.

From the point of view of cost, four complete analysis models are classically described:

- *Cost minimization analysis:* Cost minimization analysis of several programs is complete only if effectiveness of the programs is equal.
- *Cost effectiveness analysis:* Evaluates comparatively in equality of costs maximal effectiveness of the programs analyzed.
- *Cost benefit analysis:* Evaluates cost and economic consequences (economic benefits/losses) of the compared programs.
- *Cost utility analysis:* Takes into account the ratio of cost of preferences of the subjects in the compared programs with respect to a health program. Utility is preference of a subject as regards his/her health status.

Although a really complete analysis should take into account all these aspects, primarily it should take into account the concrete current human (age, health status, epidemics, vaccinations …) and economical (economical superhabit, financial crisis …) factors at the time of decision making (utility, minimal costs, benefits, income ...).

With respect to the human factors, there is a possible ethical dilemma for health professionals. Commonly, medical ethics is usually *individual-based* "human life and health are invaluable, therefore costs do not matter".

Economists point of view also tends to be ethical but from a *populational point of view*, from the principle of justice for the whole population because ill-assigned resources to individuals have ill consequence to the whole population. This collective ethical point of view is sometimes conflictive with individual ethics. Those responsible for decision making in budget assignment have a responsibility in trying to make these apparent extremes compatible and functional.

Medical retribution has to be also taken into account as it has been suggested that health professionals on salary tend to diminish demand, a *per actum*.

d. Value and Validity of Health Economic Analysis - Homogeneity

From a practical point of view, at the beginning of an economic analysis two questions should be asked:

- Is the method methodologically appropriate? (internal validity).
- Is the method practically appropriate in the studied environment only? (external validity).

Once answered, analysis value and its usefulness is determined. The result of the analysis should be standardized and several guidelines have been published depending on the use of analysis (academic, political, media).

Homogeneity in health analysis is necessary due to three reasons:

1. It increases transparence in decision making as methods are understood by all evaluators.
2. Methodologically study comparison is possible and information is added to previous studies.
3. Quality of economic analysis is improved in each study as methodologically common pitfalls are solved in future similar studies.

2. PRACTICAL ASPECTS IN COST ANALYSIS

Once the type of analysis is chosen depending on the aforementioned factors the primary aim is determining cost, and even more important, which costs are relevant to our cost estimation.

A possible schema would be the following:

1. Identify direct costs attributable to the follow-up program (personal costs, drugs if necessary and complementary tests if needed).
2. Estimate the costs of other programs or services that collaborate in the development of the program (including administrative services).
3. Estimate overhead costs of the hospital per visit.

These aspects would correspond to the direct cost estimation (DC).

If indirect cost (IC) estimation is required or important in the program analysis, they should be also included and total cost (TC) of the program would be the sum of direct and indirect costs.

$$TC=DC+IC$$

With both cost sensibility analysis is required (see sensibility analysis section).

a. Direct Costs

Direct costs are mainly attributable to *personal costs* incurred in the process of the follow-up program. An easy and practical way of determining personal costs is estimating per hour cost of each professional category and approximate time per visit (distinguishing between first and consecutive visits as first visits are usually longer).

Follow-up programs usually need *complementary tests* (urinalysis, chest X-rays, etc.) that should also be taken into account as well as *drugs* prescribed in visits if necessary.

The costs of other services necessary for the development of the program should also be taken into account (eg. ophthalmologist if fundoscopy is needed) without forgetting the costs of administrative services. These costs are usually charged to the department by other services depending on the number of examinations/tests performed and are usually available in the department past budgets.

Structural or overhead costs are really difficult to estimate, but real bills are charged to the hospital for electricity, water, and landscaping. A method of calculating these overhead costs is assuming that each visit of each patient has the same overhead costs and adding these as a constant value per visit/patient. This constant can be estimated dividing costs charged to the outpatient area by the number of patients attended in the outpatient department of the hospital.

Other factors affecting overhead cost is capital cost that is the value of the building, equipment and terrain in which the program is established. As we can observe, structural costs can be infinite but the aforementioned components are a good approximation.

b. Indirect Costs

Indirect costs are usually not taken into account in regular analysis. In long term follow-up programs indirect costs may represent:

Transport costs: Depending on geographical dispersion and private or public transport this cost is relevant to both patients and society.

Cost of time lost due to follow-up: As time is spent on follow-up instead of working or leisure, this factor should also be taken into account. Working time is a good estimation of these costs and the mean salary per hour is available from the statistical bureaus of each country.

However, in the long term, health programs may collaborate to positive changes in work productivity as they are initially intended to improve workers' health. Koopmanchap (1995) has proposed frictional costs as the cost required to restore productivity due to a health program (the cost of replacing an absent worker). Positive changes are to be taken into account in the positive aspects of health follow-up programs which have an economic translation. These *changes of productivity* may be of help in demonstrating indirect economic benefits of a follow-up program.

Cost can be expressed as *mean costs* of follow-up per visit or patient dividing cost of visits or the whole follow-up cost by the number of patients. Another method of expressing costs is marginal cost that is the expenditure in follow-up needed to early detect or avoid incipient diseases.

Sometimes hospital administration estimates a mean cost per visit for all the programs running in an outpatient area. This can be useful when approximating a first schema of costs, but it is usually inaccurate and lacks factor analysis in evaluating costs.

3. TIME EFFECT IN COST ANALYSIS AND ITS ESTIMATION

What makes the difference between cost studies and long term analysis studies is time and how it influences costs. One of the most important consequences in health programs is creating a "healthy time" that has a value in itself for the patient and can be used in productive and leisure activities useful for the patient and society.

However, in the economy as in life there is a preference to receive this benefit sooner rather than later. Short term preference is the usual common preference as the future usually has an intrinsic uncertainty. This temporal preference is reinforced by the increase in life cost that is represented in the economy by the term inflation.

How can inflation affect the analysis of a long term follow-up program and how can we practically calculate it?

Generally, inflation is calculated in each country taking into account the increase of prices in a group of predetermined products considered as basic life necessities. This inflation can be expanded to all products and services as a way of homogenization. Another more complicated estimation would be making a predictive model for each item based on previous prices. This method, although more exact, requires a tedious mathematical calculation which may not be so necessary as many different costs tend to be homogeneous when considered together (what an economist calls "the law of large numbers").

If an inflation rate is assumed for all the items evaluated in the analysis we should take into account its variability with time (periods of inflation, deflation, recession). A median 10 or 20 year estimation would be suitable for most cases of unstable economies.

Together with inflation rate we have to take into account the fact that time makes money less valuable (money loses value over time). Intuitively, today's value of a dollar is much less than the value of a dollar 20 years ago. As long term analysis is usually based on cost nowadays, we should use a mathematical tool to calculate future costs from prices today. Economists name this concept *discount rate* and it is complementary to inflation and has a complex interaction with inflation (some authors estimate a common parameter to make calculations simpler).

The mathematical expression of this discount rate is:

$$P = \Sigma \, Fn \, (1+r)^{-n}$$

Fn: cost; n: years; r: discount rate

A 5% discount rate is regularly used by most health economists. However, each country usually has a discount rate for health analysis that usually is between 3% and 6%.

The decision to use both parameters in long term economic analysis or to use a combined estimator from both parameters or using one or none of them should be uniform for each cost component and should be stated in the methods section of any investigation and taken into account when comparing programs from a long term point of view.

4. ECONOMIC MODELS - MODELS OF LONG TERM COST ANALYSIS

Economic models are necessary in long term analysis as these studies are placed temporally in the future and uncertainty is a feature of the future. This is the main handicap of this kind of studies: the model should be approximate to a future reality and a future sequence of facts that we can predict, but in some cases we cannot.

However, going from the known to the unknown is an everyday reality in life and prediction models are essential in our lives to gain a certain grade of certainty about tomorrow, about what will happen in 5 or 10 years with the information available today. We are able to place ourselves in 10 years time at least in our imagination. This unconscious mechanism has to be put into numbers if we need prediction for future costs. The mathematical expression of these models is formulas and equations.

Models are as good and precise as the information used to build them. Interaction of variables and coefficients is complex and necessary if we want to use them to do the tedious task of constructing a model. Devoting time and resources to model creation is compulsory because when conducting calculations it is easy to make errors.

Information to build models usually comes from several published data sources that can be contradictory between themselves. As a result, homogenization effort is inevitable. This is the "Frankenstein monster" phenomenon (making a model from various publications and trying to make it work in a predictable way).

There are three main models:

Extrapolation models: These models allow future prediction from empirical variables extracted from known accessory studies.

Epidemiological models: These models take into account intermediate variables or midterm markers to reach final preditions (e.g. cardiovascular risk factors and myocardial infarction).

Markov Models: These are the most complex models as they assume several health statuses and the possibility of passing from one to the other depending on prevalence or incidence in a decision tree fashion analysis based on accessory publications.

The use of these models should fit the nature of the long term analysis project. If several health statuses are possible a Markov model would fit better. In binary states with very long term analysis without markers extrapolation models may be more suitable and in cases with known intermediate markers epidemiological models are preferred.

5. VALIDITY - SENSIBILITY ANALYSIS OF MODELS

Once we have designed our economic model, internal and external validity should be assessed. This "stress test" for our model consists of making variations in the parameters and checking which of them have more importance or if taken to extremes can cause our model to yield less results.

There are four sensibility analyses:

Univariate analysis: Each parameter is checked one by one, fixing the rest. It is of help if not much interaction between variables is expected.

Multivariate analysis: Multiple parameters are assessed and interactions between them are studied.

Scenario analysis: Some common clinical scenarios are assessed and checked with known results. This analysis has the advantage of determining external validity (i.e. value in application for other scenarios).

Threshold analysis: Critical threshold values (0 - infinite) are assessed for each parameter to check how it changes with respect to the rest of the variables.

Which analysis to use depends on the form of analysis and model assumed. "Trial and error" is usually the most used method in simple models, although multivariate analysis gives us more information about the concrete weakness and strength of our analysis model. Scenario analysis is a way of checking the values for analysis in other clinical settings. Threshold analysis delineates extreme limits for our model in which assumptions are not valid. So these analyses are not exclusive to a model, as each one provides us with concrete additional information.

CONCLUSION

There is a need for long term analysis of health programs as some pathologies require a long period of follow-up due to continuously present risks. Long term economical analysis should be an essential component in final decisions in health politics (local or general). The main aim of these models is making decision for those taking decisions clearer by highlighting economic aspects which sometimes only health administrative professionals know about. So it is necessary for health administrative professionals to use a systematic approach to the design of these kinds of programs and their economic impact.

The more complete and clear our analyses are the easier they are to interpret by managers and politicians. Making analysis homogeneous with other analyses gives our models the strength of the whole corpus of well designed analyses done by our predecessors. Transparence of our data and designs with their strengths and weaknesses makes our analysis valid for other scenarios and helps in improving modeling in follow-up studies.

Multiple deficiencies are still a matter of debate in these studies such as discount rate and its use, overhead costs and the difficulties in the calculation of other more subtle costs and how much would patients pay for them.

Follow-up economic analysis is increasing in importance and will probably be a standard requirement in future clinical program designs as we are increasingly conscious about the fact that resources are becoming scarce and good use of money is indispensable and an ethical obligation on health professionals, patients, and those assessing budget assignment altogether.

6. PRACTICAL EXAMPLE OF LONG TERM ANALYSIS

As an example of the concepts mentioned above, a practical case of long term analysis is presented. There is a controversy in the field of small/medium sized congenital melanocytic nevus (SMCMN), whether to excise them in children or apply long term follow-up for life. These options have different clinical implications and to date both are valid. Economic implications however have not be studied; therefore our group tried to make comparisons of both decisions to better assess the viability of the program of pediatric dermatologic surgery.

We retrospectively reviewed the medical records of children (aged 1–16) with a clinical diagnosis of SMCMN who underwent surgery between 2001 and 2007 under general anesthesia or local anesthesia with sedation. The data collected included patient characteristics, number of interventions, operating room time, recovery room time, day-hospital time and number of visits until definitive discharge. Costs of salaries, tests, consultations, and other overhead costs (OC) for 2006 were collected from our hospital's Internal Cost Control Department.

a. Cost Model for Surgical Interventions

Total costs (TC) were calculated by the sum of total direct costs (TDC; costs to the health system associated with the intervention) and total indirect costs (TIC; the opportunity costs related to the procedure for the patient's family).

TDC included personnel costs, laboratory and preoperative examination costs, and OC. Personnel costs were calculated per hour of working time of the health professionals attending the child and applied to the first visit, operating room, recovery room, day unit, and follow-up. Laboratory and preoperative examination costs were calculated for a standard preoperative examination (full blood count, basic biochemistry, coagulation) plus histopathology processing, reporting, and complementary tests if required.

Table 1. Costs

Cost Category	Cost, €
Direct	
Cost of visit to the pediatric dermatology unit	
First	121.09
Follow-up	72.65
General dermatology visit cost	
First	140.56
Follow-up	84.34
Pediatric anesthesia, preoperative visit	
First	157.75
Follow-up	94.65
Preoperative examination and histopathology	144.00
Operating room, cost per hour	198.91
Recovery room, cost per hour	155.36
Day hospital, cost per hour	40.75
Indirect	
Mean hourly salary costs, Madrid	21.40
Subway-bus combined ticket	1.00

OC were calculated using information from our hospital's Internal Cost Control Department on the costs of care of ambulatory surgery patients. These included functional costs related to activity (records, administration, stationery, materials), intermediate costs (charged by services other than the dermatology unit), and structural costs (building, repairs, electricity, security) for the period from 2004 to 2006. We assumed that pediatric ambulatory surgery would have the same OC as adult ambulatory surgery and divided the TC by the total number of patients undergoing surgery that year. Because the cost per patient was similar during the study period (Table 1), we calculated a median constant for OC, the OC constant per patient (*OCKpp*), which was added to each surgical intervention (91,465 ± 9,795).

TIC included transportation costs and working time costs. Transportation costs included a return ticket for both parents on the day of the operation and for the child if older than 4 years. The costs of the check-up visit included a return ticket for one parent and a child older than 4. Working time cost was assumed as a complete working day (8 hours) for both parents for days of surgical intervention and half a day (4 hours) for the parent for each check-up visit.

Working time cost was collected from the National Institute of Statistics and included the mean salary and social and health insurance in Madrid, irrelevant of sex or age.

Table 2. Overhead Costs

	2004	2005	2006
Overhead costs, €	81,717	79,222	100,585
Total surgical acts (children/total)	28/807	37/970	52/1,014
Overhead costs per patient, €	101.26	81.67	99.20

Table 3. Summary of Surgery Costs

Cost	€ Median ± Standard Deviation	Total Cohort n=105
Direct		
Personnel	667.38 ± 72.10	70,075.34
Laboratory and preoperative examination	142.12 ± 5.63	15,960
Overhead	91.47	9,603.83
Total direct costs	910.85 ± 155.01	95,639.16
Indirect		
Working days (8 hours)	3.53 ± 1.4	373.00
Tickets (single)	16.68 ± 3.3	1,752.00
Total indirect costs	593.88 ± 75.66	62,357.04
Total cost	1,504.73 ± 198.33	157,996.20

b. Cost Model for Long Term Follow-up

As in the previous model, TDC and TIC were taken into account. The TDC of lifelong follow-up were calculated taking into account the patient's age at diagnosis and sex, because this determines life expectancy (77 years for men and 84 for women, according to World Health Organization data for Spain), and differential costs in pediatric and adult dermatology (Table 2). The same working time costs and transport costs were taken into account to calculate TIC. These included half of a working day for one parent and for the child upon starting work (age 18) until retirement (age 65), and travel costs on public transport (1 return ticket for 1 parent and the child when older than 4 years, and only for the child when 18 years or older). Inflation and discount rates affected direct and indirect costs. A 3.5% median inflation rate for the last 10 years in Spain (National Institute of Statistics data) and a 6% discount rate (according to economic publications in Spain) were adopted for long-time estimation of correction factors.

A sensitivity analysis for follow-up intervals of 1, 2, 4, and 5 years was conducted to determine the follow-up cost that was most similar to surgical excision cost.

c. Total Costs of Surgical Intrvention

Between 2001 and 2007, a total of 113 children (53 boys and 60 girls) underwent surgery for CMN in our unit (105 single-step interventions and 8 multiple-step interventions). Mean age was 7.6 years. Mean surgery time was 49.2 ± 13.7 minutes in the operating room, 38.7 ± 27.8 minutes in the recovery room, and 137.0 ± 148.4 minutes in the day unit. A total of 221 check-up visits (excluding multiple-step interventions) were completed. The mean staff cost was 667.38 ± 72.10 per child. The mean laboratory and preoperative examination cost was 152 ± 5.63 per child. OC were assumed to be equal to *OCKpp*, as explained above. Total cohort and mean direct costs were 95,639.16 and 910.85 ± 155.01.

Parents missed 373 working days (mean 3.5 ± 1.4 days) and paid for 1,752 tickets (mean 16.7 ± 3.3 tickets). TIC was 62,357.04 for the cohort, with a median indirect cost of 593.88 ± 75.66 per child. The TDC and TIC for excision are summarized in Table 3.

d. Costs of Long Term Follow-Up

The annual, bi-annual, and 5-yearly TDC and TIC of lifelong follow-up with a discount rate of 6% and a median 3.5% inflation rate are shown in Figure 1 while Figure 2 shows the annual, biannual, 4-yearly, and 5-yearly mean lifelong follow-up costs.

Total and mean costs of lifelong follow-up every 4 years (156,679.63 and $1,482.66 \pm 34.98$) were similar to the total and mean costs of surgery (157,996.20 and $1,504.73 \pm 198.33$) in the sensitivity analysis. The follow-up periods used in the sensitivity analysis were different from those used for surgical costs (Table 4).

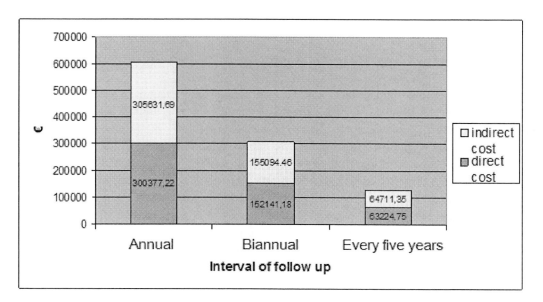

Figure 1. Cohort direct and indirect costs for the different follow-up intervals.

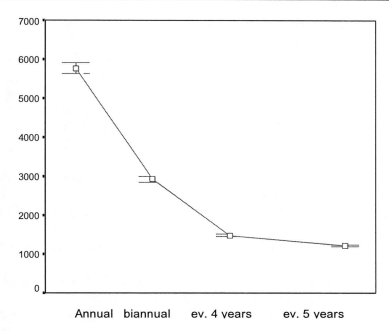

Figure 2. Median total costs for the different follow-up intervals.

Table 4. Sensitivity analysis (most similar cost in bold type)

Follow-up interval	Mean Total Costs, €	Total Cohort Costs, €
Annual	5,771.51±143.02	606,008.91
Biannual	2,926.05±71.89	307,235.64
Every 4 years	*1,482.66±34.98* (1,504.73±198.33)	*156,679.63* (157,996.20)
Every 5 years	1,218.44±28.78	127,936.10

REFERENCES

Brennan LJ, Prabhu AJ. Paediatric day-case anaesthesia. *BJA CEPD Rev.* 2003; 3: 134–9.

Briggs A, Sculpher M. Sensitivity analysis in economic evaluation: a review of published studies. *Health Economics* 1995;4:355-371.

Chouaid C. Markov models in clinical medicine. *Rev. Mal. Respir.* 2004;21:1007-9.

Drummond MF. Cost of illness studies: a major headache? *Pharmacoeconomics* 1992:2:1-4.

Drummond MF, O'Brien BO, Stodartf GL, Torrance GW. Methods for the Economic Analysis of Health Care Programmens, 2nd. Edition. New York: Oxford University Press, 1997.

Fenn P, McGuire A, Backhouse M et al. Modelling programme cost in economic analysis. *J. Health Economics* 1996:15:115-125.

Fishkin S, Litman RS. Current issues in pediatric ambulatory anesthesia. *Anesthesiol. Clin. North America.* 2003;21:305-11.

Folland S, Goodman AC, Stano M (1993): The Economics of Health and Health Care, Macmillan, Nueva York, Oxford.

García-Altés. Twenty years of health care economic analysis in Spain:are we doing well. En : Antoñanzas F, Fuster J, Castaño E (eds.) Avances en gestión sanitaria:implicaciones para la política las organizaciones sanitarias y la práctica clínica. Barcelona: Asociación de economía de la salud;2001.

http://www.oecd.org

Koopmanchap M, Rutten F, van Inveld B. The friction cost method for measuring indirect costs. *J. Health Econ.* 1995; 14: 171–189.

Liljas B. How to calculate indirect costs in economic evaluations. *Pharmacoeconomics* 1998;13:1-7.

López Casanovas G, Ortúm Rubio V (1998): Economía y salud: fundamentos y políticas", Encuentro, Madrid.

Luce BR, Elixhhauser A. Estimating costs in economic evaluation of medical technologies. *Int. J. Technology Assessment in Health Care* 1990;6:57-75.

Maarghob AA: Congenital melanocytic nevi: analysis and management. *Dermatol. Clin.* 2002 20:1-10.

McGuire A, Henderson J, Mooney G (1988): The economic of Health Care, Routledge, Londres y Nueva York.

Mejía, A.: Rev. Gerenc. Polit. Salud, Bogotá (Colombia), 7(15):91-113, junio-diciembre de 2008. "Evaluación Económica en salud: De la investigación a la toma de decisiones".

O'Brien BJ. Economic evaluation of pharmaceuticals: Frankenstein monster or vampire of trials? *Medical care* 1996;34 DS99-DS108 (Suplemento).

Ortún V (1990): La Economía en sanidad y medicina: instrumentos y limitaciones, Escola Universitaria de Trreball Social y La Llar del Llibre, Barcelona.

Phelps CE (1992): Health Economics, Harper Collings, Nueva York.

Rovira, Rev. Esp. Salud Pública 2004; 78; 293-295. "Modelos de Markov: Una herramienta útil para el análisis farmacoeconómico".

Rovira J, Antoñanzas F. Economic analysis of health technologies and programmes: a Spanish proposal for methodological standardization. *Pharmacoeconomics* 1995;8:245-252.

Rubio Terrés C. Introducción a la utilización de los modelos de Markov en el análisis farmaeconómico. *Farm. Hosp.* 2000; 24(4): 241-247.

Rubio TC, Echevarria A. Pharmaeconomics-Sapanish Research Articles . Vol 3, Suppl. 2: 71-78. "Modelos de Markov: Una herramienta útil para el análisis farmacoeconómico".

Sacristán JA, Ortún V, Rovira J, Prieto L, García-Alonso F. Evaluación económica en medicina. *Med. Clin.* (Barc) 2004;122(10);379-82.

Stigutz J. La economía del Sector Público. 2ª Edición.

Warner K, Hutton RC. Cost-benefit and cost effectiveness in health care: growth and composition of the literature. *Medical care* 1980;18:1069-1084.

Zwifel P, Breyer F (1997): Health Economics, Oxford University Press, Oxford.

In: Toward Healthcare Resource Stewardship   ISBN: 978-1-62100-182-9
Editors: J. S.Robinson, M. S.Walid et al.   © 2012 Nova Science Publishers, Inc.

Chapter 17

A REEMERGING BACTERIA: COST ANALYSIS OF CARE AND TREATMENT OF TUBERCULOSIS (TB) IN CHILDHOOD

Reka Bodnar,[1] Laszlo Kadar[2] and Agnes Meszaros[1]*

[1]Department of Pharmacy Administration,
Semmelweis University, Budapest, Hungary
[2] Pediatric Department, Pest County Pulmonological Institute,
Torokbalint, Hungary

INTRODUCTION

Epidemiology of Tuberculosis

According to a recent survey of the World Health Organization (WHO), 9.4 million new tuberculosis infections were recorded in the world in 2009. Of the 9.4 million incident cases 1.0-1.2 million (11-13%) were Human Immunodeficiency Virus (HIV)-seropositive. 1.3 million deaths in HIV-negative cases of tuberculosis (TB) were recorded in 2009 [1].

In 2009 there were 14 million prevalent cases of TB in the world, most of which occurred in Asia (55%) and Africa (30%). Fewer cases were recorded in the Eastern Mediterranean Region (7%), in the European Region (4%) and the Region of the Americas (3%).

In 2008 there were 440,000 cases of multidrug-resistant TB (MDR-TB) in the world [1].

In Europe, most of the cases occurred in Romania, Ukraine and Russia [2]. Hungary does not belong to the countries with high TB incidence. In 2009 the total number of new patients suffering from TB was 1448 (incidence: 14.4 per one-hundred-thousand), while the incidence of paediatric (children aged under 19 years old) TB infection was 3.7 per one-hundred-thousand [3] (Figure 1.).

The costs of diagnosis and treatment of the disease are significant due to the increasing number of cases with HIV co-infections, MDR-TB and the introduction of directly observed

---

* Corresponding Author: Reka Bodnar, Semmelweis Egyetem, Egyetemi Gyógyszerüg Gyógyszerügyi Szervezési Intézet 1092, Budapest, Hogyes E. u. 7-9. Hungary. E-mail: rekabodnar@freemail.hu.

therapy (DOT). Directly observed therapy means that the patients take medication under direct supervision by a health care worker.

Treatment of Tuberculosis

In Hungary, patients with drug-susceptible pulmonary TB are usually treated with isoniazid (INH), rifampicin (RMP), pyrazinamide and ethambutol for 2 months then the treatment continues with INH and RMP for 4 months. The total period of treatment of TB lasts for 6 months in Hungary. MDR-TB is defined as resistance at least to INH and RMP.

Patients are usually hospitalized at least until Acid Fast Bacillus (AFB) smear microscopy results became negative on 3 consecutive days being on adequate treatment.

Health Economic Analysis

Health economic analysis of TB can be aimed at different end-points. While the health economic studies in the developing countries focus on the cost-effectiveness of the treatment of different patient populations infected with TB, the health economic studies carried out in developed countries emphasize the cost-optimisation examinations [4-6].

Health economic analysis can be estimated according to the perspective of the health service providers or the patients. There are medical and non-medical expenses, and both with direct and indirect costs [7-10] (Table 1).

The calculation of indirect costs is complicated but important because time lost from work and early death have a significant influence on economy [11].

Table 1. Classification of type of costs

	Medical expenditures	Non-medical expenditures
Direct costs	• Medications	• Transportation
	• Hospital treatment, diagnostics, salary	• Sick pay
	• Public primary care unit	• Home care
	• Inpatient care, meal, heating and lighting charges	
Indirect costs	• Extra costs on account of won life years	• Time lost from work
		• Community loss by reason of early death

Health Economic Studies of TB in Developed Versus Developing Countries

The health economic analysis in developing countries approaches the cost of TB from a different perspective than in developed countries. Many studies examine the cost of TB from the patients' perspective because in these countries there is a significant economic burden on patients during the diagnosis and treatment of TB [12-14]. Another problem is that the availability of health care system is often limited for the patients. There are significant distances between the patients' address and the hospital, so the patients have to spend a huge amount of money on transport [12-14].

K. Floyd assessed the impact of economic studies on TB control during the period 1982-2002. The author analysed sixty-six cost-effectiveness studies and thirty-one cost studies in TB control topics. The most commonly examined topics in cost-effectiveness surveys were screening for active TB or infection with Mycobacterium tuberculosis and preventive therapy. For high-burden countries, the most frequently studied topics were the use of community-based care, the delivery of short-course chemotherapy and the comparison of short-course and standard chemotherapy. Cost studies mostly analysed the total or per patient diagnostic and treatment costs from the perspective of the patients, the health service providers and the hospitals. Investigations were carried out either in an area of a country or in the whole country. In high-burden countries, the costs incurred by patients were analysed the most frequently [15].

Suarez et al. created a cost-effectiveness analysis of second-line drug treatment for chronic TB patients in Peru between 1997 and 1999. Cost-effectiveness was assessed from the perspective of the public health sector in the year 2000 with prices in US $. The cost-effectiveness of three alternative strategies of treatment of MDR-TB was compared. The analysis focused on the increase in total costs and the effects associated with the use of second-line drugs. They found that the average cost per patients treated with second-line antituberculotics was US $ 2,381. Drugs, at US $ 824 per patient, were the greatest single cost item. Most of the money was spent on second-line drugs (35%), directly observed therapy (DOT) visits (21%) and food parcels (16%). Their results suggest that the treatment of patients with chronic TB with second-line drugs is, on average, less cost-effective than the basic DOT programme, which relies on first-line antituberculotics in low-income and middle-income countries [16].

Aspler et al. estimated patients' costs for TB diagnosis and treatment in Zambia. They compared the cost of directly observed therapy (DOT) and the cost of self-administered treatment (SAT). According to their results, the median total cost for the patients amounted to $ 24.78, of which comprised 62% indirect costs and 34% direct costs, respectively. In the pre-diagnostic period, direct costs comprised 66% of patients' costs - mostly for government health insurance fees, X-ray fees and public transport. In the post-diagnostic period, travel and time costs were the highest. The total costs incurred by patients on clinic-based DOT were four times greater compared to those who had switched to SAT (p<0.001). The total direct costs were higher for woman than men (p<0.001). Longer patient delays between first experience of symptoms and first health service encounter were also associated with higher costs [14].

Similar analysis was created in USA in 1997. Burman et al. compared costs and effectiveness of DOT versus SAT for treatment of active TB. They found that the direct costs of initial therapy with DOT and SAT were similar (US $ 1,206 vs US $ 1,221 per patient), but

DOT was more expensive when patients' time costs were included. When the costs of relapse and failure were included in the model, DOT was less expensive than SAT. The cost of hospitalization was US $ 7,820 in case of drug-susceptible patients and US $ 115,740 in case of MDR-TB. Their results suggest that despite its greater initial cost, DOT is a more cost-effective strategy than SAT because it achieves a higher cure rate after initial therapy, and decreases treatment costs associated with failure of treatment and acquired drug resistance [17].

Croft et al. measured the expenditure and loss of income incurred by TB patients in Bangladesh in 1996. In this small pilot tuberculosis study (n=21) authors determined a mean financial loss of US $ 245 to the patient. All services and medicines are free of charge (drugs are given by the Government of Bangladesh) and the only expenditure on the part of the patient is transport costs to and from the local clinic [12].

Wyss et al. determined the cost of TB from the perspective of households and health care providers in Tanzania. They found that the most popular choices for health care were governmental health services (93%), followed by private services (58%), self-treatment mainly by purchasing drugs at pharmacies (52%) and traditional therapists (28%).The average expenditure (in the year 1996 with prices in US $) of laboratory test, X-ray and other examinations was US $ 2.1 per patient, drugs and consultation costs were US $ 16.6 and hospitalization costs were US $ 0.1 from household perspective. The laboratory costs were US $ 9, drug costs US $ 40, costs for ambulatory care US $10, TB programme management costs US $ 31 from the provider's perspective. The total provider cost was US $ 90 per treated case. Despite the high cost of providers, the cost of drugs and consultations, transport costs and lost work-force put a high economic burden on patients [13].

In contrasts, in a developed country like Canada all adult immigrants undergo chest radiographic screening for TB. Schwartzman et al. compared the costs and outcomes associated with mass X-ray screening, mass tuberculin screening, and no screening in the case of immigrants. They found that tuberculin screening is more expensive than chest X-ray screening. Compared with no screening, radiographic screening cost Canadian $ 3,943 per active case prevented in the highest risk cohort, and $ 236,496 per case prevented in the lowest risk group. Compared with radiographic screening mass tuberculin skin testing cost $ 32,601 per additional case prevented in the highest risk group, and $ 68,799 per additional case prevented in the lowest risk group. The results suggest that chest radiographic screening is a low-cost preventive intervention for young immigrants with a high probability of TB infection. Tuberculin skin testing prevents additional TB cases, but it is more expensive than radiographic screening, making its routine use difficult. For low-prevalence population, both screening strategies have little impact but a high cost, because of false-positive screening tests, low prevalence of infection, and low risk of disease [18].

Dasgupta et al. compared cost of screening examinations in immigrants and close-contacts in Canada from 1996 until 1997. They found that close-contact investigation was highly cost-effective. Immigrant applicant screening and surveillance programs had significant impact but were much less cost-effective because of substantial operational problems [19].

Diel et al. created a cost-effectiveness analysis in young and middle-aged adults with latent TB infection in Germany. Health and economic outcomes of INH chemoprevention versus no intervention were compared. In Germany, INH chemoprevention (300 mg over 9 month) were recommended for latent TB infection, limiting the range of application to contacts < 50 years of age in order to minimise possible hepatotoxic side-effects. They analysed the inpatient and outpatient costs spent by the health insurance organisation. Their results suggest, that INH chemoprevention is a highly cost-effective approach for reducing the burden of TB in recently converted young and middle-aged adults in Germany [20].

Rubado et al. used a longitudinal survey to establish the costs of DOT in Oregon in USA. Forty-two patients (median age 40-44 years) were included in the study. The mean case management cost was US $ 4,831 per patient for a standard 28-week treatment course. The greatest cost was US $ 7,542 for a case with multiple complications [21]. These results are similar to our Hungarian TB research data (Table 3).

Healthcare Reimbursement in Hungary

Reimbursement of inpatient care in Hungary is based on diagnosis-related-groups (DRG).

OBJECTIVE

The aim of the study was to determine the direct cost of paediatric TB treatment in the Paediatric Department of Pest County Pulmonological Institute in Hungary.

MATERIALS AND METHODS

Sampling Procedures

All newly diagnosed pulmonary and/or extrapulmonary paediatric TB patients < 18 years of age were retrospectively assessed at the time of diagnosis between September 2008 and March 2010. The direct costs of the treatment were determined.

Data Collection

Patient medical records were used to collect the data on treatment, diagnostic interventions and outpatient consultations.

Direct Medical Costs of TB

Medical examination, chest X-ray, basic hematology and chemistry laboratory tests, tuberculin skin test, interferon gamma test, sputum and urine sample collection on 3 consecutive days for cultivation, smear microscopy and drug-susceptibility test are used for the diagnosis of TB in Hungary.

To rule out the adverse effects of medicines, liver function testing and ophthalmology check up were performed in all patients.

All costs are reported in Hungarian Forint (HUF). Costs were calculated in US dollars on the average exchange rate of the Hungarian National Bank (2009).

The cost of diagnostic interventions and outpatient consultations was calculated according to the Reference Book of the Hungarian Health Insurance Fund [22]. First, the score of the diagnostic intervention was identified. There is a table containing the minimum charge on the website of the Hungarian Health Insurance Fund. The score of the diagnostic intervention and the minimum charge were multiplied (score x minimum charge).

Data of drug expenditures were established on the basis of patients' files. The costs of medication were calculated according to the drug use and drug expenses provided by the Hospital Pharmacy.

The cost of tuberculocidal disinfectants was determined also on the basis of the use of the inpatient department and the purchase price of the Hospital Pharmacy.

The cost of inpatient care/hospitalization included the cost of meals, heating and lighting expenses and the salary of the health care workers, too. These hospitalization data were received from the Financial Department of the Hospital.

Health service costs were analysed in our study. Patients' costs were not included in the analysis.

Reimbursement

The reimbursement of tuberculosis was based on the Hungarian Diagnosis Related Groups (DRG) [23]. First, the score of the diagnosis was established according to the Hungarian DRG Reference Book which is available on the website of the Hungarian Health Insurance Fund. Then the minimum charge of the given year, given month was determined according to the minimum charge table of the Hungarian Health Insurance Fund. The total amount paid by the Hungarian Health Insurance Fund to the hospital was the multiplication of diagnosis score and minimum charge in tuberculosis.

Statistical Analysis

Data were entered into a database created in Microsoft Excel. Data were analyzed with Statistical Programme for Social Sciences (SPSS) 16.0.

RESULTS

In the one and a half year study period, tuberculosis infection was diagnosed in the case of nine (n=9) children. Average age of the children was 11.17 ± 6.34 years. The youngest patient was 7 months old, the eldest patient was 17 years old at the establishment of the diagnosis.

Two patients were immigrants (22.23 %), two (22.23 %) had multidrug-resistant TB (MDR-TB), five patients (55.56 %) were close contacts of an index case, six (66.67%) had extrapulmonary tuberculosis and three (33.34 %) also suffered from other co-morbidities (Table 2).

Table 2. Characteristics of patients diagnosed with TB

	Study population (n)	%
Sex		
Male	2	22.23
Female	7	77.78
Immigrant	2	22.23
Contact	5	55.56
MDR-TB	2	22.23
Non drug-resistant TB	7	77.78
Extrapulmonary TB	6	66.67

Total expenditures of the health service - regarding the nine patients infected with TB - are presented in Figure 2. Among the hospital costs of TB treatment, heating and lighting expenditures (US $ 25,763) accounted for the major part of the cost given by the health service. On the second place was the cost of medicines (US $ 11,483.5) and on the third the salary of the medical staff (US $ 9,213). The total direct medical cost of the care and treatment of nine children suffering from TB was US $ 53,520.

There are significant differences between the reimbursement and the expenditures of the health service in Hungary (Table 3).

Table 3. Differences between resources of health care system and reimbursement

	Hospital	Hungarian Health Insurance Fund
Days of medical care in non MDR-TB	20-162 days mean: 94.57 days	12-55 days normative: 22 days
Days of medical care in MDR-TB	109-198 days mean: 153 days	61-227 days normative: 138 days
Average cost of treatment and care of non MDR-TB (n=7)	US $ 4,432	US $ 1,052
Average cost of treatment and care of MDR-TB (n=2)	US $ 11,349	US $ 3,982

The average cost of treatment of patients under one year old was on average US $ 7,092.67 (Table 4).

Simple pulmonary TB without extrapulmonary manifestation and drug-resistance was diagnosed in cases of two patients (Table 4: patients No. 6. and 7.). The hospital cost of their treatment was an average of US $ 3,955.

Data of patients' age, period of inpatient care, hospital costs and the amount paid by the Hungarian Health Insurance Fund are contained in Table 4.

Table 4. Hospital expenditures and reimbursement

Patient	Dg.	Age	Co-morbidity	Days of medical care	Hospital costs	Health Insurance Fund
1.	Pulm. tuberculosis Tuberculosis gonitis	12 years	Haemophilia A Hepatitis C	162 days	US $ 7,492	US $ 1,052
2.	Pulm. tuberculosis Tuberculous lymphadenitis	17 years	-	66 days	US $ 3,754	US $ 1,052
3.	Pulm. tuberculosis Urogenital TB	11 years	-	128 days	US $ 5,842	US $ 1,052
4.	Tuberculous bronchoadenitis	11 months	Pes varus Mental retardation Obstr. Sleep Apnea Syndr. Pectus excavatum	109 days	US $ 4,791	US $ 1,052
5.	Urogenital TB	11 years	Tracheal bronchus	20 days	US $ 1,233	US $ 1,052
6.	Pulm. tuberculosis	16 years	-	66 days	US $ 3,030	US $ 1,052
7.	Pulm. tuberculosis	16 years	-	111 days	US $ 4,886	US $ 1,024
8.	Tuberculous lymphadenitis MDR-TB	7 months	-	198 days	US $ 9,394	US $ 1,052
9.	Pulm. Tuberculosis MDR-TB	16 years	-	99 days	US$ 13,097	US$ 6,913

DISCUSSION

The present study retrospectively reviews inpatient utilization and charges in the health care system.

Tuberculosis was identified in case of nine children during the one and a half year study period at the Paediatric Department of Pest County Pulmonological Institute which is a regional centre for treatment of paediatric TB.

Five patients were contacts and this reflects the importance of the screening examinations. Two patients were immigrants, which calls the attention to the imported cases and to the importance of the immigrants' screening. In the United States nearly 40 percent of the TB cases were diagnosed in foreign-born persons in 1999 [24].

Hospital Costs

The total direct cost of care and treatment of nine children infected with TB was US $ 53,520. The results of the present study demonstrated that most of the money was spent on heating and lighting expenditures, followed by the cost of medications, salary, the cost of diagnostics, outpatient consultations and finally the expenditures of meals. The least money was spent on tuberculocidal disinfectants. In a previous study *Wurtz et al.*, who made a cost analysis in the United States, found similar results [25]. They also demonstrated that the cost of inpatient days and charges of medications proved to be the most significant expenditures. *Menzies et al.* obtained nearly the same results in Canada in 2004. According to their *Costs for tuberculosis care in Canada* study, the total TB related expenditures were $ 47,290 per active case. Federal government spending related to TB exceeded $ 16.3 million. The total direct costs by the provinces and territories for public health activities were $ 27.7 million. Almost half of the active TB related costs were for hospitalization; laboratory costs accounted for 20 % and public health salaries another 20 % [26].

There are significant differences between the resources of developing and developed countries. In developing countries like in the Philippines TB affects the poor, who do not have access to adequate health care. TB is a sixth leading killer in the Philippines, infecting about half the population of 84 million. A standard six-month treatment costs between US $ 18 and US $ 74 [27].

Our results reflect that care and treatment of patients with tuberculosis impose significant burden on the health service but the correction of the deficit is not enough in Hungary.

Pulmonary TB

The hospital cost of simple pulmonary TB without extrapulmonary manifestation and drug-resistance was an average of US $ 3,955. *Rubado et al.* found similar results in a previous study in the United States [28]. The Hungarian Health Insurance Fund reimbursed US $ 1,052/1,024 for the treatment of these patients (Table 4.). Our results suggest that the treatment and care of paediatric pulmonary TB caused more than three and a half times extra expenses to the health service in Hungary.

Co-Morbidity and Extrapulmonary TB

Two-thirds of the study population suffered from extrapulmonary TB. We found significant cost-rise in the cases of patients diagnosed with extrapulmonary TB. *Kik et al.* found similar results among immigrants infected with TB in the Netherlands [11]. The costs of pre-diagnostic period were higher for patients with extrapulmonary TB compared to those with pulmonary TB. The reason of the difference can be in the additional diagnostic investigations needed for the diagnosis of extrapulmonary TB and exclusion of any other disorders.

Our results demonstrated that extrapulmonary manifestation combined with serious co-morbidity causes increasing length of period of inpatient care and cost-rise, that can result in a seven times higher cost for the hospital (Table 4: patient No. 1.).

Multidrug-Resistant TB

Treatment of patients infected with multidrug-resistant TB requires a longer period of inpatient care and causes a significant cost-rise, too. Inadequate TB control is a major cause of MDR-TB. One case of MDR-TB may cost up to US $ 250,000 to treat and some cases are incurable [24]. According to our observations, the treatment of MDR-TB compared to non drug-resistant TB can increase the period of hospital care by one and a half times and the costs of the treatment by two and a half times (Figure 3.,4.). In a previous study *Burman et al.*

found similar results. In their analysis the cost of hospitalization was US $ 7,820 in drug-susceptible case and US $ 115,740 in the case of MDR-TB [17].

There are significant differences between the real hospital costs and the period of inpatient care compared to the normative period of hospital care determined by the Hungarian Health Insurance Fund and to the sum of reimbursement. On average, the time of care and costs of treatment in the case of patients with non MDR-TB cost the hospital more than four times higher expenses than the normative inpatient days and reimbursed charges determined by the Hungarian Health Insurance Fund. The treatment of MDR-TB causes three times extra expenditures to the hospital but the defined maximum length of stay can be kept.

Resch et al. examined the cost-effectiveness of treating MDR-TB in Peru in 2006. Their analysis demonstrated that standardized second-line treatment for confirmed MDR-TB cases had an incremental cost-effectiveness ratio of US $ 720 per quality-adjusted life year (QALY) (US $ 8,700 per averted death) compared to first-line drugs administered under DOT [28].

TB in Childhood as a Special Challenge

In our study, the cost of treatment of patients under one year old was on average more than US $ 7,000 (US $ 7,092.67). According to the present valid system of reimbursement in Hungary, the same amount was paid both for infants' treatment and for adult patients infected with TB (US $ 1,052). This difference caused 4.5-9 times extra costs to the hospital.

According to our results, the present method of reimbursement does not appear to be realistic because the normative charge paid for the treatment of TB in childhood is the same as the normative charge paid for the treatment of adult TB patients. It seems likely that the period of the hospital care of an infant with TB infection is longer than that is of a middle-aged or a young adult patient. A longer period in hospital care - due to the challenge of medication, the special hospital tasks - yields extra costs to the hospital compared to the adults' hospital treatment and care with a continued care in an outpatient form as a directly observed therapy (DOT) after a shorter inpatient care period. Especially if DOT is preferred during the treatment in adult TB patients as the World Bank ranked the DOTS strategy as one of the most cost-effective of all health interventions [29].

The Hungarian Health Insurance Fund

If the period of treatment of a patient is beyond the maximum defined length of stay determined by the Health Insurance Fund, the provider can compensate the health service by a special daily charge for the remaining hospital care days. The daily charge is 75% of the chronic minimum charge (remaining days x chronic minimum charge x 0.75) (23). However this amount is paid to the hospital only if there is a rehabilitation department in the institute. Nowadays there is a decreasing tendency of the number of inpatient beds in Hungary and it is complicated to establish or maintain a special paediatric rehabilitation department.

Another compensation-possibility for hospitals is to claim extra financial aid in case of outstandingly high treatment expenses.

Limitations of the Study

The present study has some limitations. First of all there was a low number of patients (n=9) participating in our study. Fortunately the incidence and prevalence of TB are low in Hungary. However, this examination was not a multi-centre analysis because the study was carried out on the basis of the direct medical cost according to TB of one Hungarian Hospital. The Paediatric Department of Pest County Pulmonological Institute is a regional centre of care and treatment of TB in Hungary.

Our direct cost results were not compared to adult Hungarian TB costs data because the costs of hospital care and treatment of paediatric TB were measured.

CONCLUSION

Our study demonstrates that the treatment of tuberculosis in childhood yields significant expenses to the hospitals, despite the fact that tuberculosis incidence and prevalence is low in Hungary.

Extrapulmonary TB combined with co-morbidity results 3-7 times extra costs to the health service [30].

Hospital care over 100 days causes 4.5-9 times extra expenses to the hospital.

Compared to the results of the studies carried out in other developed countries, we found an important difference in direct medical costs and the period of inpatient care. The period of hospitalization was 5 times longer in Hungary than in the Dutch TB cost analysis. However it must not be left out of consideration that previous publications focused on adult TB population. Our results can refer to the special cost-rising role of childhood in the treatment and care of TB. To verify this statement, more comparing cost analysis should be made among paediatric and adult population. In the focus of foreign health economic studies – carried out on adult population – the social viewpoint is more and more dominant because not only the consequence of cost of hospitalization is considered but also the time lost from work [11, 25].

ACKNOWLEDGMENTS

Authors are grateful to Zsuzsa Rudnai for checking the manuscript linguistically and to Akos Somoskovi M.D. for critical review of the manuscript.

REFERENCES

[1]   Global tuberculosis control. The global burden of TB: 5-7. *WHO report* 2010.
[2]   Hutas I. Epidemiology of tuberculosis. In: Magyar P, Somoskovi A. Pulmonary and extrapulmonary tuberculosis. *Medicina,* 1st edition, Budapest, 2007; 34-38.

[3] Strausz J, Boszormenyi Nagy Gy, Csekeo A, Csoma Zs, Herjavecz I, Kovacs G, Ostoros Gy, Zsarnoczai I. Functioning and epidemiological data of pulmonological institutes in 2009. www.koranyi.hu

[4] Baltussen R, Floyd K, Dye C. Cost-effectiveness analysis of strategies for tuberculosis control in developing countries. *BMJ* 2005; 331: 1364-1368.

[5] Wrighton-Smith P, Zellweger J-P. Direct costs of three models for the screening of latent tuberculosis infection. *Eur Respir J* 2006; 28: 45-50.

[6] Diel R, Nienhaus A, Lange C, Schaberg T. Cost-optimisation of screening for latent tuberculosis in close contacts. *Eur Respir J* 2006; 28: 35-44.

[7] Kalo Z, Inotai A. Measurement of costs. In: Kalo Z, Inotai A, Nagyjanosi L. Definitions of health technology assessment. Professional Publishing Hungary Kft., 1st edition, Budapest, 2009; 89-91.

[8] Gulacsi L, Rutten, F, Koopmanschap, M. A. Cost-calculating. In: Gulacsi L. Health Economy. *Medicina,* 1st edition, Budapest, 2005; 191-265.

[9] Szende A. Economic evaluation of health technologies. In: Vincze Z, Kalo Z, Bodrogi J. Introduction to health economy. *Medicina,* 1st edition, Budapest, 2001; 101-117.

[10] Kerpel-Fronius S. Examinations of drug-economy. In: Kerpel-Fronius S, Gyires K, Furst Zs. Pharmacology and pharmaco-therapy. II. *Medicina,* 1st edition, Budapest, 2008; 55-58.

[11] Kik S. V, Olthof S. P. J, de Vries J. T. N, Menzies D, Kincler N, van Loenhout-Rooyakkers J, Burdo C, Verver S. Direct and indirect costs of tuberculosis among immigrant patients in the Netherlands. *BMC Public Health* 2009; 9: 1-9.

[12] Croft R. A, Croft R. P. Expenditure and loss of income incurred by tuberculosis patients before reaching effective treatment in Bangladesh. *Int J Tuberc Lung Dis* 1998; 2 (3): 252-254.

[13] Wyss K, Kilima P, Lorenz N. Costs of tuberculosis for households and heallth care providers in Dar es Salaam, Tanzania. *Trop Med Int Health* 2001; 6 (I): 60-68.

[14] Aspler A, Menzies D, Oxlade O, Banda J, Mwenge L, Godfrey-Faussett P, Ayles H. Cost of tuberculosis diagnosis and treatment from the patient perspective in Lusaka, Zambia. *Int J Tuberc Lung Dis* 2008; 12 (8): 928-935.

[15] Floyd K. Costs and effectiveness-the impact of economic studies on TB control. *Tuberculosis* 2003; 83: 187-200.

[16] Suarez P. G, Floyd K, Portocarrero J, Alarcon E, Rapiti E, Ramos G, Bonilla C, Sabogal I, Aranda I, Dye C, Raviglione M, Espinal A. E. Feasibility and cost-effectiveness of standardised second-line drug treatment for chronic tuberculosis patients: a national cohort study in Peru. *Lancet* 2002; 359: 1980-1989.

[17] Burman W. J, Dalton C. B, Cohn D. L, Butler J. R.G, Reves R. R. A cost-effectiveness analysis of directly observed therapy vs self-administered therapy for treatment of tuberculosis. *Chest* 1997; 112: 63-70.

[18] Schwartzman K, Menzies D. Tuberculosis screening of immigrants to low-prevalence countries. *Am J Respir Crit Care Med* 2000; 161: 780-789.

[19] Dasgupta K, Schwartzman K, Marchand R, Tennenbaum T. N, Brassard P, Menzies D. Comparison of cost-effectiveness of tuberculosis screening of close contacts and foreign-born populations. *Am J Respir Crit Care Med* 2000; 162: 2079-2086.

[20] Diel R, Nienhaus A, Schaberg T. Cost-effectiveness of isoniazid chemoprevention in close contacts. *Eur Respir J* 2005; 26: 465-473.

[21] Rubado D. J, Choi D, Becker T, Winthrop K, Schafer S. Determining the cost of tuberculosis case management in a low-incidence state. *Int J Tuberc Lung Dis* 2008; 12 (3): 301-307.

[22] Reference book to outpatient care. www.gyogyinfok.hu/magyar/szabalykonyv.html [2009. 11. 06]

[23] Classification Handbook to instruction of Hungarian Diagnosis Related Groups. www.gyogyinfok.hu/magyar/fekvo/hbcs50/konyv/valtozasok/HBCS50_besororlo_2010 0119.pdf [2010. 02. 08.]

[24] National Foundation for Infectious Diseases 1999; http://www.nfid.org/factsheets/tb.shtml [2011. 01. 18.]

[25] Wurtz R, White W. D. The cost of tuberculosis: utilization and estimated charges for the diagnosis and treatment of tuberculosis in a public health system. *Int J Tuberc Lung Dis* 1999; 3 (5) : 382-387.

[26] Menzies D, Oxlade O, Lewis M. Costs for tuberculosis care in Canada. http://www.phac-aspc.gc.ca/tbpc-latb/costtb/pdf/cost [2011. 01. 18.]

[27] Chemonics International Projects: Philippine government uses benefits to fight tuberculosis. http://www.chemonics.com/projects/default.asp?content_id={5757e6b7-0c91-485a-a186-252a4cdb5ad2} [2011. 01. 18.]

[28] Resch S. C, Salomon J. A, Murray M, Weinstein M. C. Cost-effectiveness of treating multidrug-resistant tuberculosis. PloS Med 2006; 3 (7): e241. http://www.plosmedicine.org/article/info:doi/10.1371/journal.pmed.0030241 [2011. 01. 18.]

[29] TB Advocacy, A Practical Guide 1999, WHO Global Tuberculosis Programme http://www.theunion.org/download/factsheets/tb/facts_cost [2011. 01. 18.]

[30] Bodnar R, Meszaros A, Kadar L. Analysis of direct costs during the treatment of tuberculosis in childhood. *Acta Pharmaceutica Hungarica* 2010; 80 (2): 67-73.

In: Toward Healthcare Resource Stewardship
Editors: J. S.Robinson, M. S.Walid et al.

ISBN: 978-1-62100-182-9
© 2012 Nova Science Publishers, Inc.

Chapter 18

PHYSICIAN-HOSPITAL RELATIONS: CURRENT REALITIES AND PARTNERSHIP POSSIBILITIES

Aaron C. M. Barth[1]* *and Louis Goolsby*[1]

[1]Medical Center of Central Georgia, Macon, GA, US

ABSTRACT

As American healthcare costs continue to soar, healthcare providers face their own sets of internal and external challenges. Regulatory and economic pressures often exacerbate communication and accountability difficulties that have the potential to drive wedges between physicians and hospital leaders. Fundamental philosophical differences between the hospital and physician cultures can often intensify existing problems. In the face of what often seem to be daunting realities, there is a need for collaboration between physicians and hospitals if they are to remain true to their mission of providing optimal patient care. Joint Ventures, Hospital Employment of Physicians, and Clinic Models are three of the many partnership models pursued in recent years and explored in this paper. Although physicians and hospitals face pressures from every side, their decision to collaborate appears essential for the long term well-being of not only their institutions, but also the patients for which they care.

BACKGROUND

Healthcare issues have garnered considerable attention throughout the 2008 United States presidential election cycle, particularly as the costs of healthcare continue to soar. National healthcare expenditure crossed the $2 trillion mark in 2005, and this figure is expected to balloon beyond $4 trillion by the year 2016 (CMS 2006). As solutions to the many problems facing the American healthcare industry are continually debated, healthcare providers face

---

[*] Corresponding Authors: Aaron Barth. The Medical Center of Central Georgia, 777 Hemlock St, MSC 72, Macon, GA 31201, Phone: (478) 633-7707, Fax: (478) 633-7879. E-mail: barth.aaron@mccg.org.

their own sets of internal and external challenges. One dynamic of particular interest is the ever-evolving relationship between hospitals and the physicians who serve within these health systems. While the mutual goal of providing excellent patient care generally unites both parties, the pressures associated with healthcare delivery in a hospital environment often create discord. External regulatory, legal, and economic pressures often exacerbate internal communication and accountability difficulties that have the potential to drive wedges between physicians and hospital leaders. Nevertheless, these challenges present opportunities for the two groups to collaborate in efforts to find mutually beneficial solutions. Strong collaboration between physicians and hospitals remains essential for the welfare of patients and our nation's healthcare system.

AN EVOLVING RELATIONSHIP

The relationship between hospitals and physicians has generally been a symbiotic one that has enabled each party to achieve their missions of providing patients with high levels of care. Hospitals work to keep their doors open so that physicians can access the latest technologies and equipment, support staff and administrative infrastructure for the benefit of the patients they treat. Physicians bring the expertise, skills, and insight needed to facilitate the healing process within the hospital environment. Each party depends on the other as physicians bring a wide breadth of knowledge and skills to a hospital setting that enable it to exist, while these hospitals offer a supportive framework within which doctors may optimally provide their services.

As the delivery of health care has evolved over the years, so has the nature of the interaction between physicians and the hospitals in which they practice. Healthcare Strategic Advisor Nate Kaufman (2008) provides a noteworthy description of how hospital-physician interactions have evolved from a "social" to a "market" relationship. Whereas in the past physicians and hospital leaders may have been able to interact and depend on one another in more informal and collegial manners, the regulatory and economic realities of the current healthcare system have forced them to relate in a more business-like fashion. Kaufman argues that physicians and hospitals continue to wrestle with the uncertainties of collaborating within the context of this newfound relationship.

EXTERNAL PRESSURES

A host of external pressures face healthcare providers as they attempt to perform the daily duties associated with treating patients. Legislative mandates from state and federal governments are often set in place with the hope of ensuring that patients receive optimal care and are not financially or otherwise harmed in times of need. Healthcare providers within the highly-regulated domain of healthcare can subsequently face a large number of lawsuits when questions of malpractice or undesirable outcomes result from clinical care. As a result, hospitals and physicians both face enormous legal restraints that can add a great deal of tension to their relationships with patients and with each other. When treatment has failed for a patient, both the hospital and physician can often be held liable regardless of which party has committed the error. The federal government's National Practitioner Data Bank (NPDB) reveals that from September 1990 to May 2008, 319,173 medical malpractice payments were reported in the United States for healthcare professionals, a figure equivalent to 17,253 cases per year. 234,242 (73.4%) of these represent payments made for Medical Doctor malpractice claims (NPDB 2008). Although debate persists as to the extent to which medical malpractice issues truly impact healthcare providers (see Public Citizen 2007), they can certainly act as daunting psychological and financial concerns for those involved.

The regulatory and legal matters that surround healthcare are only two of the many economic concerns facing hospitals and physicians on a regular basis. Dr. Robert Wachter (2004) lists a number of the countless pressures hospitals currently face, which include high patient censuses, shortages in nursing and clinical staff, pressures to improve quality and safety, and the successful implementation of technologies required for keeping in step with healthcare advances. These factors place immense economic strain on institutions and often threaten their viability. From the physician standpoint, Medicare reimbursement has remained predominantly flat in spite of the rising costs and demands for the provision of their expertise and services (Kaufman 2008). This reality hinders the ability of physicians to both provide maximum patient care and remain economically secure. Using information from the national survey conducted by Mitretek Healthcare as his basis, author Robert McGowan (2004) succinctly states the dilemma facing many healthcare providers: "both hospital leadership and physicians reported that they are working harder than ever, yet making less money."

In the face of mounting external pressures, physicians and hospitals can occasionally become pitted against one another. In some instances, physicians have abandoned the traditional reliance on hospital infrastructure and technology and developed their own competing facilities as a result of disagreements or in efforts to capture more revenue. Dr. Richard Rohr (2006) explains, "now that physicians have found ways to secure those technologies on their own and with the help of outside investors, the model no longer works." Further, in the face of declining reimbursements for many of their services, many physicians have elected to withdraw from providing hospital care and choose instead to focus their time on treating patients in their offices in order to maximize their resources and energies. Whereas in the past, physician participation in hospital affairs was generally considered a standard component of their duties, this involvement has steadily declined. Wachter reports that, "In this environment, it is not surprising that many hospitals report that 'volunteerism is dead' among high rank-and-file medical staff members. Most physicians are too busy in their offices to willingly participate in hospital committees or emergency department call schedules."(Wachter 2004). In many instances, hospitals have discovered that they have lost both business and physician input as the relationship between the two parties has reshaped itself in light of the realities of the healthcare environment.

INTERNAL TENSIONS

Not all of the tensions between physicians and hospitals come as a reaction to external pressures. Fundamental philosophical differences between the hospital and physician cultures can often intensify existing problems. Differing priorities even within the physician community can also complicate matters, as individual physicians may place different values on income, flexibility, and life-work balances, with these differences often varying greatly between generations and genders (AAMC 2006). Healthcare consultant David Shipman (2005) provides an insightful list of eighteen fundamental differences between the hospital culture and the physician practice culture that can create gaps in communication between physicians and hospital executives. At the heart of these differences, Shipman argues, is the philosophical mindset that "to many hospital executives, business is business and business has nothing to do with relationships. For many physicians all business is personal." As a result, Shipman further notes, hospital executives too often attempt to "solve" relationships with physicians, and do not recognize that these relationships can never be solved because of vastly different priorities and approaches toward patient care. Rather, these relationships should be managed by addressing concerns of physicians and recognizing their aversion to having medical care seen as a business enterprise (Shipman 2005).

These fundamental differences in priorities and expectations can sometimes lead to poor interactions within a health system. While communication problems can spell disaster in any organization, this is certainly the case in regards to physician dialogue with hospital administrators and staff. Misunderstandings regarding patient care may lead to serious medical errors, while disagreements regarding expectations or standards can lead to ongoing friction between hospital workers and their physician counterparts. McGowan points out an example of the disparities in perceptions between physicians and hospital leaders, noting that "While 73 percent of the participating CEOs rated their hospital-physician relationships quite positively, only 44 percent of the participating physicians shared this view." (McGowan 2004). This difference in opinion may reflect the reality that communication problems often taint attempts at improving interaction between the two groups.

FORGING AHEAD TOGETHER

In the face of what often seem to be daunting external and internal realities, there is a need for collaboration between physicians and hospitals if they are to remain true to their mission of providing optimal patient care together. Generally, hospitals have access to a greater pool of resources and support staff, and thus have the opportunity to initiate potential partnerships with interested physicians. The way in which they do this can impact the success or failure of a potential partnership. Shipman argues that "The attitude of the hospital's top executives toward their physicians will permeate all the business and financial arrangements with physicians and will be the indirect key to success or failure of the ventures." (Shipman 2005). Hospital leaders should nonetheless be careful about overextending in efforts to attract physician loyalty. Providing a cautionary warning, The Healthcare Advisory Board Company contends that in the past many hospitals and health systems have failed to respond effectively to the challenges facing them, sometimes to their own long-term determinant. They explain that "Facing an onslaught of pressure from multiple specialist groups, many CEOs have defaulted to reactive and defensive physician strategy – scrambling to address each threat as it arises, often bargaining away hospital surplus in exchange for (tenuous) specialist loyalty." (Advisory Board Company, 2005, Introduction).

The American Medical Association produced a list of guidelines they view as a sturdy framework of ideas and norms that might facilitate healthy physician-hospital interactions.

These guidelines emphasize several points, including the notion that "Everything depends on mutual accountability, interdependence, and both parties meeting respective obligations." (AMA 2008). The guidelines also emphasize that leaders of an organized medical staff at the hospital should be empowered to "develop goals to address the healthcare needs of the community and [be] involved in hospital strategic planning." Finally, the AMA guidelines stress that effective communication and allowing physician self-governance are essential elements to successfully engaging medical staff. Kaufman similarly promotes ideas for encouraging physician engagement by promoting physician participation in leadership, creating physician advisory group, forming physician-administrative dyads, and including physician leaders in management retreats, meetings, budgeting, planning and leadership development. On the flip side, Kaufman argues, expectations also rest on the physicians' shoulders to honor accountability guidelines and performance expectations set before them in exchange for involvement in hospital leadership (Kaufman 2008).

Certainly, each situation may call for different measures and approaches to dealing with the specific physician-hospital issues that have arisen. Some healthcare settings, such as academic medical centers, may be more conducive to positive physician-hospital partnerships than others. Wachter (2004) explains that "In [academic medical center] environments, the shared mission dissonance is created more by the pressure on the faculty physicians to publish and teach in addition to their clinical care, rather than overt conflict with the hospital." In settings where the collaborative opportunities are not as straightforward, both physicians and hospitals must ensure that they understand and can articulate their own concerns and reasons for seeking a partnership.

JOINT VENTURES

The "Joint Venture" arrangement is a type of partnership that has gained popularity over the past several decades. In this model physicians act as independent contractors in a formalized relationship with a particular health system. Physicians might agree, for example, to partner with a hospital in opening a joint clinic, or to bring a certain volume of their patients to receive care at one hospital in exchange for a financial return of some sort. Many hospitals consider joint ventures with key private physician groups in hopes of securing patient volume that the physicians might otherwise take to competing healthcare facilities. These joint ventures are theoretically beneficial for both parties from a financial standpoint.

Joint venture propositions have faced mix reviews in recent years, however, as their efficacy in achieving desired financial outcomes has been called into question. Philip Betbeze, finance editor for HealthLeaders magazine, analyzes the shift in attitude toward joint ventures, noting that financial problems have arisen for hospitals because they lose many of the profits they hoped for as a result of lower reimbursement rates for joint ventures and higher taxation for revenues earned (Betbeze 2008). He notes that these joint ventures can also potentially be more fragmentary among medical staff than uniting. Hospitals can usually only afford to enter joint ventures with physician specialists who bring in a large amount of revenue. Thus, physicians whose services are less lucrative are often left out of such partnerships, which can lead to resentment or conflict.

A large reason for the souring attitude of some observers regarding joint ventures is that regulatory restrictions have made gain-sharing arrangements between physicians and hospitals less feasible and attractive. In his article discussing the legal issues surrounding physician-hospital relations, David Manko (2005) explains the regulatory statutes that should be considered before joint ventures are finalized. He warns of the anti-kickback and anti-referral statues that limit the terms to which physicians and hospitals can agree, explaining that "For example, hospitals may not agree to pay a physician income based on the volume or value of referrals the doctor makes to the hospital." The legal restrictions on physician-hospital partnerships lead to both positive and negative results. The established statutes help to curb any collusive attempts of hospitals and physicians to make financial gains at the expense of patients or insurers. On the other hand, these regulations also create barriers to those physicians and hospitals who genuinely seek to collaborate to improve system inefficiencies or work together to improve patient care.

HOSPITAL EMPLOYMENT

Betbeze concludes his article on joint ventures by explaining that such partnerships are becoming and will become less useful as physicians increasingly become employed by hospitals. "The idea of hospitals employing more of their physicians," Betbeze explains, "has been touted as a potential solution to the problem of declining physician income and interest in specialty centers in many markets" (Betbeze 2008). The notion of hospitals employing physicians is certainly not a new idea, but one that runs counter to the private practice model that physicians have generally preferred in the past. As Wachter (2004) explains, "Physicians have been trained and socialized to be fiercely independent," and the private practice model has certainly always seemed to provide physicians with the maximum opportunity for independence. However, in light of the many pressures and uncertainties facing physicians from a financial and regulatory standpoint, the option of hospital employment has become a more secure and attractive option for some physicians (Kaufman 2008). Although regulatory cautions exist in situations where physicians are considering hospital employment options (Manko 2005), there are successful models that have proven to be valuable not only from the perspective of physician-hospital interaction, but also from a patient care standpoint.

The "hospitalist" model of physician employment has gained positive reviews as its popularity has grown over the past decade. Health systems who recognize that physicians from primary care specialties have less incentive to provide patient care in hospital settings, may choose to hire "hospitalists" to oversee the medical care and management of patients who enter the hospital facilities. Rohr presents a rationale as to how these physicians can partner to help hospitals in providing strong patient care: "Hospitalists are in the forefront of efforts to improve clinical outcomes, promote patient safety and reduce cost. Caring for unassigned patients, participating on hospital committees and improving throughput are some of the other ways hospitalists can support hospitals." (Rohr 2006). It can be argued that because hospitalists are the physicians that spend the largest portion of their time in the hospital, partnership with these types of physicians are of paramount importance.

The presence of hospitalists may also improve relationships with non-employed physicians as they can partner together in patient care or work on mutually beneficial ventures. Wachter (2004) places high value on the hospitalist model explaining, "Their presence and immersion in their practice environments creates fertile soil for alignment of incentives with the hospital and for the creation of high-functioning teams involving these physicians, the other hospital-employed professionals, and the physicians who are comfortable with the precepts of systems thinking." The notion of collaboration and teamwork are certainly vital for any successful hospital venture with physicians.

In addition to the employment of hospitalists, hospitals have increasingly sought to hire other physician specialists as a way to counteract some of the economic pressures facing physicians. Some hospitals have chosen to hire specialized physicians or surgeons as part of a mission to provide comprehensive care for a particular disease, or in hopes of attracting more patients and improving their bottom line. In some instances, hospitals may employ specialists to perform cases that are less financially profitable in order to relieve the burden on private practitioners. This type of arrangement allows for the hospital to continue providing care to all members of the community, while providing private physicians with a positive incentive to continue practicing at the hospital facility (Advisory Board 2005, 88-89). In any physician employment scenario, it would be important to honor the fundamental philosophical differences between hospitals and physicians outlined by Shipman. Hospitals should honor the physician values of independence and not seek to "solve" relational problems from a purely business-minded standpoint. Similarly, physicians should be expected to respond to performance metrics & accountability structures, recognizing that the hospital's financial viability is a foundational element for providing excellent patient care.

CLINIC MODELS

Although there are countless opportunities for physician-hospital partnership (see Advisory Board 2005), the "clinic model" is one final example of physician-hospital partnership worth discussing. This model is perhaps the oldest and most traditional, but one that has been disregarded at times due to the lack of financial incentives for hospitals and physicians to participate within this structure. Traditionally, the clinic model has allowed for patients with a particular condition to be screened, triaged and treated in one setting by appropriate specialists. In his article "Keep 'Em Close," Betbeze (2007) gives special attention to hospital teams attempting to shift clinical care back toward clinic-style arrangements. The leaders he quotes have sought to shift their hospital infrastructure away from resembling independent businesses and working instead to integrate physicians into the system. "The essence of the clinic model is that hospitals stop becoming independent businesses and start becoming ancillary services to the physician practice," says Edward G. Murphy, CEO of Carilion Clinic in Virginia (Betbeze 2007). The Advisory Board further notes that this clinic model can be a "Highly effective and inexpensive model for optimizing surgeons' time and increasing hospital procedural volume," noting however that it is primarily "applicable only for programs with sizeable volume of referrals, for surgeons with high burden of patient evaluations, and for hospitals that can overcome potential turf battles by ensuring equitable distribution of patients across clinic-affiliated surgeons" (Advisory Board 2005, 81). The great advantage of the clinic model is that all players are focused on delivering integrated patient care into one setting, which is arguably ideal from the patient perspective. To date, however, financial realities have inhibited such ventures from gaining widespread popularity. Nonetheless, as federal insurers study the quality and efficiency of care that may result from such models, payment structures may shift to favor the clinic approach.

CONCLUSION

Physicians and hospitals fundamentally strive to achieve the common goal of excellent patient care in spite of the tensions and philosophical differences that can frequently divide them. If physicians and hospitals are able to maintain a commitment to collaboration, each can work toward the common goals of long-term economic viability and integrated patient care. Wachter provides his vision of the future, postulating that "The high functioning hospitals of the future…will operate as if the doctors, nurses, administrators, and others recognize their complete interdependency in a shared effort to achieve a single, overarching goal: the provision of the highest-quality, safest, and most-satisfying care to patients at the lowest possible cost" (Wachter 2004). McGowan provides a blunt warning that "Given the financial challenges of today's healthcare environment, hospitals and physicians will become either more collaborative partners or more active competitors, with few in the neutral zone" (McGowan 2004). These healthcare providers should proactively pursue mutually beneficial interaction if both parties hope to survive and thrive in the ever-changing U.S. healthcare environment. Although physicians and hospitals face pressures from every side, their decision to collaborate appears essential for the long term well-being of not only their institutions, but also the patients for which they care.

REFERENCES

American Medical Association. Principles for strengthening the physician-hospital relationship." (May 27 2008). Accessed June 1, 2008: http://www.ama-assn.org/ama1/pub/upload/mm/21/principlesprintable.pdf

Association of American Medical Colleges. AAMC 2006 survey of physicians under 50 (2006). Accessed June 25, 2008: http://www.aamc.org/members/gsa/coa/pdcpres/gwen.pdf

Betbeze, Philip. (June 2007). Keep 'Em Close. *HealthLeaders*, 22-27.

Betbeze, Philip. (May 2008). Are JVs losing some luster? *HealthLeaders*, 55-56.

Center for Medicare and Medicaid Services. National Health Expenditure Projections 2006-2016. (2006). Accessed on June 20, 2008: http://www.cms.hhs.gov/National health expenddata/downloads/proj2006.pdf

Health Care Advisory Board. (2005) Overcoming Ruinous Competition: Emerging Models for Hospital-Physician Alignment. Washington DC: The Advisory Board Company.

Kaufman, Nate. (May 20, 2008). General overview of healthcare field and predictions: "Facts vs. Fads." [Kaufman Strategic Advisors, LLC, PowerPoint Slides]. Presentation to the Medical Center of Central Georgia. Macon, GA.

Manko, David A. (May 9, 2005). Hospital-physician relationships growing more complex. *New York Law Journal*. Accessed June 11, 2008: http://www.rivkinradler.com/rivkinradler/Publications/newformat/200505manko.shtml

McGowan, Robert A. (December 2004). Strengthening hospital-physician relationships. Healthcare Financial Management. Accessed June 5, 2008: http://findarticles.com/p/articles/mi_m3257/is_12_58/ai_n8574803

National Practitioner Data Bank. 2008 NPDB Summary Report (June 2008). Accessed June 25, 2008: http://www.npdb-hipdb.hrsa.gov/pubs/stats/NPDB_Summary_Report.pdf

Public Citizen. The Great Medical Malpractice Hoax: NPDB Data Continue to Show Medical Liability System Produces Rational Outcomes (January 2007). Accessed: June 25, 2008: http://www.citizen.org/documents/NPDB%20Report_Final.pdf

Rohr, Richard. (May 1, 2006). Changing the physician-hospital relationship: hospitalists are the levers. Physician Executive. Retrieved June 11 from Goliath database: http://goliath.ecnext.com/coms2/summary_0199-5567152_ITM

Shipman, David. (July 2005). The solution to hospital/physician relations is management. Practice Support Resources. Accessed June 9, 2008: http://www.practicesupport.com/attitude.pdf

Wachter, Robert M. (July 2004). Physician–hospital alignment: The elusive ingredient. The Commonwealth Fund. Accessed June 11, 2008: http://www.commonwealthfund.org/usr_doc/Meyer_hopital_quality_commentary_wachter.pdf?section=4039

In: Toward Healthcare Resource Stewardship
Editors: J. S.Robinson, M. S.Walid et al.

ISBN: 978-1-62100-182-9
© 2012 Nova Science Publishers, Inc.

Chapter 19

BUREAUCRACY AND COST-INEFFICIENCY IN THE HEALTHCARE SYSTEM

Richard L. Heaton[1] and M. Sami Walid[2]*

[1]Heart of Georgia Women's Center, Warner Robins, GA, US
[2]Medical Center of Central Georgia, Macon, GA, US

Cost-efficiency is one of the necessary attributes for a high performance healthcare system. Over the years, the US health care has undergone progressive government interference that has had the unintended consequence of leading to a storm of overutilization (Emanuel EJ, 2008) and increasing healthcare cost by steadily eroding the impact of free market forces in the relationship between providers of care and patients. In 2001 the Institute of Medicine (IOM) called upon the healthcare system to focus on Six Aims for Improvement: care that is safe, timely, effective, efficient, equitable, and patient-focused (Richardson, 2001). Yet evidence is compelling that the health care system is far from being superior. The United States of America rank 37th in the overall health system performance according to the World Health Organization statistics (The World Health Report 2000 – Health systems: Improving performance). This ranking may arguably be useless due to the anti-American bias of all UN-related organizations and is a tool used by some politicians to push for nationalized health care. Interestingly, however, many wealthy people come from all over the world to access our "poorly rated system" when they have significant health issues.

Healthcare providers should play a very decisive role in defining healthcare efficiency. Providers engaging in dialogue with payers and patients can have a significant input in the dynamic interplay between efficiency and quality in the healthcare system in a proactive constructive manner. In order to excel in this ever changing system, incentive structures will have to evolve to take full advantage of the potential synergies between efficiency and quality(Butala, 2010).

In this paper, we put forth examples of healthcare inefficiency from our experience and suggest solutions for the rampant bureaucracy in the healthcare system.

---

* Corresponding Author: Richard L. Heaton, MD, FACOG, Heart of Georgia Women's Center, 209 Green Street, Warner Robins, GA 31093-2727. E-mail: riclheaton@yahoo.com.

INPATIENT HYSTEROSCOPY: AN EXAMPLE OF COST-INEFFICIENCY

We have been doing hysteroscopy with D and C (dilatation and curettage) as an office procedure for over twenty years. Over a thousand of patients underwent this procedure uneventfully. Patients were given minimum anxiolytics and paracervical-parametrial block and the procedure was very well tolerated similar to any kind of dental procedure. Approximately two out of each hundred (2%) patients had the procedure in hospital because of increased cardiovascular risk. We had only two cases that were admitted to stay in hospital overnight because of uterine perforation. The overwhelming majority of cases were treated without any significant complications.

We believe that hysteroscopy has no place in the hospital; it should be an office procedure. There is no incentive for physicians, however, to convert hysteroscopy to an office procedure even though it very clearly is. The reason for that is lack of proper oversight by the government allowing monopolistic behavior by the insurance companies to the detriment of patients and the providers of care.

As an inpatient procedure, the anesthesia charges the payor, the OR (Operation Room) charges, the recovery room charges and everything under the sun has charges. When we do hysteroscopy as office procedure, physicians get paid only $400 despite the fact that we are providing our own equipment, our own personnel, and our own supplies, none of which we get reimbursed for. Physicians simply get paid for the procedure code and that is it. If patients go to hospitals we know from the EOBs (Explanation of Benefits) that hospitals are charging for the procedure around $14,000-15,000. They do not get paid all requested amount but they receive around $8,500-9,500 a case.

Does $8,500-9,500 compare to $400, economically? If insurance companies double the payment for office hysteroscopy as opposed to hospital hysteroscopy, then instead of probably 5% of hysteroscopies in the country being done in the office we will have 95% of hysteroscopies done in the physician's office which will save a tremendous amount of money and healthcare resources for other care indications. And that is just one procedure in one specialty. Why does it not happen? We do not know! It may be that insurance companies do not decrease the cost of care because if they do they would have to decrease their premiums and therefore the amount of money they hold and invest for profit. Insurance companies make their money from the money they hold. So do they have any particular interest in dropping the cost of hysteroscopy which is a frequent gynecological procedure that they deal with everyday? Insurance companies say they have interest in decreasing cost but it seems they are not ready to promote it by offering hysteroscopies and many other minor procedures for a fraction of cost as office procedures by a relatively small increase in reimbursement for physicians and coverage of related supplies. We have been doing office hysteroscopy for over twenty years saving the system millions of dollars and have had no reward for it whatsoever.

The prime cause of high U.S. health care costs is the failure of the third party payor system to provide sufficient incentives to providers (physicians and hospitals) to be value–conscious in the management of their clients (patients) to promote rational use of healthcare resources (Angrisano C, 2007). We have thus been doing office hysteroscopy for over twenty years saving the system a considerable amount of money and got no reward for it whatsoever.

Reintroducing free market principles with proper regulation preventing monopolies will drastically drop cost as it has in any area where it is allowed to function. Competition between providers with the improvement in technology will drive cost down just as it does in all service industries. Technology linked with provider competition will lead to transfer of many procedures to the doctor's office away from high cost inefficient bureaucratic hospitals.

INSURANCE COMPANIES AND ANTITRUST LAW

We think the problem with healthcare efficiency originally comes from government interference in people's healthcare. We are amazed to hear that the government officials want to fix what they themselves have broken. Where does this entire problem we have with "Managed Care" start from? It comes from very progressive tax rates in the forties and fifties that at the highest income levels took the majority of a taxpayers' income. When this started to affect factory workers, due to higher wages and inflation pushing them into higher tax brackets and affecting their income, business companies started giving workers health care insurance and other nontaxable perks instead of giving them higher salaries effectively increasing their real income without adverse tax increases (Friedman, 2001). As a result, business companies took charge of their workers' insurance which was the end of free medicine market where the consumer had an interest in keeping cost down and the provider had an interest in being competitive with other providers to maintain market share. Now, the relationship is between the insurer and the business company, not between the insurer and the patient. The insurer is no longer responsive to the patient; they are only responsive to the business company they have a contract with. Provider reputation has been devalued because if you are not on the patients insurance plan no matter how good you are in your profession the patient will be forced by their insurance companies to see other providers. This transfer of power to third party payers defused the power of free market principles to control cost and promote efficiency and excellence and unfortunately prompted the downfall of American medicine.

Most of these health insurance companies were non-profit in the beginning then they were allowed to go for profit and to "manage care" by the government If this is truly what they were doing and it reduced cost and increased services resulting in our economy being more competitive internationally then perhaps these government interventions would be justified. But the only thing they managed was to change who got the money to the detriment of patients who have their choices in health care providers limited, their indicated care delayed, and indicated care not paid for by using a myriad of excuses to refuse to pay. It has also been to the extreme detriment of physicians transferring their rightful income to insurance companies via "contracts" that are nothing but legalized extortion. Physicians take all the risk, do the work, loose the sleep and die younger than the rest of the population due to stress related illnesses and the insurance companies with the willing collusion of the government steal their earned income. A contract is an agreement willingly entered into by two or more parties after a negotiation of terms. This does not describe the onerous one-sided documents drawn up by insurance company lawyers which physicians are told to "take it or leave it!" There is no realistic ability of unprotected individual physician practices to negotiate with monopolistic antitrust-exempted insurance companies. If we take there "contracts" we have trouble staying in business due to low and delayed reimbursement; if we do not we have no patients to see because they control where the insured go for care. Their contracts would more appropriately be called articles of indentured servitude which they more closely resemble. The only thing the health insurance manages is to swallow up health care dollars better spent elsewhere.

The CEOs (chief executive officers) of these companies get without merit a big share of the insurance money that is supposed to go for patient care. Why we left the original nonprofit insurance system, we do not understand! Certainly, the managed care healthcare system has not been more beneficial to the patient, has not been more beneficial to the provider of care and certainly has not cost less. They hire far more personnel in order to obstruct payment, to obfuscate and claim they need more information and delay, delay and delay in order to hold on to the money. One study estimated some 64% of administrative costs incurred by private insurance companies are due to underwriting health risks, and marketing(Angrisano C, 2007).

Another problem is, if insurance companies are now for-profit companies, why do they have antitrust exemption?! Why are they allowed to talk to one another about how not to pay patient's claims, about how to "rob" providers ...? How come that when an insurance company finds a way to delay payment or not pay the physician at all, all the other insurance companies learn about it and they are all doing it? None of this makes any sense. If allowing insurance companies monopoly protection that they have is actually decreasing the cost of medicine to the patient then perhaps that makes sense; but that is not the case. All that is done is change who wins and who loses. The patients and the providers of care lose and the high-level executives of insurance companies win. So the government has created winners and losers and they have stolen the free market from medicine; there is no free market.

If this would have been in any other sector of the economy where the government was not egregiously biased in its behavior these people would have been investigated by the FBI (Federal Bureau of Investigation) for code fraud charges. And they should be, because what they are doing is fraudulent behavior. But nothing is done because the government started the mess in the first place.

FREE MARKET HEALTHCARE SYSTEM

To give an example of exactly what we are talking about; if we went back to the standard free market insurance system we used to have where people pay 20% of their bill and the insurance pays the rest then even if the physician charges $800 for an office hysteroscopy and the hospital charges $14,000 the patients certainly will choose to pay 20% of $800 instead of 20% of $14,000 and the additional doctor's $400. That is why we do not have a free market in medicine.

We do not have free market in medicine for over fifty years. Once the insurance companies were permitted to go for profit but were allowed to maintain antitrust exemption they simply abused that monopolistic tool in order to just basically rape the providers of medicine of their livelihood and the due reimbursement for their work and redistribute the money to executives, who do nothing in medicine. So people at the top of the insurance business receive ridiculous compensation packages taking a lot of the money out of the healthcare system; they are simply corporate tax collectors who take the money and go. It is legalized thievery that has been put on us by our own government and our government now tells us they are going to fix the problem! They created the problem! They created the antitrust protection for insurance companies! They created the providers being paid by third parties because of a very high individual incremental tax rate that was confiscating the income of factory workers so the business companies went on giving nontaxed perks instead of paying higher wages. The government created that situation; the free market at that point quit existing and the destruction of American medicine began.

If you want healthcare to be readily available and want it to reach the cost level that it should be at, let the market take effect, let the people have free market medicine which we did not have in this country in our lifetime. All the problems the government is complaining about have been created by the government itself. Now they say they are going to fix it with socialism. Socialism has worked nowhere. The basic tenet of socialism is that people would do the right thing even when it is bad for them. The fact is that it is not human nature; people do not behave like that. If it is bad for them and bad for their families they do not cooperate, they simply try to work around the system and do as little as they can and the system becomes extremely inefficient. So socialized system is always a medical rationing system; it delays diagnosis, it delays care, it makes people so fed up with the system they do not even try to get care unless they are desperately ill. And when they are desperately ill they find out they cannot be seen by the doctor soon enough to do them any good.

You know in this country if you have a severe new headache and you go to the emergency room you get an MRI that night. In Canada with its socialized system, you cannot come to see your family doctor in a week, and then the primary care doctor says you need to see a neurologist, and the neurologist says you need an MRI, so now you are four months out and your brain cancer is inoperative whereas it would have been curable probably four months before (Man's penis amputated following misdiagnosis, 2010). So the system saved the surgery, saved the radiation, saved the chemotherapy and they can simply send the patient home with a bottle of pain elixir that is fairly cheap; that is socialized medicine. That is a cost-saving system also but it is not equal to a system that pushes the cost down by competition.

Why cannot we work the efficient way? Why does the food cost remain so low? Why do so many things and services have low cost? Because we let the market decide the price, but in medicine we let the government, the insurance companies, and hospitals decide what it is going to be. We regulate things to the degree that the providers of care have no saying in anything. Doctors are prevented from creating their own surgery centers by CON (Certificate of Need) requirements; they are prevented from getting a DNE number so they can be reimbursed for their supplies and equipment as hospitals and surgery centers are. Otherwise, these practices have to take the loss on supplies to offer office procedures without any increase in reimbursement. It is nearly impossible without jumping through exhaustive bureaucratic hoops. You have to hire a consultant and pay a lawyer and work nearly two years to get it. So it is not a free market and it is bad for the patients, bad for the provider and bad for the system.

You would get the most care for the least money if you establish a system that works by the market rules. The system we have now shifts large amounts of money from the hospitals, which are politically connected and have a good lobby; it shifts a big amount of the ability to control things to insurance companies, who have similarly good lobbies. So, do they really "manage care"? Of course not; they spend their time delaying and preventing payment and wasting money on checking physician's credentials instead! The government has already checked our credentials and given us a license to practice medicine and the hospital has checked our credentials and given us hospital privileges. That is all a worthless waste of time. It has nothing to do with anything except for controlling what they pay doctors. Why would an insurance company say to a licensed physician who has hospital privileges that he is unacceptable! It is ridiculous on the face of it. But they want you to jump all over their hoops and fill their paper work. To what end? If we are that bad why are we licensed by the state and why do we have hospital privileges? All this has nothing to do with quality and is just pretending to be "managing care" because what they are really doing is managing to shift the revenue. For example, we have one case that we are trying to collect on for over eight months now that has been deliberately incorrectly paid; it has been appealed and appealed and appealed. The patient had extensive laparoscopic procedures and hysteroscopy done at the same time. They paid the hysteroscopy as primary and bundled the rest into it which does not meet the coding regulations; and they have dragged their feet over nearly a year unfairly. If this is an isolated incidence, fine, but this is routine behavior by the insurance companies. They are able to treat providers like this because the providers have no protection and the government is doing nothing to help them. We are continuously hammered by the insurance companies who actually work as a monopoly and tell us what they will pay and the government is not following its responsibility to regulate the industry and to investigate the routine fraudulent behavior of insurance companies, all without exception.

The insurance companies have an exemption from antitrust law, it is not clear why?! Perhaps because they need to share actuarial data. So, by allowing insurance companies to go for profit and having exemption from antitrust law, the insurance companies have now totally different motivation. They are responsible to the stockholders; they have a motivation at the top to rip off the system and make a lot of money. Even people at the second and third echelons in insurance companies are taking home large paychecks, far more than you think they would deserve for the work they are doing. What makes it so valuable? They are skimming the money out of system, they are taking the money that should go to take care of patients and utilizing large bureaucracies that are set up to delay reimbursement and not pay and not pay and hope the physician would give up then deflect all that money to the company and its stockholders and its layers of executives. And that is exactly what is happening. They do not have "Managed Care;" they have done nothing to improve care in this country. Arguably, they made it a lot worse, because they made it very difficult to get procedures and screening tests done. "Managed care maims and kills patients" as Dr. Linda Peno said in her testimony before the Congress on May 30th 1996 (Moore, 2007). This is the "dirty" work of managed care (Moore, 2007). It is also ironically amusing! There was a time when it was almost impossible to get a hysterectomy approved. Physicians, however, found a way in order to do it. You do not get a hysterectomy approved; so you do a diagnostic hysteroscopy and you prove the patient has a hypertrophic enlarged uterine cavity causing the heavy flow and you show it to the insurance company; you do an endometrial ablation and the patient continues to have cyclic pelvic pain and enlarged uterus due to adenomyosis; now you have two procedures that would have been saved if the initial hysterectomy was initially approved. Now, they have reversed themselves on all that, because they found out they were paying out a lot of money. Now if the patient is over thirty and has symptoms that are documented, it is fairly easy to get approved for a hysterectomy. It is all just a big game and they change the game rules regularly. It has nothing to do with what is good for the patient. It has to do with holding on to the money. They do not care about care. This whole concept of "Managed

Care" is ludicrous! What interest does an insurance company have in dropping the cost of medicine?! Remember, they make their money by how much money they hold. So the higher the premium the market can bear the higher the amount of money they hold. Why would they want the premium to go any lower than the number of working people who can afford to pay for it? They hold less money they make less money. The other part is they want to delay the payment of legitimate claims as long as they can because they want to hold the money as long as they can. That is a bureaucracy that is employed to eat up patients' money and deny providers reimbursement for legitimate procedures. That is what is going on and they are protected still by these antitrust laws because they have an exemption!

Physicians on the other hand are completely unprotected. If we do anything to try protect ourselves as a group, because we are competing businesses and we are covered completely by the antitrust laws, we get fined or we go to jail. It is not a fair game, why do antitrust laws apply to doctors and not insurance companies if they are all for profit?! When insurance companies originally were not for profit, antitrust protection made sense but when the government allowed them to go for profit they should have taken their antitrust exemption away which they have not. So insurance companies dictate to us and we are powerless.

We will never have a constructive change in the delivery of and cost efficiency of our health care system until community healthcare providers and patients have an equal seat at the table with third party payers and hospitals. The federal government is the entity that has disempowered providers and patients via regulation and law creating winners and losers and disabling the free market impact on medical care that would otherwise with improving technology drive down the cost of care.

HOSPITALS EMPLOYING DOCTORS

Late people might think that hospitals employing doctors is a good thing. In certain areas where hospital-based doctors are present doing things for other doctors it is useful. They do not have to fight for the patients' rights, they are just responding to a physician's order. So, I order an X-ray study, I get a good X-ray read from the hospital-employed radiologist; this does not negatively affect the patient. The pathologist, the same thing, employed by the hospital; they give me a good read, it is done. It is not affecting the patient's care adversely. Now we start to get to the point where we have physicians that are actually doing the evaluation and the direct the care of the patient, the hospital can tell them this is not schematic or according to the protocol for the care of that patient. It becomes the bureaucrats are telling the physician how to take care of the patient. I have more than a quarter a century experience in what I do, I am good at what I do, I know how to work up patients; but I am going to be pushed towards either doing what the hospital wants or lose my hospital privileges. As we are now, separate entities, we are able to advocate for the patient; the patient does not want to lose the independent patient advocate because whatever the government, lawyers and everybody else think or try to say about us, the majority of physicians do a good job taking care of their patients, and they try, when the hospitals interfere with that, to make the hospitals behave and take care of their patients. If physicians become hospital employees, we are disempowered completely. We already have a system put in place where they have what is called the "Disruptive Physician" policy which on the face of it sounds good because it says we are going to deal with physicians who break out and start cursing and throwing things or come in drunk or come in with other aberrant behavior. But that is not the only way the policy is used. The policy is used to go after doctors who are righteously angry about bad care in the hospital. Now already they disempowered us to some degree even without us being employed by them, because if we get angry and express that anger to the wrong level person we are then called "disruptive" and no longer is the problem the problem, the physician becomes the problem, and we get threatened with anger management. So what does that do with your ability to advocate for the care of the patient? It is extremely suppressing of our ability as patient advocates. If you get threatened a couple of times with things that will go on your permanent record it very much disinclines you from actively trying to make the people at the working level do their job. You are still responsible for the patient; that person is doing improper care for your patient; but now if you direct your criticism to that person who is doing the care and state that what they are doing is wrong then you are "disruptive." Now if we, doctors, want to express our unhappiness with the work of a hospital employee we have to go to several levels higher in management and explain our frustration to that high-level person and we often get a letter back that there was actually no problem. So, doctors essentially have been "castrated" already in hospitals by limiting their direct input on hospital work appraisal. Now they want to finish the process by making us employees. If we are employed by hospitals we can no longer advocate for the patient if we want to keep our job. If we lose the job and hospital privileges because we are not a "team player" with one hospital what is the possibility of us getting hospital privileges at another hospital with a tarnished record. When we say the patient needs this other care but it costs a little more we are advocating for a better patient care which is more economically viable in the long term. So, what you lose when you have a nonindependent physician is you lose the ability to confront the bureaucracy and advocate for the care of the patient. Many doctors will not be able to tolerate a system that is so much bureaucratic and lose hope of working in such system effectively.

REFERENCES

Angrisano C, F. D. (2007). *Accounting for the.* San Francisco, CA: McKinsey Global Institute.

Butala, N. (2010). Perspectives on Efficiency and Quality in an Ever Changing System. *Yale J. Biol. Med. 83(2)*, 93–95.

Emanuel EJ, F. V. (2008). *The perfect storm of overutilization. JAMA.* ;299(23):2789-91.

Friedman, M. (2001). How to cure health care. *The Public Interest.*

Man's penis amputated following misdiagnosis. (2010). *The Local.*

Moore, M. (Director). (2007). *Sicko* [Motion Picture].

Richardson, W. e. (2001). *Crossing the Quality Chasm: A New Health System for the 21st Century.* Committee on Quality of Health Care in America, Institute of Medicine.

The World Health Report 2000 – Health systems: Improving performance. World Health Organization.

In: Toward Healthcare Resource Stewardship
Editors: J. S.Robinson, M. S.Walid et al.

ISBN: 978-1-62100-182-9
© 2012 Nova Science Publishers, Inc.

Chapter 20

AN ECONOMIC ANALYSIS OF THE PHYSICIAN WORKFORCE SHORTAGE

Don K. Nakayama[*]

Department of Surgery, Medical Center of Central Georgia,
Macon, GA, US

ABSTRACT

The physician shortage reflects issues that involve supply and demand, and so have economics as its foundation. The interactions of supply, demand, and prices, create shortages and surpluses. Traditionally economists plot supply and demand curves, with the intersection indicating the point of equilibrium where both match at the market clearing price. Keeping prices artificially low describes a situation where suppliers are unwilling to provide goods at a quantity sufficient to meet demand. This situation exists in medicine, where there is a perceived physician shortage. One way to resolve this situation is through market based mechanisms that more accurately reflect the shortage in physician supply. Another mechanism through which a shortage arises is through entry barriers, a situation that has evolved through licensure, board accreditation, and restriction of immigration. Thus another solution involves decreasing entry barriers and broadening supply of providers through physician extenders and relaxed immigration restrictions. Economic analyses provides insights into the nature of workforce shortages, focuses on the issues of supply, demand and prices, and suggests rational solutions to their solutions.

INTRODUCTION

The shortage of medical providers in the U.S. is a central issue of health policy [1, 2] and extends into all specialties, including surgery [3]. Issues of supply and demand in physician workforce thus inform important decisions regarding the education and accreditation of

[*] Don K. Nakayama, MD, MBA. Department of Surgery, Medical Center of Central Georgia, 777 Hemlock St., H.B. 140, Macon, GA 31201. Phone: 478-633-1367. Fax: 478-633-5153. E-mail: nakayama.don@mccg.org.

physicians and surgeons and affect policies regarding immigration of foreign-trained providers. Proposals for health reform attempt to address the some 50 million U.S. residents presently without health insurance coverage. Integration of millions into the demand side of the health care equation will make supply issues worse. Physician education and training takes several years, so decisions that focus solely on increasing supply through traditional educational tracks will not have immediate effects.

Discussions on health care supply and demand have economics as a foundation. Traditional issues regarding physician education and training have centered on educational content, caseload, knowledge, and clinical judgment. Economics, however, is better suited as an analytic decision tool when the subject turns to numbers of physicians, demand for services, and compensation for practitioners. Just as recombinant DNA technology forced many scientists to educate themselves in molecular genetics as a basis for their research, current health policy issues require an understanding of supply, demand, and prices, and how their interactions create shortages and surpluses.

The issue of the physician workforce shortage is a textbook illustration of these economic principles. Our discussion follows *Health Care Economics* (6th edition, Clifton Park, NY, Thomson Delmar Learning, 2005), an excellent text by Paul J. Feldstein [4].

SUPPLY, DEMAND AND PRICE

Economists plot supply and demand with quantity on the horizontal axis and price on the vertical (Figure 1), different from the scientific and mathematical convention of placing the independent variable on the abscissa and the dependent variable on the ordinate. Suppliers will increase their goods as the price increases, so the supply line slopes upward to the right (S1). Conversely, consumers will buy less with higher prices, so the demand line slopes downward to the right (D1). Where the two lines intersect is known as the market-clearing price (P1), the point where supply matches demand at quantity Q1. At a lower price there is excess demand, so suppliers increase supply; higher prices decrease demand, so suppliers produce less. P1 is the point of equilibrium between supply and demand.

Prices set below this equilibrium point result in an economic shortage in the world of health care economics. The dominant purchasing power of the federal and state government Medicare and Medicaid programs result in prices (P2 in Figure 1) being set below the market-clearing price (P1; in economic terminology, the government has a monopsony). At lower price P2 the demand Q2 is higher, but supply Q3 falls short of meeting the demand and there is a shortage. This phenomenon (lower reimbursement leading to compensation issues) thus contributes a shortage of any product, including the numbers of providers of health care.

NON-ECONOMIC AND ECONOMIC SHORTAGES
OF PHYSICIANS AND SURGEONS

The shortage described above is a true economic shortage: Monopsony price pressure holds supply below demand levels. This is in contradistinction to non-economical shortages. Feldstein notes there are several non-economical assessments of shortages, usually embedded in declarative statements without an economic basis: "We need more physicians," and, "Prices are too high." An example of a noneconomic analysis is using a physician-to-population ratio to judge whether there are enough doctors for a community, with the implication that a certain ratio reflects an ideal situation. Another example is comparison of per capita spending on health care, again implying there is a level where spending is excessive. While the first involves numbers of providers, or supply, and the second gives an index of expenditure, or price, neither can be considered to give an economic analysis whether a shortage exists.

However well-informed by surveys, census data, and expert opinion, these determinations of need are arbitrary and do not reflect either the supply or demand curves. This is the situation we face today. The various accrediting bodies that educate medical students (the Liaison Committee on Medical Education and the Association of American Medical Colleges), train resident physicians (Accreditation Council of Graduate Medical Education), and fund physician training (Centers for Medicare and Medicaid Services) have determined that more doctors must be trained to meet future supply. An arbitrary number thereby is set that the agencies believe will satisfy demand in the future independent of market forces such as physician compensation and costs of training. Figure 2 illustrates the situation: line N sets the quantity of services thought to be needed independently of where lines S1 and D1 exist. N is a vertical line because it is independent of price.

Thus wherever line N is set will result in either an excess or deficit of pediatric surgeons. N to the right of the intersection of S1 and D1 will result in supply greater than demand (see where N intersects with S1 and D1); to the left, demand will exceed supply. It is unlikely that N will be set exactly where S1 and D1 intersect. Real-life examples and consequences abound: Every year there is a shortage of popular toys during Christmas shopping seasons (N to the left the intersection of S1 and D1). Flu seasons where there are excess doses of vaccine reflect the opposite situation. Both result from non-economic decisions where to place line N.

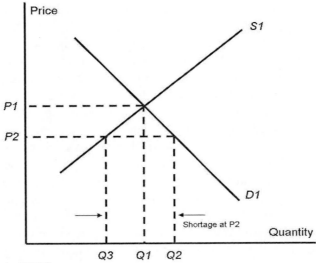

Adapted from Feldstein (2005).

Figure 1. Supply and demand relationships. At price P1 Supply S1 is in equilibrium with demand D1 at quantity Q1. At price P2 demand Q2 exceeds supply Q3 and a shortage exists.

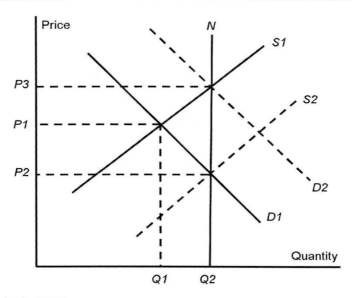

Adapted from Feldstein (2005).

Figure 2. Non-economic determination of a workforce shortage. Supply, demand, and price relationships are given as S1, D1, P1 and quantity Q1. A determination of need Q2 and is defined by line N. Meeting the desired quantity Q2 can be met by increasing supply, S2, with a corresponding decrease in price, P2. Alternatively, Q2 can also be met by increasing demand, D2, with an increase in price, P3.

Figure 2 shows the economic solutions to reach the desired quantity of providers, Q2, determined by line N. First is to increase supply, shifting the supply line to S2, which lies below and to the right of the original line S1. In fact this is already happening: in addition to the increased numbers of positions in U.S. allopathic medical schools and residencies, the numbers of osteopathic positions are increasing at an even faster rate. Foreign medical graduates take unfilled positions in many residency training programs. In addition non-physicians, such as nurse practitioners, are gaining increasing acceptance as independent providers of care. Osteopathic and foreign trained physicians and nurse practitioners, known as substitutes in economic terms, respond to the economic shortage and increase supply.

The effect of increasing supply on price is also shown in Figure 2. The market clearing price P2 in this situation rests at the intersection between S2 and D1. P2 falls below P1, meaning that with increased supply salaries and compensation will fall. While many osteopathic and foreign trained providers command the same levels of compensation as U.S. educated and trained allopathic physicians, they often take jobs in less desirable areas of the country such as remote rural areas and areas of poverty. Nurse practitioners are low cost providers of care and also reflect the effects on provider price when supply curves are shifted rightward. Figure 2 shows that N also intersects at that point, but we have discussed already that setting N requires a degree of forecasting and planning impossible to achieve.

A second means of increasing supply is to increase demand, shifting the demand curve D1 upward and to the right to D2. Without a change in the position of the supply line S1, the market clearing price moves to price P3, above P1. Again, whether that matches with the predicted need line N is a matter of luck. A shift in demand can be induced by a demand subsidy, such as increasing insurance coverage for surgical services, so that more surgeons are attracted to the practice. In a freely operating market, surgeons, attracted by the increased price, would begin to shift their practice into that area. A current example is the trauma surgeon subsidy offered by hospital trauma centers or state-wide trauma systems to make taking trauma call more lucrative and palatable to general surgeons.

In the field of pediatric surgery there also appears to be a true economic shortage. Pediatric surgical practices have had to increase the size of their groups to eight to ten from four to five. Hospitals with large pediatric volumes need pediatric surgeons on staff to cover neonatal and pediatric intensive care units in addition to providing operative services to children and infants. Pediatricians, trained hospitals where pediatric surgeons are readily available, expect the same back-up in their new positions. General surgeons who care primarily for adult conditions are less available and less willing to perform basic general surgery operations on pediatric patients. So there are several indications that there is a true shift in the demand curve to position D2.

In a freely operating market, the supply will move up curve S1 to meet the new demand curve D2 and set a higher market-clearing price P3. But in economic terms the supply curve for pediatric surgery is inelastic: quantity does not change significantly with any price change because supply is constrained. The constrained supply of pediatric surgeons is a legacy of having a limited number of training programs, the long training period necessary for board certification, and the long-standing view that the ideal pediatric surgical practice was in a specialty children's hospital that could attract the necessary case mix of index operations, the complicated cases like congenital corrective surgery and tumor cases, that define the specialty. In fact the Residency Review Committee, the group responsible for approving training programs in the specialty, requires that a program provide trainees with a minimum number of index cases during the course of training. Once trained the surgeon must pass examinations by the American Board of Surgery. These administrative hurdles constrain the supply of pediatric surgeons, to the economic benefit of the group, by keeping supply low, demand high, and prices high. The myriad job listings on professional web sites (e.g., the American Pediatric Surgical Association), the individual hospital advertisements, and job bulletin boards at national pediatric surgical conferences attest that a shortage of pediatric surgeons exists.

The true situation is illustrated in Figure 3. The short-term supply curve is S1, illustrated here as a vertical line because the supply is Q1 at any price, or in the Figure, wages: in economic terms the supply of pediatric surgeons is completely inelastic. Wages W1 are the intersection between the demand line D1 and S1. If surgeons were free to enter pediatric surgery regardless of education and certification, the supply line would be SL (L for long-term, the situation that will exist once enough pediatric surgeons enter the market and can freely decide to practice depending on the wage level). The intersection between D1 and SL shows both the expected market-clearing wage W0, and the quantity of services provided Q0. The difference between W1 and W0 are the excess wages given to pediatric surgeons currently in practice, and results from their monopoly power on the market. The graph illustrates is the difference in quantity of services provided under circumstances where the short term inelastic supply curve S1 and the long term curve SL after entry of sufficient numbers of pediatric surgeons. The difference between Q0 and Q1 is the true economic shortage of pediatric surgery.

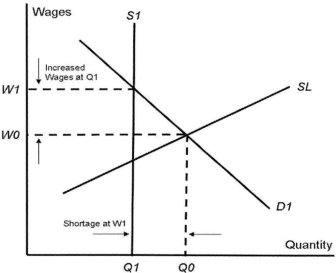

Adapted from Feldstein (2005).

Figure 3. Shortage created by restriction of supply. The supply curve S1 over the short term is inelastic and therefore vertical, i.e., insensitive to changes in price. If there were no shortage of pediatric surgeons, or when the supply eventually eliminates shortage, the supply line would be SL (L for long term). Market clearing wages would be W0 and the quantity provided would be Q0. With a shortage of surgeons created by entry barriers, the intersection between S1 and D1 gives the quantity Q1 and wages W1. Quantity provided is therefore lower and wages are higher.

DYNAMIC AND STATIC SHORTAGES

According to Feldstein, a dynamic shortage occurs when there is an increase in demand but the new price has not increased to reflect the new equilibrium point. Prices are an important signal to the market: increased prices are a signal that increased profits are available. Suppliers therefore increase the quantity of goods produced to meet increased demand. Thus dynamic shortages are temporary and are nearly instantaneous for commodities like aspirin and bread. Static shortages occur because supply does not increase in respond to increased demand. In the case of adult general surgery, prices are controlled and prevented from rising to the equilibrium level. If prices cannot rise, general surgeons cannot cover their expenses and pay for increased staff necessary to accommodate the increased patient load. At some point they choose free time or retirement to more work.

In the case of pediatric surgery, there is a fixed constraint in the pipeline of new pediatric surgeons. Practice patterns and professional credentialing prevent other surgeons from freely entering the practice of pediatric surgery. Thus we see excess profits come to pediatric surgeons in practice, and limited entry of more pediatric surgeons into the market. Increased subsidies to the few new entrants and those already in practice will not alleviate the static shortage because these changes do not address the entry barriers, and only serve to increase the returns to a specialty already earning excess profits. Increasing the number of pediatric surgical training programs will increase the number of practitioners, but the response will be 'sticky' insofar as their effect will be years in coming until the new fellows graduate in significant numbers to affect supply.

The most direct way to address a static shortage is to ease entry barriers. Feldstein asks whether professional associations and medical board accreditation requirements serve to preserve physicians' monopoly power (reflected in pediatric surgery as excess profits or wages), or as a means of consumer (patient) protection. In economic terms such requirements are entry barriers that prevent free entry into the field. Examples abound: graduation from an approved medical school, training requirements, state licensure, and board certification. In surgery trainees choose to enter general surgical practice than devote the extra years required to gain acceptance in a surgical residency like pediatrics. Entry barriers, especially in medical professions, are easy to rationalize. The public interest is served by assuring that a surgeon has complete training, with qualifications certified by an impartial professional board. But in economic terms it is still an entry barrier that creates an economic shortage to the financial benefit of members of the profession, illustrating perfectly the view of economics as the "dismal science" of 19th century historian Thomas Carlyle.

SOLUTIONS

Solutions must address monopsony pricing and entry barriers, the underlying economic causes that have led to shortages of physicians and surgeons. Single payment systems where the government acts as the agent for consumers will only exacerbate shortages by giving it monopsony pricing power, as discussed above. Patients will pay in the form of decreased access to medical and surgical care (supply) and longer wait times for necessary care (time, the other form of "payment" in short supply besides money). Placing resources back in the hands of patients through medical savings accounts will return them as consumers who respond to market signals and make independent decisions regarding providers, quality, and other considerations including proximity and ease. Consumers will also be able to purchase insurance based upon their perceived risk of needing care, the consequences to themselves and their families should they become sick, and the value they place on health. In a free market system such decisions require transparency of information, so outcome data for providers is necessary. Such a system depends on consumers able to make informed decisions, so primary providers of care, nurses or physicians, must act as educators or consumers' (i.e., patients') agents in complicated situations. They, too, would receive market-based compensation based upon the value they deliver to their patients.

Strategies that address entry barriers must address the bona fide need to protect the public from unqualified practitioners. Quality measures should be based upon outcome and not solely educational and training processes. Measures to ease licensure requirements of qualified domestic- and foreign-trained surgeons would increase supply, as would decreasing the overall time required for training. Having a tiered training paradigm, where general surgeons would receive additional training to provide community hospital-level pediatric surgery services, is another means of addressing supply. Removing the requirements that high-level neonatal intensive care nurseries have on staff pediatric surgeons may be an additional means of lessening the demand.

In summary, the workforce problem in medicine and surgery illustrates basic economic principles of supply and demand. Decisions made today – the numbers and lengths of training, licensure and certification requirements – will have effects on workforce, medical and surgical practice, and reimbursement that likely will last for decades. Solutions must address two economic bases of the current workforce shortage: the monopsony power of government pricing and physician and surgeon monopolies created by entry barriers. Market-based solutions that address these causes will be more likely to be successful than command and control manipulations. In the words of Steven Levitt, author of *Freakonomics* (New York, HarperCollins, 2005), "Incentives are the cornerstone of modern life. 'Experts' use informational advantages for their own agenda. Knowing what to measure and how to measure it make a complicated world much less so [5]."

REFERENCES

[1]   Cooper RA. The coming era of too few physicians. *Bull. Amer. Coll. Surg.* 2008;93:11-18.

[2]   Cooper RA, Getzen TE, McKee HJ, and Laud P. Economic and demographic trends signal an impending physician shortage. *Health Affairs* 2004;21:140-54.

[3]   Sheldon GF and Schroen AT. Supply and demand – surgical and health workforce. *Surg. Clin. N. Am.* 2004; 84:1493-1509.

[4]   Feldstein PJ. *Health Care Economics*, 6th edition. Clifton Park, NY, Thomson Delmar Learning, 2005.

[5]   Levitt S. *Freakonomics*. New York, HarperCollins, 2005.

In: Toward Healthcare Resource Stewardship   ISBN: 978-1-62100-182-9
Editors: J. S.Robinson, M. S.Walid et al.   © 2012 Nova Science Publishers, Inc.

Chapter 21

COST AWARENESS IN CLINICAL RESEARCH: LACK OF COST INCLUSION IN THE CLINICAL METHODOLOGY IN SPINE FUSION LITERATURE

M. Sami Walid,[1]* *Joe Sam Robinson III*[2] *and Joe Sam Robinson Jr.*[1,2,3]

[1]Medical Center of Central Georgia, Macon, GA, US
[2]Mercer University School of Medicine, Macon, GA, US
[3]Georgia Neurosurgical Institute, Macon, GA, US

ABSTRACT

Background. Some observers have highlighted the relative lack of level one clinical evidence supporting the increasing trend in spine fusion procedures (Resnick et al. 2005). To better specify this issue we conducted a review of the available clinical evidence upon which such practices are based.

Methods. Firstly, the Nationwide Inpatient Sample (NIS) database was probed for fusion rates and cost. Secondly, employing the PubMed search engine (January 2011) the keywords: *spine fusion degenerative, clinical trials, English, Humans* were assessed between 1978 and 2011. Seventy four papers were indexed, all of which were reviewed to access clinical methodology.

Results. Spine fusion procedures more than tripled in number from 1997 to 2008 while corresponding hospital charges increased more than ten times.

The 74 clinical trials accounted for only 5.5% of all papers on spine fusion for degenerative disease. Of these, 71 (96%) somewhat nebulously defined degenerative spine disease with or without myelopathy as the main inclusion criterion, 50 papers had preoperative radiographic evaluation, 47 papers quantified pain and function preoperatively, 21 papers mentioned failure of conservative treatment, and 12 papers mentioned the duration of disease/pain from 6 weeks to 6 years. Thirty four (46%) papers had exclusion criteria, the most frequent of which were prior spine surgery (N=17), neoplasia (N=10), infection (N=8), trauma/fracture (N=8) and myelopathy (N=2).

---

[*] Corresponding Author: M. Sami Walid. Medical Center of Central Georgia, 840 Pine Street, Suite 880, Macon, GA 31201, (478) 743-7092 ex. 266. E-mail: mswalid@yahoo.com.

Comorbidities were included as confounding variable in only 11 (15%) papers of 74. The least used outcome variables were consumption of healthcare resources, long-term mortality and reoperation on a distant spine region (N=7, N=6, N=1 respectively). The total number of patients in the extracted papers was 245,422. The average age of these patients was 53 years. The average percentage of females was 55% and the average follow-up period was 3.5 years.

Conclusion. Outcome analysis in spine fusion research would benefit from methodological standardization with better attention to consumption of healthcare resources.

INTRODUCTION

Over the last several decades, among other factors, new technologies and approaches have dramatically increased the frequency of operative spine fusion interventions. Parallel to this, there was no apparent increase in high-grade clinical evidence supporting this trend (Resnick et al. 2005).

In this paper we study the specifics of research methodology related to spine fusion and the comprehensiveness of outcome parameters used in clinical investigation with an insight into the aggregate cost of this major and expensive procedure.

METHODS

The study consists of three branches:

1. The national cost of spine fusion was extracted from the Nationwide Inpatient Sample (NIS) website.
2. Level I or II evidence papers related to spine fusion for degenerative disease were extracted using the biomedical search engine PubMed (January 2011) and the following criteria: English, Studies on Humans, and Clinical trials. The following methodological elements were investigated:

    1) Inclusion criteria of the cohorts in the extracted papers were studied as regards preoperative pain, duration of pain and failure of conservative treatment.
    2) Exclusion criteria were studied regarding history of previous spine surgery and others.
    3) Average age of patient cohort.
    4) Percentage of females in the cohort.
    5) Average follow-up period.
    6) Outcome parameters were categorized as follows:
        *   Pain (visual analog scale).
        *   Function (Oswestry disability scale, arm/leg function, return to work).
        *   Radiography (angle/range of motion, fusion).
        *   Complications (postoperative).
        *   Mortality during follow-up.
        *   Reoperation on the same or distant spine region.

- Patient satisfaction.
- Consumption of healthcare resources as reflected by length of stay (LOS) or cost.

7) Comorbidities, as a confounding variable, were also recorded because of the important relationship between comorbidities and fusion outcome as well as complications and mortality.

3. U.S. population life expectancy was obtained from the Social Security Website. Average age of patients in the literature is compared with the average age of fusion patients in country.

For comparison purposes the total number of papers indexed in PubMed using the criteria "Humans" and "English" and keywords "spine fusion degenerative" is recorded.

The average age of the patient cohorts in the extracted papers was calculated using the formula:

Average age = $(\sum N*M)/\sum N$ where N is the number of studies and M is the average age in each study.

The average percentage of females and average follow-up period for all extracted papers were calculated using the simpler formulas:

Average percentage of females = $\sum M/\sum N$

Average follow-up = $\sum M/\sum N$

RESULTS

Spine Fusion Prevalence and Cost

In 2008, hospital charges related to lumbar fusion procedures amounted to $34 billion. The average age of lumbar fusion patients was 54 years in 2008. There were 413,171 lumbar fusion procedures in USA in the same year. More females (54.4%) than males underwent spinal fusion procedures in the same year (Figures 1 and 2).

Probing Spine Fusion Literature

Using PubMed and the keywords *spine fusion degenerative* 74 clinical trials dated from 1978 to 2011 were indexed as "English" and on "Humans". All papers underwent further investigation on inclusion/exclusion criteria and outcome analysis. For comparison purposes, search of papers on PubMed using the criteria "Humans" and "English" and keywords "spine fusion degenerative" yields 1348 papers, 203 reviews, 154 case reports/series and 13 meta-analysis papers. Thus, trials made only 5.5% of all papers on spine fusion for degenerative disease (Figure 3). None of them were blinded.

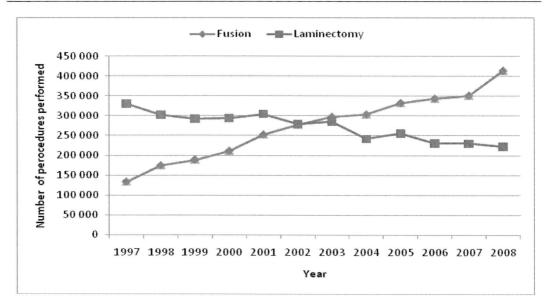

Figure 1. Total number of laminectomies and lumbar fusions performed in US per year 1997-2008.

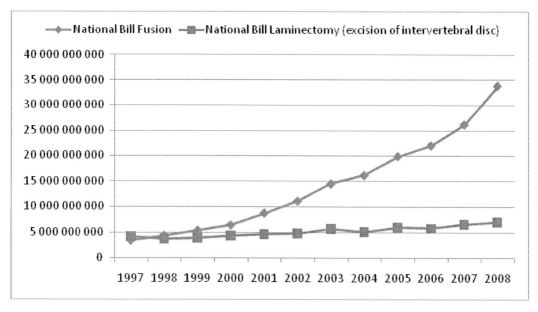

Figure 2. Hospital charges associated with lumbar fusion and laminectomy procedures per year 1997-2008.

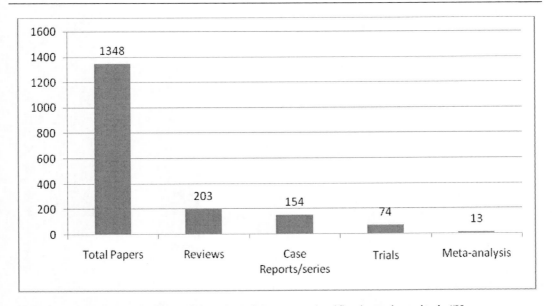

Figure 3. Number of papers indexed in PubMed per paper classification using criteria "Humans, English" and keywords: spine fusion degenerative.

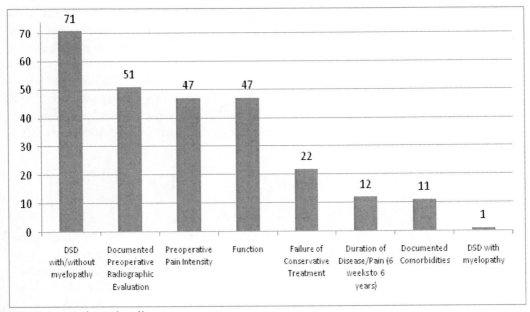

DSD: Degenerative spine disease.

Figure 4. The number of papers reporting preoperative spine indications and comorbidities.

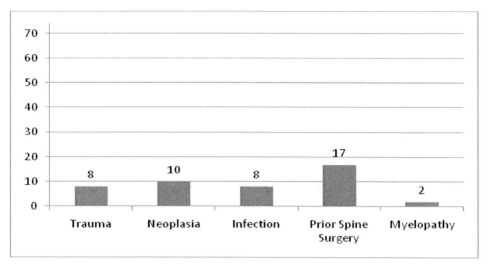

Figure 5. The number of papers with exclusion criteria.

Inclusion and Exclusion Criteria

71 (96%) papers mentioned degenerative spine disease with/without myelopathy as the main inclusion criterion. Among these, 50 papers had preoperative radiographic evaluation, 47 papers quantified pain and function preoperatively, 21 papers mentioned failure of conservative treatment, and 12 papers mentioned the duration of disease/pain from 6 weeks to 6 years (Figure 4). Thirty four (46%) papers had exclusion criteria (Figure 5), the most frequent of which were prior spine surgery (N=17), neoplasia (N=10), infection (N=8), trauma/fracture (N=8) and myelopathy (N=2). Comorbidities were included as confounding variable in only 11 (15%) papers of 74. No paper mentioned the amount of disease-modifying medications at the time of the study.

Outcome Parameters

Fiver papers used 5 outcome parameters, 10 papers used 4 parameters, 34 papers used 3 parameters, 12 papers used 2 parameters, and 13 papers used one parameter. Pain and function were the most commonly used parameters (N=47, N=47, respectively), followed by radiography, complications, reoperation and patient satisfaction (N=40, N=21, N=19, N=16, respectively). Among papers studying reoperation, only one paper mentioned reoperation on a different site. The least used variables were consumption of healthcare resources and mortality (N=7, N=6, respectively, Figure 6).

Age, Female Percentage and Follow-Up Periods in Spine Fusion Literature

The total number of patients in the extracted papers was 245,422. The average age of these patients was 53 years. The average percentage of females was 55% and the average follow-up period was 3.5 years (Figure 7). The follow-up period in the 81% of these papers is <5 years.

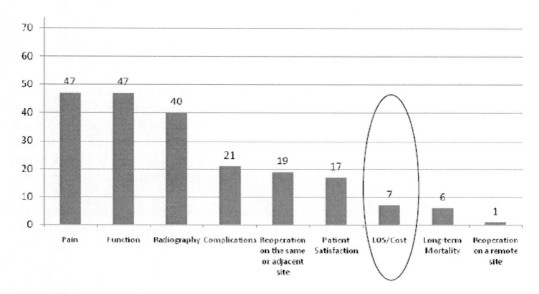

Figure 6. Outcome variables used in 74 spine fusion papers (notice lack of cost inclusion!).

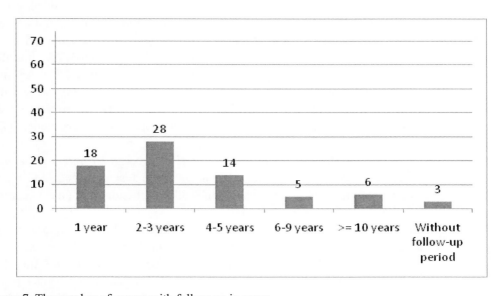

Figure 7. The number of papers with follow-up in years.

DISCUSSION

A review of national data demonstrates that spine fusion procedures have more than tripled in numbers since 1997 while corresponding hospital charges for such procedures have increased more than ten times. An aging population, advances in spine surgical technology, improved diagnostic modalities, better access to spine surgery, and possibly compensation issues may explain to some degree such an impressive increase.

While in our assessment of the literature some supportive papers germane to the subject may have been excluded by our strict selection criteria, rigorous and expansive clinical support for such an increase in fusion rates is a bit sparse. Reasonably, randomized controlled trials account for only a small percentage of spine surgery literature. For after all, blinded randomization and outcome analysis is often ethically and logistically difficult to implement; as well as being expensive. Also of difficulty with this cohort of patients is their relative older age associated with many secondary clinical afflictions – factors often defeating appropriate subcategorization for effective clinical analysis. Additionally sufficient numbers of patients to support statistical validation are often difficult to obtain and may require several institutions to join together in a cooperative study, a process fraught with difficulties. Nevertheless, our literature review extracted level I evidence papers on spine fusion with a summated cohort of around 250,000 patients.

Among the reviewed studies, inclusion criteria were not unified or homogenous. Most papers fail to describe the indications for surgery while the boundaries of the disease are poorly defined in terms of severity and duration. Additionally, confounding variables such as comorbidity and medication protocols were missing in the majority of patients.

Similar problems existed in outcome analysis. Most papers assessed mainly pain, function, and radiographic results. On a positive note, the use of visual analog scale and Oswestry disability scale commencing rather universally in our literature review at about 1999 did usefully enhance clinical comparisons. Substantially less interest was displayed in costs, mortality, and re-operation on different spine regions. Long-term mortality and cost are basic elements of cost effectiveness analysis. An example of how important the long-term mortality parameter is: a study from 2005 showed a 10-year survival rate of 67.7% (mortality 32.3%) among patients enrolled in the study with an average age of 65.6 years [1]. Absence of therapeutic cost assessment is particularly troubling in light of the present-day unsustainable rise in national healthcare expenditures; and particularly so considering the major increase in the amount of healthcare resources devoted to spine fusion procedures ($30 billion in 2008).

Reoperation rates, both at close-by spine level and distant levels were rarely mentioned despite the causal relationship existing between the index spine fusion surgery and repeat surgery at adjacent level due to biochemical disturbance and progression of adjacent segment instability [3].

Another problem in the literature was the absence of extended follow-up. Improved life expectancy in the United States has increased the risk of degenerative spine disease and postoperative complications due to comorbidities. Demographic data in the literature corresponded with the national data regarding average age (53-54 years) and gender (more females). However, the follow-up period in the overwhelming majority (81%) of these papers is short (<5 years) and did not reach the average life expectancy of an American citizen at age 54, based on the average patient age of 53-54 years (Table 1).

For objective analysis of spine fusion outcome, larger clinical trials on de novo and recurrent patients, from younger and older age groups, with and without comorbidities, and for longer follow-up periods, with inclusion of cost of care, mortality, and reoperation rates on a distant site in the outcome analysis are needed. Ideally, pursuant to differences in cohort comorbidity status and drop-out rates, studies on younger populations should focus on long-term clinical outcome while studies in older populations focus on complications, mortality, and cost-effectiveness of surgical intervention.

In the United States, there has been a huge increase in fusion rates and corresponding expenses. One would hope that there is substantial base of evidence data to support such an increase. Our review of the subject indicates that evidence is somewhat diffuse. One may well ask the question what is it that influences changes in healthcare practice patterns? It may be local customs, CPT (Current Procedural Terminology) codes, malpractice concerns, or insurance policies. Because of the vagaries in the formulations of the healthcare system, it would be in the nation's best interest if the above-mentioned categories respond to evidence-based practice guidelines (our literature review finds no such guidelines present). Unifying the methodology of clinical research and employment of a checklist of inclusion criteria, exclusion criteria, and outcome parameter would help standardize outcome analysis of spine fusion and related disciplines. Funding for such improved clinical inquiries would be a useful adjunct to national healthcare policy.

Table 1. Life Expectancy per age 54 in USA

	Males	Females
Life Expectancy at age 54 in 2006	25.14	28.68

CONCLUSION

The massive increase in the United States spine fusion rates mandates appropriate clinical trials with particular attention to economic issues.

REFERENCES

[1]   Atlas SJ, Keller RB, Wu YA, Deyo RA, Singer DE. Long-term outcomes of surgical and nonsurgical management of lumbar spinal stenosis: 8 to 10 year results from the maine lumbar spine study. *Spine* (Phila Pa 1976). 2005 Apr 15;30(8):936-43.

[2]   Kanayama M, Togawa D, Hashimoto T, Shigenobu K, Oha F. Motion-preserving surgery can prevent early breakdown of adjacent segments: Comparison of posterior dynamic stabilization with spinal fusion. *J. Spinal Disord. Tech*. 2009 Oct;22(7):463-7.

[3]   Anand N, Baron EM, Thaiyananthan G, Khalsa K, Goldstein TB. Minimally invasive multilevel percutaneous correction and fusion for adult lumbar degenerative scoliosis: a technique and feasibility study. *J. Spinal Disord. Tech*. 2008 Oct;21(7):459-67.

[4]   Berg S, Tullberg T, Branth B, Olerud C, Tropp H. Total disc replacement compared to lumbar fusion: a randomised controlled trial with 2-year follow-up. *Eur. Spine J*. 2009 Oct;18(10):1512-9.

[5]   Bertalanffy H, Eggert HR. Clinical long-term results of anterior discectomy without fusion for treatment of cervical radiculopathy and myelopathy. A follow-up of 164 cases. *Acta Neurochir*. (Wien). 1988;90(3-4):127-35.

[6]   Bhadra AK, Raman AS, Casey AT, Crawford RJ. Single-level cervical radiculopathy: clinical outcome and cost-effectiveness of four techniques of anterior cervical discectomy and fusion and disc arthroplasty. *Eur. Spine J.* 2009 Feb;18(2):232-7.

[7]   Bridwell KH, Baldus C, Berven S, Edwards C 2nd, Glassman S, Hamill C, Horton W, Lenke LG, Ondra S, Schwab F, Shaffrey C, Wootten D. Changes in radiographic and clinical outcomes with primary treatment adult spinal deformity surgeries from two years to three- to five-years follow-up. *Spine* (Phila Pa 1976). 2010 Sep 15;35(20): 1849-54.

[8]   Burkus JK, Haid RW, Traynelis VC, Mummaneni PV. Long-term clinical and radiographic outcomes of cervical disc replacement with the Prestige disc: results from a prospective randomized controlled clinical trial. *J. Neurosurg. Spine.* 2010 Sep;13(3):308-18.

[9]   Cho CB, Ryu KS, Park CK. Anterior lumbar interbody fusion with stand-alone interbody cage in treatment of lumbar intervertebral foraminal stenosis : comparative study of two different types of cages. *J. Korean Neurosurg. Soc.* 2010 May;47(5):352-7.

[10]   Chou YC, Chen DC, Hsieh WA, Chen WF, Yen PS, Harnod T, Chiou TL, Chang YL, Su CF, Lin SZ, Chen SY. Efficacy of anterior cervical fusion: comparison of titanium cages, polyetheretherketone (PEEK) cages and autogenous bone grafts. *J. Clin. Neurosci.* 2008 Nov;15(11):1240-5.

[11]   Ciol MA, Deyo RA, Kreuter W, Bigos SJ. Characteristics in Medicare beneficiaries associated with reoperation after lumbar spine surgery. *Spine* (Phila Pa 1976). 1994 Jun 15;19(12):1329-34.

[12]   Ciol MA, Deyo RA, Howell E, Kreif S. An assessment of surgery for spinal stenosis: time trends, geographic variations, complications, and reoperations. *J. Am. Geriatr. Soc.* 1996 Mar;44(3):285-90.

[13]   Coric D, Cassis J, Carew JD, Boltes MO. Prospective study of cervical arthroplasty in 98 patients involved in 1 of 3 separate investigational device exemption studies from a single investigational site with a minimum 2-year follow-up. Clinical article. *J. Neurosurg. Spine.* 2010 Dec;13(6):715-21.

[14]   Crandall DG, Revella J. Transforaminal lumbar interbody fusion versus anterior lumbar interbody fusion as an adjunct to posterior instrumented correction of degenerative lumbar scoliosis: three year clinical and radiographic outcomes. *Spine* (Phila Pa 1976). 2009 Sep 15;34(20):2126-33.

[15]   Deyo RA, Ciol MA, Cherkin DC, Loeser JD, Bigos SJ. Lumbar spinal fusion. A cohort study of complications, reoperations, and resource use in the Medicare population. *Spine* (Phila Pa 1976). 1993 Sep 1;18(11):1463-70.

[16]   Dufour T, Huppert J, Louis C, Beaurain J, Stecken J, Aubourg L, Vila T. Radiological analysis of 37 segments in cervical spine implanted with a peek stand-alone device, with at least one year follow-up. *Br. J. Neurosurg.* 2010 Dec;24(6):633-40.

[17]   Faldini C, Leonetti D, Nanni M, Di Martino A, Denaro L, Denaro V, Giannini S. Cervical disc herniation and cervical spondylosis surgically treated by Cloward procedure: a 10-year-minimum follow-up study. *J. Orthop. Traumatol.* 2010 Jun; 11(2): 99-103.

[18]   Faldini C, Pagkrati S, Leonetti D, Miscione MT, Giannini S. Sagittal segmental alignment as predictor of adjacent-level degeneration after a Cloward procedure. *Clin. Orthop. Relat. Res.* 2011 Mar;469(3):674-81.

[19]   Freudenberger C, Lindley EM, Beard DW, Reckling WC, Williams A, Burger EL, Patel VV. Posterior versus anterior lumbar interbody fusion with anterior tension band plating: retrospective analysis. *Orthopedics.* 2009 Jul;32(7):492.

[20]   Frymoyer JW, Hanley E, Howe J, Kuhlmann D, Matteri R. Disc excision and spine fusion in the management of lumbar disc disease. A minimum ten-year followup. *Spine* (Phila Pa 1976). 1978 Mar;3(1):1-6.

[21]   Fu KM, Smith JS, Polly DW, Ames CP, Berven SH, Perra JH, McCarthy RE, Knapp DR, Shaffrey CI; the Scoliosis Research Society Morbidity and Mortality Committee. Correlation of higher preoperative American Society of Anesthesiology grade and increased morbidity and mortality rates in patients undergoing spine surgery. *J. Neurosurg. Spine.* 2011 Feb 4. [Epub ahead of print]

[22]   Garrido BJ, Taha TA, Sasso RC. Clinical outcomes of Bryan cervical disc arthroplasty a prospective, randomized, controlled, single site trial with 48-month follow-up. *J. Spinal Disord. Tech.* 2010 Aug;23(6):367-71.

[23]   Hamilton DK, Smith JS, Sansur CA, Glassman SD, Ames CP, Berven SH, Polly DW Jr, Perra JH, Knapp DR Jr, Boachie-Adjei O, McCarthy RE, Shaffrey CI; Scoliosis Research Society Morbidity and Mortality Committee. Rates of New Neurological Deficit Associated with Spine Surgery Based on 108,419 Procedures: A Report of the Scoliosis Research Society Morbidity and Mortality Committee. *Spine* (Phila Pa 1976). 2011 Jan 6. [Epub ahead of print]

[24]   Heary RF, Kheterpal A, Mammis A, Kumar S. Stackable Carbon Fiber Cages for Thoracolumbar Interbody Fusion After Corpectomy: Long-term Outcome Analysis. *Neurosurgery.* 2011 Mar;68(3):810-9.

[25]   Hermansen A, Hedlund R, Vavruch L, Peolsson A. A comparison between the carbon fiber cage and the Cloward procedure in cervical spine surgery: A 10-13 year follow-up of a prospective randomized study. *Spine* (Phila Pa 1976). 2011 Jan 5. [Epub ahead of print]

[26]   Howe CR, Agel J, Lee MJ, Bransford RJ, Wagner TA, Bellabarba C, Chapman JR. The Morbidity and Mortality of Fusions from the Thoracic Spine to the Pelvis in the Adult Population. *Spine* (Phila Pa 1976). 2011 Jan 10. [Epub ahead of print]

[27]   Hu RW, Jaglal S, Axcell T, Anderson G: A population-based study of reoperations after back surgery. *Spine* (Phila Pa 1976). ;22(19):2265-70; discussion 2271, 1997.

[28]   Ito Z, Matsuyama Y, Sakai Y, Imagama S, Wakao N, Ando K, Hirano K, Tauchi R, Muramoto A, Matsui H, Matsumoto T, Kanemura T, Yoshida G, Ishikawa Y, Ishiguro N. Bone union rate with autologous iliac bone versus local bone graft in posterior lumbar interbody fusion. *Spine* (Phila Pa 1976). 2010 Oct 1;35(21):E1101-5.

[29]   Jansson KA, Németh G, Granath F, Blomqvist P. Spinal stenosis re-operation rate in Sweden is 11% at 10 years--a national analysis of 9,664 operations. *Eur. Spine J.* 2005 Sep;14(7):659-63.

[30]   Jiya TU, Smit T, van Royen BJ, Mullender M. Posterior lumbar interbody fusion using non resorbable poly-ether-ether-ketone versus resorbable poly-L: -lactide-co-D: ,L: -lactide fusion devices. Clinical outcome at a minimum of 2-year follow-up. *Eur. Spine J.* 2010 Sep 15. [Epub ahead of print]

[31] Jones AA, Stambough JL, Balderston RA, Rothman RH, Booth RE Jr. Long-term results of lumbar spine surgery complicated by unintended incidental durotomy. *Spine* (Phila Pa 1976). 1989 Apr;14(4):443-6.

[32] Katz JN, Stucki G, Lipson SJ, Fossel AH, Grobler LJ, Weinstein JN. Predictors of surgical outcome in degenerative lumbar spinal stenosis. *Spine* (Phila Pa 1976). 1999 Nov 1;24(21):2229-33.

[33] Katz JN, Lipson SJ, Chang LC, Levine SA, Fossel AH, Liang MH. Seven- to 10-year outcome of decompressive surgery for degenerative lumbar spinal stenosis. *Spine* (Phila Pa 1976). 1996 Jan 1;21(1):92-8.

[34] Katz JN, Lipson SJ, Larson MG, McInnes JM, Fossel AH, Liang MH. The outcome of decompressive laminectomy for degenerative lumbar stenosis. *J. Bone Joint Surg. Am.* 1991 Jul;73(6):809-16.

[35] Keskimäki I, Seitsalo S, Osterman H, Rissanen P. Reoperations after lumbar disc surgery: a population-based study of regional and interspecialty variations. *Spine* (Phila Pa 1976). 2000 Jun 15;25(12):1500-8.

[36] Kim JS, Choi WG, Lee SH. Minimally invasive anterior lumbar interbody fusion followed by percutaneous pedicle screw fixation for isthmic spondylolisthesis: minimum 5-year follow-up. *Spine J.* 2010 May;10(5):404-9.

[37] Kim DH, Jeong ST, Lee SS. Posterior lumbar interbody fusion using a unilateral single cage and a local morselized bone graft in the degenerative lumbar spine. *Clin. Orthop. Surg.* 2009 Dec;1(4):214-21.

[38] Kim JS, Kim DH, Lee SH, Park CK, Hwang JH, Cheh G, Choi YG, Kang BU, Lee HY. Comparison study of the instrumented circumferential fusion with instrumented anterior lumbar interbody fusion as a surgical procedure for adult low-grade isthmic spondylolisthesis. *World Neurosurg.* 2010 May;73(5):565-71.

[39] Kim SW, Limson MA, Kim SB, Arbatin JJ, Chang KY, Park MS, Shin JH, Ju YS. Comparison of radiographic changes after ACDF versus Bryan disc arthroplasty in single and bi-level cases. *Eur. Spine J.* 2009 Feb;18(2):218-31.

[40] Kim KH, Park JY, Chin DK. Fusion criteria for posterior lumbar interbody fusion with intervertebral cages: the significance of traction spur. *J. Korean Neurosurg. Soc.* 2009 Oct;46(4):328-32.

[41] Koakutsu T, Morozumi N, Ishii Y, Kasama F, Sato T, Tanaka Y, Kokubun S, Yamazaki S. Anterior decompression and fusion versus laminoplasty for cervical myelopathy caused by soft disc herniation: a prospective multicenter study. *J. Orthop. Sci.* 2010 Jan;15(1):71-8.

[42] Kwon YM, Chin DK, Jin BH, Kim KS, Cho YE, Kuh SU. Long Term Efficacy of Posterior Lumbar Interbody Fusion with Standard Cages alone in Lumbar Disc Diseases Combined with Modic Changes. *J. Korean Neurosurg. Soc.* 2009 Oct;46(4):322-7.

[43] Lee DY, Lee SH, Maeng DH. Two-level anterior lumbar interbody fusion with percutaneous pedicle screw fixation: a minimum 3-year follow-up study. *Neurol. Med. Chir.* (Tokyo). 2010;50(8):645-50.

[44] Lee CK, Park JY, Zhang HY. Minimally invasive transforaminal lumbar interbody fusion using a single interbody cage and a tubular retraction system : technical tips, and perioperative, radiologic and clinical outcomes. *J. Korean Neurosurg. Soc.* 2010 Sep;48(3):219-24.

[45] Li J, Dumonski ML, Liu Q, Lipman A, Hong J, Yang N, Jin Z, Ren Y, Limthongkul W, Bessey JT, Thalgott J, Gebauer G, Albert TJ, Vaccaro AR. A multicenter study to evaluate the safety and efficacy of a stand-alone anterior carbon I/F Cage for anterior lumbar interbody fusion: two-year results from a Food and Drug Administration investigational device exemption clinical trial. *Spine* (Phila Pa 1976). 2010 Dec 15; 35(26):E1564-70.

[46] Lian XF, Xu JG, Zeng BF, Zhou W, Kong WQ, Hou TS. Noncontiguous anterior decompression and fusion for multilevel cervical spondylotic myelopathy: a prospective randomized control clinical study. *Eur. Spine J.* 2010 May;19(5):713-9.

[47] Liebensteiner MC, Jesacher G, Thaler M, Gstoettner M, Liebensteiner MV, Bach CM. Restoration and preservation of disc height and segmental lordosis with circumferential lumbar fusion: a retrospective analysis of cage versus bone graft. *J. Spinal Disord. Tech.* 2011 Feb;24(1):44-9.

[48] Lied B, Roenning PA, Sundseth J, Helseth E. Anterior cervical discectomy with fusion in patients with cervical disc degeneration: a prospective outcome study of 258 patients (181 fused with autologous bone graft and 77 fused with a PEEK cage). *BMC Surg.* 2010 Mar 21;10:10.

[49] Löfgren H, Engquist M, Hoffmann P, Sigstedt B, Vavruch L. Clinical and radiological evaluation of Trabecular Metal and the Smith-Robinson technique in anterior cervical fusion for degenerative disease: a prospective, randomized, controlled study with 2-year follow-up. *Eur. Spine J.* 2010 Mar;19(3):464-73.

[50] Malter AD, McNeney B, Loeser JD, Deyo RA: 5-year reoperation rates after different types of lumbar spine surgery *Spine* (Phila Pa 1976) ;23(7);814-20, 1998.

[51] Marshman LA, Kasis A, Krishna M, Bhatia CK. Does Symptom Duration Correlate Negatively With Outcome After Posterior Lumbar Interbody Fusion for Chronic Low Back Pain? *Spine* (Phila Pa 1976). 2010 Feb 26. [Epub ahead of print]

[52] McAfee PC, Cappuccino A, Cunningham BW, Devine JG, Phillips FM, Regan JJ, Albert TJ, Ahrens JE. Lower incidence of dysphagia with cervical arthroplasty compared with ACDF in a prospective randomized clinical trial. *J. Spinal Disord. Tech.* 2010 Feb;23(1):1-8.

[53] Meisel HJ, Schnöring M, Hohaus C, Minkus Y, Beier A, Ganey T, Mansmann U. Posterior lumbar interbody fusion using rhBMP-2. *Eur. Spine J.* 2008 Dec;17(12):1735-44.

[54] Möller H, Hedlund R. Instrumented and noninstrumented posterolateral fusion in adult spondylolisthesis--a prospective randomized study: part 2. *Spine* (Phila Pa 1976). 2000 Jul 1;25(13):1716-21.

[55] Ntoukas V, Müller A. Minimally invasive approach versus traditional open approach for one level posterior lumbar interbody fusion. *Minim. Invasive Neurosurg.* 2010 Feb;53(1):21-4.

[56] Ohnmeiss DD, Bodemer W, Zigler JE. Effect of adverse events on low back surgery outcome: twenty-four-month follow-up results from a Food And Drug Administration investigational device exemptiontrial. *Spine* (Phila Pa 1976). 2010 Apr 1;35(7):835-8.

[57] Park SH, Park WM, Park CW, Kang KS, Lee YK, Lim SR. Minimally invasive anterior lumbar interbody fusion followed by percutaneous translaminar facet screw fixation in elderly patients. *J. Neurosurg. Spine.* 2009 Jun;10(6):610-6.

[58] Peolsson A, Vavruch L, Hedlund R. Long-term randomised comparison between a carbon fibre cage and the Cloward procedure in the cervical spine. *Eur. Spine J.* 2007 Feb;16(2):173-8.

[59] Ploumis A, Albert TJ, Brown Z, Mehbod AA, Transfeldt EE. Healos graft carrier with bone marrow aspirate instead of allograft as adjunct to local autograft for posterolateral fusion in degenerative lumbar scoliosis: a minimum 2-year follow-up study. *J. Neurosurg. Spine.* 2010 Aug;13(2):211-5.

[60] Prolo DJ, Oklund SA, Butcher M. Toward uniformity in evaluating results of lumbar spine operations. A paradigm applied to posterior lumbar interbody fusions. *Spine* (Phila Pa 1976). 1986 Jul-Aug;11(6):601-6.

[61] Rodgers WB, Gerber EJ, Patterson J. Intraoperative and early postoperative complications in extreme lateral interbody fusion: an analysis of 600 cases. *Spine* (Phila Pa 1976). 2011 Jan 1;36(1):26-32.

[62] Rouben D, Casnellie M, Ferguson M. Long-term Durability of Minimal Invasive Posterior Transforaminal Lumbar Interbody Fusion: A Clinical and Radiographic Follow-up. *J. Spinal Disord. Tech.* 2010 Oct 21. [Epub ahead of print]

[63] Sandén B, Försth P, Michaëlsson K. Smokers show less improvement than non-smokers 2 years after surgery for lumbar spinal stenosis: A study of 4555 Patients from the Swedish Spine Register. *Spine* (Phila Pa 1976). 2011 Jan 8. [Epub ahead of print]

[64] Sethi A, Lee S, Vaidya R. Transforaminal lumbar interbody fusion using unilateral pedicle screws and a translaminar screw. *Eur. Spine J.* 2009 Mar;18(3):430-4.

[65] Shin HC, Yi S, Kim KN, Kim SH, Yoon do H. Posterior lumbar interbody fusion via a unilateral approach. *Yonsei Med. J.* 2006 Jun 30;47(3):319-25.

[66] Silvers HR, Lewis PJ, Suddaby LS, Asch HL, Clabeaux DE, Blumenson LE. Day surgery for cervical microdiscectomy: is it safe and effective? *J. Spinal Disord.* 1996 Aug;9(4):287-93.

[67] Skidmore G, Ackerman SJ, Bergin C, Ross D, Butler J, Suthar M, Rittenberg J. Cost-effectiveness of the X-STOP® Interspinous Spacer for Lumbar Spinal Stenosis. *Spine* (Phila Pa 1976). 2011 Mar 1;36(5):E345-56.

[68] Topuz K, Colak A, Kaya S, Simşek H, Kutlay M, Demircan MN, Velioğlu M. Two-level contiguous cervical disc disease treated with peek cages packed with demineralized bone matrix: results of 3-year follow-up. *Eur. Spine J.* 2009 Feb;18(2): 238-43.

[69] Tsai TH, Huang TY, Lieu AS, Lee KS, Kung SS, Chu CW, Hwang SL. Functional outcome analysis: instrumented posterior lumbar interbody fusion for degenerative lumbar scoliosis. *Acta Neurochir.* (Wien). 2010 Dec 16. [Epub ahead of print]

[70] Videbaek TS, Bnger CE, Henriksen M, Neils E, Christensen FB. Sagittal Spinal Balance After Lumbar Spinal Fusion: The Impact of Anterior Column Support Results From a Randomized Clinical Trial With an Eight- to Thirteen-Year Radiographic Follow-up. *Spine* (Phila Pa 1976). 2011 Feb 1;36(3):183-91.

[71] Villavicencio AT, Burneikiene S, Roeca CM, Nelson EL, Mason A. Minimally invasive versus open transforaminal lumbar interbody fusion. *Surg. Neurol. Int.* 2010 May 31;1:12.

[72] Wang J, Zhou Y, Zhang ZF, Li CQ, Zheng WJ, Liu J. Comparison of one-level minimally invasive and open transforaminal lumbar interbody fusion in degenerative and isthmic spondylolisthesis grades 1 and 2. *Eur. Spine J.* 2010 Oct;19(10):1780-4.

[73] Watanabe K, Yamazaki A, Morita O, Sano A, Katsumi K, Ohashi M. Clinical Outcomes of Posterior Lumbar Interbody Fusion for Lumbar Foraminal Stenosis: Preoperative Diagnosis and Surgical Strategy. *J. Spinal Disord. Tech.* 2010 Jul 14. [Epub ahead of print]

[74] Yamashita T, Steinmetz MP, Lieberman IH, Modic MT, Mroz TE. The Utility of Repeated Postoperative Radiographs Following Lumbar Instrumented Fusion for Degenerative Lumbar Spine. *Spine* (Phila Pa 1976). 2011 Feb 7. [Epub ahead of print]

[75] Zencica P, Chaloupka R, Hladíková J, Krbec M. Adjacent segment degeneration after lumbosacral fusion in spondylolisthesis: a retrospective radiological and clinical analysis. *Acta Chir. Orthop. Traumatol. Cech.* 2010 Apr;77(2):124-30.

In: Toward Healthcare Resource Stewardship
Editors: J. S.Robinson, M. S.Walid et al.

ISBN: 978-1-62100-182-9
© 2012 Nova Science Publishers, Inc.

Chapter 22

PHYSICIANS AS GUARDIANS OF HEALTHCARE RESOURCES

M. Sami Walid,[1,] Aaron C. M. Barth,[1] Edward R. M. Robinson[2] and Joe Sam Robinson Jr.[3]*

[1]Medical center of Central Georgia, Macon, GA, US
[2]Sewanee: The University of the South, Sewanee, TN, US
[3]Georgia Neurosurgical Institute, Macon, GA, US

Bound by medical ethics and the obligations of the Hippocratic Oath, physicians have historically focused on practicing the art of medicine without regard to the cost of medical care. However, the rising and unsustainable increases in healthcare expenditure along with prospective government regulations suggest a mandate for an evolutionary revision of the traditional medical oath to incorporate the need for appropriate physician stewardship of healthcare resources (See figure 1).

In common parlance, the taking of a public oath is not a trivial affair. "Oath" is defined by the Merriam-Webster dictionary as *a solemn usually formal calling upon God ... to witness that one sincerely intends to do what one says.* [1] Indeed, since biblical times, an oath made public was deemed a binding commitment that cannot be annulled ("*And the children of Israel smote them not, because the princes of the congregation had sworn unto them by the LORD, the God of Israel.*"). [2] Reasonably, as protectors and defenders of the welfare of their patients, physicians have taken an oath to obey the high calling of their profession binding themselves to the high principles of conduct toward teachers, patients, colleagues, and society. Unsurprisingly, most American medical schools require their students to take the oath either on entry or upon graduation.[I cut the part about other countries because it weakens our argument, suggesting that other countries don't care about oaths] [3-5]

---

* Corresponding Author: M. Sami Walid, 840 Pine Street, Suite 880, Medical Center of Central Georgia, Macon, GA 331201. E-mail: mswalid@yahoo.com.

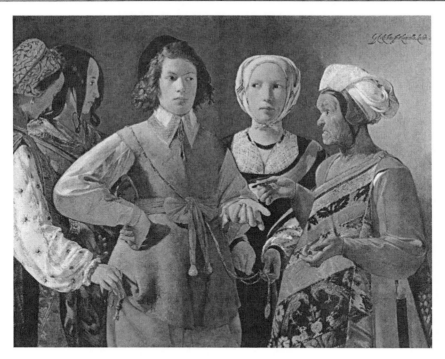

Figure 1. "The Fortune Teller" – Georges de La Tour (c.1630). (Many patients imagine that rising healthcare costs metaphorically are picking their pockets).

HISTORICAL REVIEW

Oaths ensuring ethical restraint were common in ancient cultures and civilizations (ancient India, Seventh-Century China, Middle-Century Arab Caliphate, …), and contained many similar principles. [6] The Hippocratic Oath, with its origin in the 4th century B.C., golden period of classic Hellenic civilization, has remained the prototype of medical ethics in the Western World – though not in a fixed fashion. The Hippocratic Oath faded toward obscurity with the 4th century spread of Christianity in Europe. It did not entirely disappear however, as some Christian physicians, not wanting to recite the oath and swear by pagan gods, omitted the heading and kept the text, or modified the oath so as to swear by the Holy Trinity. [7] The oath resurfaced again during the Age of Enlightenment of Western civilization with the proclaimed principles of reason, liberty, and individual rights. These principles impacted the moral, social, and political structure of that era and required an oath to bind physicians to high morals. The Hippocratic Oath, as it were, experienced its own renaissance.

With the arrival of the Twentieth Century, the world witnessed two horrific World Wars suborning some physicians into connivance with infamous immoral atrocities, including experimentation on living humans in the name of a dictator or national cause. After World War II the World Medical Association (WMA) was established as an international forum wherein national medical associations could debate the ethical challenges left from the war and the postwar social structure. The Declaration of Geneva Physician's Oath was written as a secular, updated form of the Hippocratic Oath and a 20th century restatement of the medical profession's commitment to the priority of the patient care. [8] This revision focused on social justice in the context of the Modern West-European social system.

CONTEMPORARY PERSPECTIVE

While the principles of beneficence and nonmalfeasance were set forth in the ancient text of the Hippocratic Oath, no mention was made of the need for stewardship of healthcare resources. Nor have the subsequent revisions of the Hippocratic Oath remedied this oversight (Table 1). Unfortunately, such ethical indifference does not comport with the present and impending financially-driven crisis in the American healthcare system. [17-19] Physicians have generally abstained from the grand national debate reshaping the American healthcare system. For instance, less than 10% of peer-reviewed clinical papers in PubMed incorporate cost in their outcome analysis. [20] Instead, fuelled by malpractice concerns, a competing and often observed paradigm has arisen mandating that a physician should obtain maximum diagnostic and therapeutic resources for patient care regardless of cost and occasionally in defiance of common sense. Such a viewpoint has caused other generally nonphysician interested parties to suggest and institute healthcare changes (often quite theoretic) focusing on healthcare cost reduction often at the expense of healthcare quality.

Table 1. Medical oaths and physician responsibility in managing healthcare resources

Oath	Reference to Resources Custodianship
Hippocratic Oath [9] 5th century B.C.	No
Declaration of Geneva [9,10] Physician's Oath World Medical Association 1948, 1968, 1983, 1994, 2005, 2006	No
The Oath of a Medical Student [11] Education Department of the People's Republic of China, 1991	No
Modern Hippocratic Oath [9] Louis Lasagna 1962	No
The Oath of the Healer [12] Louis Weistein 1991	No
Soviet Medical Oath [9] 1971, 1983	No

One may reasonably recognize that opinions, advice and guidance should be sought from any knowledgeable quarter; however, excessively leaving formulation of healthcare policy arrangements to distracted bureaucrats fails to honor the traditional physician covenant with these patients to defend their rights and maximize their care. One remedy would be to directly incorporate into physician professional oath those reforms which have already found their way into codes of ethics (Table 2). Such a change would empower physicians with substantial moral authority and obligation to help fashion an efficient and caring American healthcare system.

Table 2. Codes of Ethics and physician responsibility in managing healthcare resources

Code of Ethics	Reference to Resources Custodianship
World Medical Association [9] 1949, 1968, 1983, 2006	*A physician shall strive to use health care resources in the best way to benefit patients and their community*
American Medical Association [13] Principles of Medical Ethics 2001	--------------
American Medical Association [13] Opinions on Social Policy Issues Costs 2001	*While physicians should be conscious of costs and not provide or prescribe unnecessary medical services, concern for the quality of care the patient receives should be the physician's first consideration. Physicians should encourage health care plans to develop mechanisms to educate and assist physicians in cost-effective prescribing practices, ... The organized medical staff has an obligation to avoid wasteful practices and unnecessary treatment that may cause the hospital needless expense.*
Canadian Medical Association 1996 [14]	*Use health care resources prudently.*
General Medical Council [15] Duties of a Doctor United Kingdom	--------------
Australian Medical Association [16] 2004, 2006	*Use your special knowledge and skills to minimize wastage of resources, but remember that your primary duty is to provide your patient with the best available care. Make available your special knowledge and skills to assist those responsible for allocating healthcare resources.*

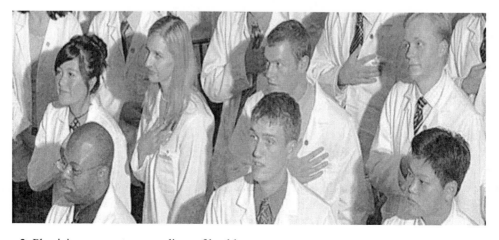

Figure 2. Physicians can act as guardians of healthcare resources.

Moreover, it may be argued that other advantages would occur from such an assertion of a physician role in custodianship of healthcare resources:

1. The doctor-patient relationship would be encouraged as patients realize physician involvement and concern with unsustainable healthcare cost.
2. Perhaps it is not too far of an extreme viewpoint to suggest that many physicians have higher than usual cognitive ability. Channeling such meritorious qualities into resolution of a great national crisis would be in the national interest.
3. Physicians, living their lives and practicing their profession as they do, possess special insight into appropriate healthcare efficiency and resources allocation.
4. An effective system of checks and balances would be encouraged as physicians become more knowledgeable in healthcare economics making arbitrary usurpation of patient rights under the guise of government or third party cost savings scheme less likely.

Of course, nothing implicit in oath-directed physician concern over appropriate healthcare economic efficiency should be construed as obviating physician's primary role as caregiver and patient defender. Physician's great oath-given responsibility stands far above artificial bureaucratic or insurance company regulations and should remain intact (Figure 2). It may be feared that unless physician culture becomes altered to obtain maximum healthcare economic efficiency, utopian cost reduction schemes - experimental and centrally directed - will worsen an already difficult situation.

CONCLUSION

We suggest that an obligation for custodianship of healthcare resources be added to the traditional oath undertaken upon the receipt of a Doctor of Medicine degree.

REFERENCES

[1] Merriam-Webster Dictionary. Yount, Lisa. The History of Medicine. Lucent Books Inc. 2002. San Diego.
[2] Joshua Chapter 9. http://bibleresources.bible.com/passagesearchresults.php?passage1= joshua+9andpassage2=andpassage3=andpassage4=andpassage5=andversion1=9andvers ion2=0andversion3=0andversion4=0andversion5=0andSubmit.x=38andSubmit.y=10
[3] Tyson P. The hippocratic oath today: meaningless relic or invaluable moral guide? Nova Online 2009. http://www.pbs.org/wgbh/nova/doctors/oath.html
[4] Weller DP, Heller RF, Jamrozik K. Jeopardising a Hippocratic tradition. *Med. J. Aust.* 2004 Dec 6-20;181(11-12):660-1.
[5] McNeill PM, Dowton SB. Declarations made by graduating medical students in Australia and New Zealand. *Med. J. Aust.* 2002 Feb 4;176(3):123-5.
[6] Yount, Lisa. The History of Medicine. Lucent Books Inc. 2002. San Diego.

[7]   Helidonis ES, Prokopakis EP. The contribution of Hippocratic Oath in third millennium medical practice. *Am. J. Otolaryngol.* 2001 Sep-Oct;22(5):303-5.

[8]   Declaration of Geneva (1948). Adopted by the General Assembly of World Medical Association at Geneva Switzerland, September 1948.

[9]   Physician oaths. Association of American Physicians and Surgeons. http://www. aapsonline.org/ethics/oaths.htm

[10]   World Medical Association. International Code of Medical Ethics. http://www.wma.net/en/30publications/10policies/c8/index.html

[11]   Qing L. Chinese Oath of a Medical Student. *Eubios Journal of Asian and International Bioethics (EJAIB)* Vol 9 (3) May 1999.

[12]   Weinstein L. The Oath of the Healer. *JAMA.* 1991;265(19):2484.

[13]   Code of Medical Ethics. American medical Association. http://www.ama-assn.org/ama/ pub/physician-resources/medical-ethics/code-medical-ethics.shtml

[14]   Code of Ethics of the Canadian Medical Association. *CMAJ.* 1996 October 15;155(8): 1176A–1176D.

[15]   Good Medical Practice: Duties of a doctor. General Medical Council 2009. http://www.gmc-uk.org/guidance/good_medical_practice/duties_of_a_doctor.asp

[16]   Australian Medical Association Code of Ethics - 2004. Editorially Revised 2006. http://www.ama.com.au/node/2521

[17]   Budget deficit to hit $1.2 trillion in fiscal 2009. Reuters. Accessed 1/12/2009. URL: http://www.reuters.com/article/businessNews/idUSN0643708720090107?feedType=RS SandfeedName=businessNewsandsp=true

[18]   Medicare "drifting towards disaster": U.S. official. Reuters. Accessed 6/15/2009. URL: http://www.reuters.com/article/healthNews/idUSN2936521220080429?pageNumber=1 andvirtualBrandChannel=0

[19]   Emanuel EJ, Fuchs VR. The perfect storm of overutilization. *JAMA* 2008 Jun 18; 299(23):2789-91.

[20]   Robinson JS, Sevin C., Fountas KN, Feltes CH, Nikolakakos LG, Robinson JS. Neurosurgeons' Role in Cost Control. *AANS Bulletin* 2006;15(3):16-17.

ABOUT THE EDITORS

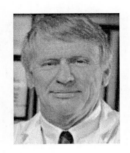

Dr. Joe Sam Robinson Jr is one of Georgia's most experienced neurosurgeons. After graduation from Harvard College with honors in 1967, he continued his studies at the University of Virginia from which he received his doctorate in medicine in 1971. Further training included rotations in London, England; an internship and a general surgery residency at Emory University in Atlanta; and a neurosurgical residency at Northwestern University, Chicago. During this period, he was also involved in research programs at the National Institute of Health.

In 1981, Dr. Robinson began his neurosurgical practice in Central Georgia and is currently the Chief of the Neurosurgery Department at the Medical Center of Central Georgia.

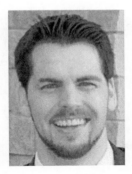

Mr. Aaron C.M. Barth, MBA served as the Program Support Manager of the Georgia Neuro Center and the Emergency Center at the Medical Center of Central Georgia from 2006-2010. He completed his undergraduate studies at Harvard University in 2004 and earned a Master of Business Administration Degree at Wesleyan College (Macon, GA) in 2009.

Mr. Barth has presented at both national and international scientific conferences on topics addressing the socioeconomic aspects of modern healthcare. He seeks to apply his experience and insights within developing world healthcare contexts.

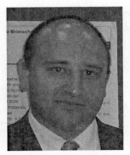

Dr. M. Sami Walid has authored numerous articles in such noted periodicals as the Journal of Hospital Medicine, the Journal of Neurosurgery, and the International Journal of Gynecology and Obstetrics. His wide-ranging clinical and socioeconomic research have been featured at regional and national conferences throughout the United States. Dr.Walid's poster presentation "Earlier spine surgery as a marker for additional spine surgery at a distant site" was awarded first place in the category of socioeconomic studies at the 2011 American Association of Neurological Surgeons Annual

Meeting in Denver, Colorado.

Dr. Walid graduated from Tishreen University School of Medicine in Syria and received his PhD degree from Kuban State Medical University in Russia. He has served as a clinical researcher at the Medical Center of Central Georgia since 2006.

INDEX

A

abuse, 87
access, 4, 24, 46, 47, 49, 51, 63, 64, 65, 83, 100, 128, 146, 157, 164, 169, 192, 197, 227, 234, 236, 243, 257, 259, 266
accessibility, 186, 207
accommodation, 122
accountability, 233, 234, 237, 239
accounting, 20, 38, 52, 177, 183, 201
accreditation, 251, 257
actuality, x
acute renal failure, 127, 128, 145
adaptation, 172
adenomyosis, 248
adipose, 151
adjustment, 174
administrators, 4, 96, 136, 162, 236, 240
adult obesity, 142
adults, 20, 25, 38, 71, 138, 141, 142, 143, 152, 157, 158, 159, 160, 161, 162, 163, 164, 165, 166, 167, 168, 170, 171, 172, 174, 175, 176, 177, 178, 179, 180, 182, 222, 228
advancement, 45, 119
adverse effects, 166, 223
adverse event, 137, 165, 271
advertisements, 255
advocacy, 25
Africa, 219
African Americans, 38
age, ix, 25, 38, 85, 86, 89, 91, 100, 106, 114, 119, 130, 133, 150, 157, 158, 159, 160, 161, 167, 169, 176, 181, 182, 202, 205, 206, 208, 214, 215, 216, 222, 223, 224, 225, 260, 261, 264, 266, 267
agencies, 24, 166, 253
agility, 177
aging population, 186, 265
agranulocytosis, 114

air traffic control system, 23
Alaska, 30
Alaska Natives, 30
alcohol use, 159
algorithm, 203
alteplase, 49, 73, 74
American culture, 3
American Healthcare System, 4
American Heart Association, 45, 47, 48, 49, 63, 70, 71, 136
amniotic fluid, 145
anaesthesiologist, 204
anemia, 86, 87, 113, 114, 115
anesthesiologist, 22
anger, 250
angiography, 49, 189
anti-angiogenic agents, 153
antidepressant, 163, 165, 166
antidepressant medication, 165, 166
antidepressants, 85, 167, 172
antitrust, 245, 246, 248, 249
anxiety, 159, 161, 167, 168, 171, 174, 175, 178, 179
anxiety disorder, 175
arrest, 145, 192
arterial blood gas, 124, 128, 191
artery, 75, 128
arthritis, 85, 158
arthroplasty, 268, 269, 270, 271
Asia, 219
aspirate, 272
aspiration, 77, 80, 81, 145, 146
aspiration pneumonia, 77, 80, 146
assault, 8
assessment, 13, 47, 49, 74, 78, 80, 116, 124, 128, 147, 167, 174, 175, 178, 181, 185, 192, 203, 230, 266, 268
assessment tools, 167
atelectasis, 87
atrial fibrillation, 75, 188

atrocities, 276
Austria, 56, 58, 140
authorities, 167
authority, 4, 277
autonomy, 124
autopsy, 150
average costs, 56, 66, 166
average revenue, 52, 67
aversion, 236
avoidance, 111, 192
awareness, 5, 46, 63, 74, 87, 115, 130, 194, 195, 196, 197, 198, 204

B

baby boomers, 119
back pain, 89, 90, 151
bacteria, 77
bad habits, 5
bandwidth, 65
Bangladesh, 222, 230
bankruptcy, 4
bargaining, 236
barriers, 4, 159, 163, 238, 251, 256, 257, 258
base, 62, 121, 125, 136, 143, 165, 200, 267
behaviors, 161, 162, 168, 169, 179, 180
benchmarking, 126
beneficiaries, 34, 160, 182, 268
benefits, 46, 47, 63, 100, 108, 123, 131, 165, 166, 173, 207, 208, 210, 231
benign, 148, 154
bias, 108, 243
bible, 9, 279
biochemistry, 213
biomarkers, 168
birth control, 151
births, 144, 147
Blacks, 30, 142
bleeding, 148, 150, 191
blood, 12, 35, 62, 86, 114, 115, 127, 141, 143, 145, 146, 150, 159, 170, 191, 200, 213
blood clot, 141
blood flow, 170
blood pressure, 62, 145, 159
blood transfusion, 86, 115, 150
bloodstream, 122
blueprint, 180
BMI, 141, 142, 143, 145, 151
body fat, 141
body mass index, 85, 86, 91, 141, 142, 145, 153
body weight, 151
bone, 99, 100, 101, 106, 107, 108, 110, 111, 138, 144, 268, 269, 270, 271, 272

bone marrow, 138, 272
bone marrow transplant, 138
bone morphogenic proteins (BMP), 106, 108
bones, 104
bowel, 148
brachial plexus, 144
brain, 48, 60, 62, 63, 73, 80, 82, 97, 144, 170, 173, 177, 180, 247
brain cancer, 247
brainstem, 80
Brazil, 72
breakdown, 15, 121, 170, 267
break-even, 34, 52, 68
breast cancer, 206
breathing, 128, 175
bronchus, 226
bureaucracy, 243, 249, 250
burn, 13, 14, 19, 122, 138
burn care, 14, 19
business model, 70
businesses, 239, 249
Butcher, 76, 272

C

cadaver, 99, 100, 101
campaigns, 63
cancer, 30, 38, 52, 141, 147, 148, 151, 152, 154, 155
candidates, 70, 85, 90, 91, 92, 95, 96, 146
capillary, 200
carbon, 269, 271, 272
cardiac surgery, 20
cardiovascular disease, 35, 63, 160
cardiovascular risk, 212, 244
care model, 52, 65, 117, 118, 122, 166, 172, 174
caregivers, 6, 7, 34, 45, 121, 162, 172, 178
caregiving, 172, 181
case study, 11, 13, 14, 19, 26, 137
catastrophes, 193
category a, 209
catheter, 120, 122, 146
Caucasian population, 119
Caucasians, 114
causal relationship, 266
CBS, 87
CCNC networks, 167
CDC, 38, 47, 142
cell phones, 124
Census, 74, 119, 138
Centers for Disease Control and Prevention (CDC), 38, 47, 142
central nervous system, 160
cerebrovascular disease, 62, 168

certification, 64, 127, 136, 255, 257, 258
cervical radiculopathy, 267, 268
cervical spondylosis, 101, 110, 268
cesarean section, 144, 146, 147, 152, 154
challenges, 11, 19, 26, 47, 63, 64, 81, 117, 135, 136, 166, 170, 172, 233, 234, 236, 240, 276
Chamber of Commerce, 13
checks and balances, ix, 7, 279
chemoprevention, 222, 230
chemotherapy, 221, 247
Chicago, 74, 281
childhood, 153, 161, 228, 229, 231
children, 1, 25, 145, 147, 158, 186, 213, 215, 216, 219, 224, 225, 226, 255, 275
China, 276, 277
cholecystectomy, 154
cholesterol, 85
cholinesterase, 172
cholinesterase inhibitors, 172
Christianity, 276
chronic diseases, 35, 92, 152, 158, 176
chronic illness, 161, 171
chronic obstructive pulmonary disease, 77, 85, 96
circulation, 128
cities, 39
citizens, 37, 46
City, 8
civilization, 276
classes, 5, 38, 128
classification, 263
classroom, 128
clients, 161, 244
clinical assessment, 63
clinical diagnosis, 213
clinical examination, 64
clinical judgment, 127, 252
clinical presentation, 167
clinical trials, 166, 259, 261, 266, 267
closure, 122
CNS, 117, 165, 173
coding, 248
coercion, 5
cognition, 161, 166, 167, 172, 174
cognitive ability, 279
cognitive activity, 165, 170
cognitive deficit, 170
cognitive deficits, 170
cognitive dysfunction, 159
cognitive function, 173, 181
cognitive impairment, 165, 167, 168, 170, 175, 178
cognitive performance, 174
cognitive system, 173

collaboration, 7, 46, 118, 124, 130, 162, 165, 233, 234, 236, 239, 240
collateral, 174
collusion, 245
Colombia, 218
colon, 141
combined effect, 161
commercial, 20
common sense, 168, 277
communication, 14, 23, 25, 26, 46, 62, 64, 121, 122, 126, 164, 169, 233, 234, 236, 237
communication technologies, 169
communities, 11, 25
community, 2, 12, 34, 49, 53, 64, 71, 72, 74, 75, 122, 159, 163, 182, 187, 201, 207, 221, 235, 237, 239, 249, 253, 257, 278
Community Care of North Carolina (CCNC), 166
community service, 53, 201
comorbidity, 90, 91, 92, 93, 97, 147, 160, 179, 180, 266
compensation, 2, 8, 22, 34, 38, 128, 228, 246, 252, 253, 254, 257, 266
compensation package, 246
competing interests, 4
competition, 245, 247
competitors, 121, 240
complement, 175
complexity, 168, 173
compliance, 61, 64, 78, 79, 80, 131, 176
complications, 53, 62, 81, 86, 87, 96, 97, 98, 107, 108, 111, 116, 118, 142, 143, 145, 146, 148, 150, 152, 153, 154, 155, 186, 187, 188, 223, 244, 261, 264, 266, 267, 268, 272
composition, 37, 218
computed tomography, 46, 49
computer, 80, 173, 174
computerized tomography (CT), 148
Concise, 197
conference, 194
confidentiality, 122, 171
conflict, 237
confounding variables, 39, 266
Congress, 87, 139, 140, 248
connectivity, 170
consciousness, 77, 204
consensus, 54
consent, 123, 129, 131
constituents, 5
consulting, 1, 96, 137, 166
consumers, ix, 252, 257
consumption, 80, 90, 260, 264
contraceptives, 151
contradiction, 206

control group, 197, 198
controlled trials, 61, 266
controversial, 148
convention, 252
coordination, 45, 46, 126, 134
COPD, 176, 192
coronary artery bypass graft, 123
coronary artery disease, 141
correction factors, 215
correlation, 92, 191, 194, 195
correlations, 89, 91, 163, 194
corruption, 7
cortisol, 177
cost effectiveness, 24, 51, 54, 55, 56, 61, 64, 65, 109, 218, 266
cost saving, 52, 61, 62, 64, 65, 85, 95, 97, 98, 108, 166, 167, 172, 177, 279
cost-benefit analysis, 92
coughing, 77
covering, 95, 96, 194
CPT, 267
credentials, 247
crises, 6
critical analysis, 111
critical thinking, 127, 128
criticism, 115, 250
CRR, 17
cultivation, 223
culture, ix, 167, 236, 279
cure, 87, 170, 206, 222, 250
currency, 73
curriculum, 124, 127, 128, 130
cycles, 3

D

daily living, 159, 167, 172
data collection, 54, 129, 131
database, 54, 63, 81, 150, 161, 224, 241, 259
death rate, 30, 38
deaths, 30, 38, 48, 141, 152, 159, 219
decision makers, 47
decision trees, 178
decision-making process, 109
defects, 144
deficiencies, 213
deficit, 106, 227, 253, 280
deflation, 205, 210
Delta, 171
demand curve, 251, 253, 254, 255
dementia, 165, 168, 172, 173, 178, 179, 180, 181, 182
demographic transition, 30

demography, 204
demyelination, 170
Department of Health and Human Services, 26, 47
dependent variable, 252
depression, 141, 159, 161, 163, 164, 165, 166, 167, 168, 169, 170, 171, 172, 174, 175, 178, 179, 181, 182
depressive symptoms, 159, 165, 166, 175, 178, 180
dermatology, 214, 215
designers, 136
destruction, 247
detectable, 192
detection, 49, 180, 192
developed countries, ix, 54, 142, 206, 220, 221, 227, 229
developing countries, 54, 220, 221, 227, 230
deviation, 4, 195
diabetes, 35, 38, 63, 85, 96, 133, 134, 143, 144, 145, 147, 153, 159, 166, 168, 170, 171
diabetic patients, 134
diagnosis-related group (DRG), 87
dialysis, 119, 128
diarrhea, 137
dichotomy, 168
diet, 122, 143, 162
dieting, 176
diffusion, 74
dilatation and curettage, 244
direct cost, 38, 95, 97, 104, 105, 106, 120, 132, 148, 187, 209, 213, 215, 216, 221, 223, 226, 229, 231
direct costs, 38, 104, 105, 106, 120, 148, 187, 209, 213, 215, 216, 221, 223, 227, 231
disability, 1, 38, 39, 45, 48, 52, 62, 72, 107, 159, 163, 164, 167, 172, 175, 177, 179, 206, 207, 260, 266
disaster, 14, 23, 204, 236, 280
discharges, 87, 119
discomfort, 120
discrimination, 141
disease model, 177
disease progression, 162
diseases, ix, 4, 45, 70, 85, 127, 142, 160, 164, 210
disinfection, 185
disorder, 160, 175, 177, 181
dispersion, 210
dissatisfaction, 188
dissonance, 206, 237
distillation, 168
distress, 145, 172
distribution, 39, 70, 89, 90, 91, 183, 186, 189, 197, 239
District of Columbia, 141
divergence, 43

diversity, 162
dizziness, 114
DOC, 60, 66, 76
doctors, 3, 23, 194, 195, 196, 197, 199, 204, 205, 234, 240, 248, 249, 253, 279
DOI, 35, 203
donors, 128
doppler, 144
dosing, 159, 166
DOT, 220, 221, 223, 228
drug interaction, 176
drug reactions, 159
drug resistance, 222
drug therapy, 34, 38
drug treatment, 221, 230
drugs, 3, 142, 159, 165, 166, 186, 204, 209, 221, 222, 228
dysphagia, 77, 79, 80, 81, 82, 271
Dysphagia Screen, 78, 81

E

earnings, 34, 38, 180
Eastern Europe, 22
eating disorders, 165
economic consequences, 207
economic development, 6, 206
economic efficiency, 196, 279
economic evaluation, 205, 218
economic resources, 185
economic status, 30, 38
economics, 30, 47, 155, 251, 252, 257, 279
economies of scale, 19
ecosystem, 172
ectopic pregnancy, 154
edema, 145
editors, x
education, 3, 12, 26, 49, 64, 74, 124, 125, 127, 143, 163, 166, 167, 169, 181, 189, 194, 196, 197, 199, 251, 252, 255
educational attainment, 161
educators, 257
effusion, 192
elderly population, 163
elders, 158, 159, 164, 165, 167, 170, 180
election, 233
electives, 122
electricity, 209, 214
electrolyte, 118, 128, 191
electrolyte imbalance, 128
embolism, 87, 150, 192
embolus, 150

emergency, 4, 11, 12, 13, 14, 18, 22, 23, 24, 25, 26, 38, 39, 45, 46, 48, 49, 52, 73, 74, 76, 119, 123, 128, 144, 159, 166, 183, 184, 185, 186, 187, 188, 189, 190, 191, 192, 193, 194, 196, 197, 198, 199, 200, 201, 202, 203, 204, 235, 247
emergency communications, 14
Emergency Medical Services (EMS), 39
emergency physician, 12, 22, 183, 188, 189, 190, 193, 202, 203
emergency rooms (ERs), 39
emotional disorder, 175
emotional distress, 6
employees, 185, 249
employment, 85, 91, 138, 238, 239, 267
employment status, 85, 91
EMS, 13, 14, 21, 23, 24, 25, 26, 39, 40, 41, 42, 43, 44, 46, 49, 184
encephalopathy, 145
endocrine, 88, 93
endometritis, 146
end-stage renal disease, 118, 127, 130
energy, 162
England, 7, 83, 195, 203, 281
enrollment, 131
environment, ix, 27, 52, 64, 118, 124, 126, 137, 138, 169, 170, 196, 208, 234, 235, 240
epidemiology, 74, 155
epilepsy, 145, 153
episodic memory, 178
equality, 207
equilibrium, 251, 252, 253, 256
equipment, 19, 20, 25, 67, 87, 105, 118, 137, 148, 191, 209, 234, 244, 247
estrogen, 151
ethical issues, 128
ethics, 208, 275, 276, 277, 280
etiology, 165
Europe, 65, 219, 276
everyday life, 170
evidence, 16, 63, 64, 118, 125, 126, 136, 152, 157, 160, 163, 164, 166, 171, 174, 175, 177, 181, 202, 243, 259, 260, 266, 267
evidence-based practices, 126, 163
examinations, 209, 220, 222, 226, 255
excess demand, 252
exchange rate, 73, 223
excision, 215, 216, 269
exclusion, 130, 227, 260, 261, 264, 267
execution, 64, 65
executive function, 174
executive functioning, 174
exercise, 35, 127, 143, 159, 162, 165, 170, 171, 173, 176, 179

exercise programs, 171
expenditures, 4, 38, 47, 83, 92, 146, 159, 161, 175, 182, 183, 185, 220, 224, 225, 226, 228, 266
expertise, 52, 62, 63, 76, 97, 234, 235
exposure, 121, 175, 197
external validity, 208, 212

F

factor analysis, 210
false positive, 167
families, 118, 175, 181, 247, 257
family history, 206
family members, 118
family physician, 159
family support, 168
FBI, 246
FDA, 54
FDA approval, 54
fears, 175
Federal Bureau of Investigation, 246
federal government, 234, 249
Federal Government, 7
feelings, 124
fertility, 119, 151
fertility rate, 119
fertilization, 152
fetal growth, 144
fetus, 144, 145
fever, 86, 87, 98, 119
fiber, 269
fibroids, 148
financial, 2, 3, 4, 5, 13, 14, 18, 20, 24, 45, 47, 87, 96, 97, 98, 147, 166, 203, 208, 222, 228, 235, 236, 237, 238, 239, 240, 257
financial crisis, 208
financial data, 96
financial incentives, 14, 24, 239
financial performance, 13, 18, 20
financial stability, 87
fitness, 173
fixation, 99, 100, 101, 108, 110, 270, 271
fixed costs, 52, 67, 70
flexibility, 119, 122, 167, 189, 236
fluid, 118, 127, 128, 146
food, 9, 77, 221, 247
force, 21, 45, 181, 222
Ford, 50
forecasting, 254
foreign-born population, 230
formation, 120
formula, 55, 261
fractures, 110, 192

France, 83, 194
fraud, 246
friction, 218, 236
frontal lobe, 174
fundamental needs, 167
funding, 3, 11, 13, 17, 18, 24, 26, 27, 34, 45, 46, 64, 166, 185, 186
fusion, 85, 86, 89, 90, 99, 101, 110, 111, 113, 114, 115, 259, 260, 261, 262, 263, 265, 266, 267, 268, 269, 270, 271, 272, 273

G

gait, 167
gallbladder, 141
gallbladder disease, 141
gate-keeping, 64
GDP, 83, 159
gender differences, 206
general anesthesia, 146, 213
general practitioner, 203
general surgeon, 188, 255, 256, 257
general surgery, 255, 256, 281
genetics, 170, 252
genotype, 30, 35
Georgia, 1, 11, 13, 14, 15, 16, 17, 18, 19, 20, 23, 24, 25, 26, 27, 29, 30, 37, 38, 39, 40, 41, 42, 43, 44, 45, 46, 47, 48, 49, 60, 66, 77, 83, 86, 88, 89, 95, 99, 113, 157, 233, 240, 243, 251, 259, 275, 281, 282
Georgians, 25, 26, 27
Germany, 56, 57, 58, 194, 222
gestation, 153
gestational diabetes, 143, 145
global village, 119
glucose, 35, 143, 144, 145, 159, 171
glucose tolerance, 143
glucose tolerance test, 143
glycosylated hemoglobin, 85, 88, 98
GNP, 4
God, 7, 275
governance, 124, 237
government intervention, 245
government spending, 227
GPS, 23, 24
grades, 272
grants, 64
graph, 97, 161, 255
grassroots, 63
Greece, 99
gross domestic product, 159, 183
Gross National Product (GNP), 4, 83
growth, 6, 87, 144, 158, 177, 218

growth factor, 177
guidance, 46, 49, 192, 277, 280
guidelines, 45, 49, 53, 61, 62, 63, 78, 87, 127, 152, 153, 157, 177, 186, 205, 208, 236, 267

H

harvesting, 101, 106, 107
hazards, 177
haze, 1
HE, 154
headache, 217, 247
healing, 3, 8, 101, 118, 125, 126, 136, 234
health care costs, 158, 202, 244
health care sector, 25
health care system, 24, 172, 175, 185, 186, 203, 221, 225, 226, 243, 249
health condition, 124, 160
health effects, 181
health expenditure, 9
health information, 163, 170
health insurance, 4, 178, 214, 221, 222, 245, 252
health policy issues, 252
health problems, 141, 159, 160, 164, 170, 184
health promotion, 163
health risks, 246
health services, 19, 76, 155, 167, 178, 180, 206, 222
health status, 147, 207, 208, 212
healthcare consumers, ix
healthcare cost reductions, x
healthcare costs. Diffuse, ix
healthcare technologies, ix
heart attack, 23, 25
heart disease, 30, 38, 48, 52, 85, 158, 171
height, 18, 141, 271
hematology, 223
hematoma, 109, 145
hemorrhage, 130, 145, 146
hemorrhagic stroke, 29, 30, 38, 63
hepatitis, 133, 134
high blood pressure, 145, 170
high school, 142
high school diploma, 142
Hippocratic tradition, 279
Hispanics, 30, 38, 142
history, 9, 86, 132, 161, 260
HIV, 132, 219
holistic care, 177
homes, 159, 171
homogeneity, 124
hormones, 177
hospital death, 80

hospitalization, 4, 48, 65, 72, 73, 85, 87, 92, 97, 105, 107, 108, 109, 126, 145, 152, 154, 222, 224, 227, 228, 229
host, 4, 234
House, 16, 180
household income, 158
hub, 52, 65, 66, 67, 70
human, 54, 83, 84, 97, 110, 131, 152, 155, 188, 205, 208, 247
human nature, 247
human resources, 188, 205
Hungary, 219, 220, 223, 225, 227, 228, 229, 230
hybrid, 117, 118, 124, 135
hypercholesterolemia, 141
hyperglycemia, 143, 144, 145, 147
hypertension, 38, 141, 143, 145, 147, 158, 168
hypoglycemia, 145
hypothesis, 30, 80, 174, 189
hypothesis test, 174
hypothyroidism, 85
hypoxia, 144
hysterectomy, 148, 152, 154, 248

I

icon, 7
ideal, 62, 108, 151, 157, 239, 253, 255
ideals, 171
identification, 70, 152, 171
iliac crest, 101, 107, 110
image, 64
imagination, 211
immersion, 127, 239
immigrants, 4, 222, 224, 226, 227, 230
immigration, 119, 251, 252
immune activation, 169
impairments, 38
implants, 100, 101, 106, 151, 155
improvements, 47, 98, 109, 171, 172
in utero, 144
in vitro, 152
incidence, 30, 38, 47, 48, 76, 81, 87, 109, 122, 143, 146, 153, 212, 219, 229, 231, 248, 271
income, 5, 49, 87, 158, 161, 208, 221, 222, 230, 236, 238, 245, 247
income inequality, 49
incremental cost effectiveness ratios (ICER), 56
independence, 54, 238, 239
independent variable, 252
index case, 224, 255
India, 81, 276
Indians, 30
individual rights, 276

individuals, ix, 6, 81, 157, 160, 161, 163, 167, 170, 172, 175, 177, 179, 208
induction, 146, 153
industrialization, 184
industrialized countries, 184
industry, 4, 119, 121, 136, 233, 248
inefficiency, 5, 175, 243
inequity, 66
infants, 144, 145, 152, 228, 255
infection, 88, 107, 108, 118, 120, 122, 123, 125, 131, 133, 136, 138, 144, 147, 185, 192, 219, 221, 222, 224, 228, 230, 260, 264
infertility, 142, 147, 151, 152
inflammation, 177
inflation, 186, 205, 210, 211, 215, 216, 245
infrastructure, 20, 23, 24, 46, 52, 54, 62, 63, 119, 126, 167, 184, 234, 235, 239
inhibition, 173
initial state, 13
initiation, 49, 52, 147
injections, 143
injuries, 12, 15, 118, 126, 144, 148, 151, 159, 184, 189, 192, 203
injury, 12, 14, 15, 19, 20, 23, 24, 46, 48, 144, 148, 155, 170, 192
injury prevention, 14, 24
insecurity, 196
Institute of Medicine (IOM), 175, 243
institutions, 4, 6, 34, 37, 108, 123, 124, 126, 186, 233, 235, 240, 266
insulin, 143, 144, 145, 177
insulin signaling, 177
integration, 80, 163, 169
integrity, 169, 170, 185
intensive care unit, 53, 81, 121, 128, 138, 144, 145, 153, 204, 255
interdependence, 237
interference, 243, 245
interferon, 223
interferon gamma, 223
internal validity, 208
internist, 95, 96, 97, 98
internists, 85, 95, 98
internship, 281
interpersonal relations, 127, 162
interpersonal relationships, 162
intervention, 45, 70, 80, 165, 166, 169, 171, 172, 174, 175, 176, 178, 180, 181, 182, 197, 198, 199, 200, 205, 213, 222, 224
intervention strategies, 171
intracranial pressure, 192
intrinsic value, 19
investment, 6, 46, 47, 52, 64, 68, 125, 126

investments, 45
investors, 235
ischaemic heart disease, 35
ischemia, 29, 30, 73, 81, 145
isolation, 124, 138, 168, 175
isoniazid, 220, 230
Israel, 275
issues, ix, 8, 13, 25, 44, 47, 75, 87, 100, 107, 108, 109, 118, 159, 164, 168, 169, 170, 171, 175, 176, 177, 181, 188, 196, 217, 233, 235, 237, 243, 251, 252, 266, 267
Italy, 56, 57, 58, 59, 195

J

Japan, 83
jaundice, 145
Joint Commission, 39, 53, 77, 78, 81
joint ventures, 237, 238
jumping, 247
jurisdiction, 4, 184

K

kidney, 117, 118, 126, 127, 128, 131, 134
Kidney Transplant Nursing CORE Curriculum (KTNCC), 130
kidneys, 128

L

laboratory tests, 223
laceration, 145
laminectomy, 262, 270
landscape, 119
laparoscopy, 148
laparotomy, 148
laptop, 129
later life, 145, 161, 176
Latin America, 119
laws, 128, 249
lawyers, 245, 249
lead, 6, 8, 97, 106, 127, 128, 141, 148, 158, 160, 170, 177, 236, 237, 238, 245
leadership, 126, 130, 235, 237
leadership development, 237
learning, 124, 169, 171, 175, 178
learning process, 171
Lebanon, 203
legal issues, 184, 238
leisure, 158, 165, 170, 173, 210
length of stay (LOS), 65, 96, 100, 101, 261

leukemia, 138
liberty, 276
life expectancy, 4, 97, 119, 158, 163, 205, 215, 261, 266
lifetime, 34, 38, 53, 138, 247
ligament, 110
light, 45, 119, 128, 235, 238, 266
literacy, 170, 176
litigation, 145
liver, 145, 223
local anesthesia, 213
logistics, 126
longevity, 83, 161
lordosis, 271
Louisiana, 141
low risk, 222
loyalty, 236
lumbar spine, 267, 268, 270, 271, 272
lupus, 85
lying, 39
lymphadenitis, 226

M

macrosomia, 144
magnet, 129
magnetic resonance, 74, 148
magnetic resonance imaging, 74, 148
magnitude, 63, 160
major depression, 160, 164, 167, 180
major issues, 197
majority, 38, 39, 142, 186, 187, 189, 193, 194, 202, 244, 245, 249, 266
malaise, 201
malnutrition, 159
mammogram, 207
management, 5, 45, 49, 51, 52, 53, 56, 61, 63, 64, 71, 72, 74, 95, 96, 97, 120, 121, 124, 127, 128, 147, 153, 154, 163, 165, 166, 169, 170, 171, 172, 177, 181, 182, 203, 204, 218, 222, 223, 231, 237, 238, 241, 244, 250, 267, 269
market share, 21, 245
marketing, 246
Maryland, 60
mass, 132, 152, 154, 185, 222
materials, 86, 109, 111, 214
matrix, 272
matter, 84, 128, 173, 208, 213, 245, 254
measurement, 121, 167
meconium, 145
media, 208
median, 122, 192, 202, 210, 214, 215, 216, 221, 223

Medicaid, 3, 4, 16, 17, 20, 27, 34, 64, 66, 83, 142, 160, 161, 166, 175, 178, 180, 182, 240, 252, 253
medical care, 19, 23, 64, 83, 97, 142, 147, 157, 164, 165, 166, 170, 177, 184, 203, 204, 225, 226, 236, 238, 249, 275
Medicare, 3, 16, 17, 20, 30, 34, 45, 64, 66, 71, 76, 83, 87, 142, 159, 161, 175, 178, 181, 235, 240, 252, 253, 268, 280
medication, 107, 120, 121, 122, 125, 133, 136, 158, 159, 162, 165, 170, 177, 186, 220, 224, 228, 266
medication compliance, 170
medicine, 3, 9, 18, 46, 49, 84, 95, 155, 165, 168, 186, 189, 190, 194, 196, 197, 198, 204, 206, 207, 217, 245, 246, 247, 248, 249, 251, 258, 275, 281
Mediterranean, 219
melanoma, 206
mellitus, 35, 85, 143
memory, 168, 173, 174, 178, 181, 182
memory loss, 181
memory performance, 173
menstruation, 147
mental disorder, 160, 161, 179, 180
mental health, 157, 159, 160, 161, 162, 164, 165, 167, 171, 175, 176, 177, 179
mental illness, 84, 160, 165, 175, 177, 179
messages, 172
meta-analysis, 52, 61, 110, 161, 162, 167, 181, 261
methodology, 16, 164, 259, 260, 267
metropolitan areas, 39
microscopy, 220, 223
Microsoft, 224
migration, 4
military, 11
minorities, 38
mission, 45, 233, 236, 237, 239
missions, 234
Missouri, 60, 139, 141, 144
modelling, 35, 48
models, x, 64, 66, 67, 68, 69, 165, 169, 171, 172, 176, 177, 181, 183, 207, 211, 212, 213, 217, 230, 233, 238, 240
modifications, 162
modules, 128
monopoly, 246, 248, 255, 257
monopoly power, 255, 257
monopsony, 252, 257, 258
mood disorder, 159, 169
morbidity, 37, 39, 41, 42, 100, 101, 107, 108, 110, 137, 144, 145, 152, 154, 163, 177, 183, 226, 227, 229, 269
mortality, 29, 35, 37, 38, 39, 41, 42, 46, 47, 48, 49, 53, 54, 72, 80, 81, 119, 141, 143, 145, 146, 150, 161, 180, 183, 200, 202, 260, 261, 264, 266, 269

mortality rate, 29, 38, 39, 41, 42, 46, 47, 53, 119, 269
motivation, 162, 248
MRI, 97, 148, 247
multidrug-resistant tuberculosis, 231
multimedia, 65
multiplication, 224
multivariate analysis, 212
multivariate data analysis, 110
muscles, 145
music, 178
music therapy, 178
myocardial infarction, 188, 191, 212

N

narcotic, 1
national expenditure, 6
national identity, 2
National Institute for Occupational Safety and Health, 151
National Institute of Health Budget for Drug and Biological Product Development, 3
National Institutes of Health, 75
national product, 5, 83
NCS, 160, 178, 180
negative affective (NA), 175
neglect, 45
nephropathy, 127, 128
nerve, 144
Netherlands, 48, 56, 58, 59, 62, 188, 227, 230
networking, 46, 64
neurologist, 63, 247
neurosurgery, 12, 18, 96
neutral, 187, 240
nevus, 213
New England, 178
New Zealand, 279
Nobel Prize, 3, 9
non-smokers, 272
normal aging, 167
normal distribution, 70, 91
North America, 65, 217
Norway, 56, 58, 59
NSA, 35
nurses, 4, 11, 12, 13, 20, 62, 78, 96, 118, 119, 122, 123, 124, 125, 126, 127, 129, 130, 134, 137, 165, 166, 185, 186, 188, 201, 205, 240, 257
nursing, 12, 34, 38, 53, 62, 65, 72, 80, 117, 118, 119, 120, 121, 124, 126, 127, 129, 130, 131, 134, 137, 138, 158, 159, 174, 177, 187, 235
nursing care, 53, 120, 129, 131, 158
nursing home, 34, 38, 65, 72, 159, 174, 177

nutrition, ix, 143, 170, 171, 174

O

Obama, x
obesity, 88, 96, 141, 142, 143, 144, 147, 148, 150, 152, 153, 154, 159, 170
obstruction, 133, 187
OCD, 165
oedema, 192
oesophageal, 192
officials, 245
Oklahoma, 141
old age, 1, 169, 182
operating data, 131
operations, 45, 52, 62, 69, 70, 105, 118, 255, 269, 272
ophthalmologist, 209
opportunities, 14, 26, 123, 234, 237, 239
opportunity costs, 213
opt out, 24
optimization, 204
organ, 126, 169
organs, 148
orthostatic hypotension, 114
ossification, 110
out-of-state treatment, 19
outpatient ACDF procedures, 108
Outpatient surgery, 96
outpatients, 150, 206
outsourcing, 187
ovarian cysts, 148
overhead costs, 205, 209, 213
overlay, 167
oversight, 4, 244, 277
overweight, 143, 145, 152
oxidative stress, 169, 177
oxygen, 126, 129, 145

P

Pacific, 30
Pacific Islanders, 30
pain, 1, 100, 101, 105, 107, 110, 120, 147, 148, 155, 167, 168, 174, 188, 247, 248, 259, 260, 264, 266
palliative, 46
pallor, 114
paradigm shift, 53
parallel, 25, 39, 175
parents, 205, 214
parity, 153
participants, x, 9, 121, 131, 147

password, 129
pathologist, 249
pathology, 148, 168, 169, 192, 206
pathways, 73, 160, 167
patient care, 13, 16, 19, 20, 54, 61, 87, 107, 109, 117,
    118, 119, 120, 122, 125, 126, 134, 137, 139, 168,
    233, 234, 235, 236, 238, 239, 240, 246, 250, 277
patient rights, 279
PCP, 166, 167
penalties, 88
penis, 250
per capita cost, 34, 38
per capita income, 30, 39
perforation, 244
perfusion, 49, 74
perinatal, 143, 145, 152
perineum, 145
peripheral smear, 114
permit, 66, 185
personal responsibility, 3, 157
personal welfare, ix
personnel costs, 67, 213
Peru, 221, 228, 230
PET, 97
pharmaceutical, 3, 151
pharmaceuticals, 218
pharmacology, 127
pharmacotherapy, 157, 166
phenotype, 170
Philadelphia, 137, 138
Philippines, 227
physical environment, 138
physical health, 177
physical therapist, 62
physician assistant (PA), 130
physician involvement, 279
Physiological, 133
physiology, 3, 194
pilot study, 72, 82, 129, 130, 134
pitch, 119
placenta, 144, 145
plasmapheresis, 128
plasminogen, 49, 72, 75
plasticity, 173, 179, 181
platform, 76
playing, 24, 173, 175
pleasure, 7
PM, 279
pneumonia, 77, 80, 81, 120
police, 24, 25, 26
policy, 6, 21, 46, 47, 50, 160, 162, 166, 249, 251,
    267, 277
policy makers, 162

policymakers, 47
politics, 4, 202, 212
population, ix, 4, 41, 42, 44, 46, 47, 48, 63, 68, 76,
    80, 83, 118, 119, 123, 131, 137, 142, 143, 148,
    151, 159, 162, 164, 170, 178, 182, 206, 207, 208,
    222, 225, 227, 229, 245, 253, 261, 268, 269, 270
population density, 44
population group, 47
population growth, 4
Portugal, 56, 58
positive correlation, 47
post natal care, ix
post-anesthesia care unit (PACU), 130
potential benefits, 47
poverty, 38, 43, 45, 158, 159, 161, 184, 254
precedent, 65
prediction models, 211
preeclampsia, 143, 145, 153
prefrontal cortex, 174
pregnancy, 142, 143, 144, 145, 146, 147, 151, 152,
    153, 154, 155
pre-hospital care, 19
preoperative screening, 85, 92
preparation, 117, 125, 128, 134
preparedness, 14
preschool, 154
preschool children, 154
preservation, 271
President, x, 158
preventative care, 177
prevention, 20, 44, 47, 53, 75, 98, 120, 128, 152,
    162, 165, 166, 170, 171, 176, 177, 179, 182, 206
preventive programs, 207
principles, 206, 244, 245, 252, 258, 275, 276, 277
private practice, 21, 238
privation, 45
probability, 52, 69, 70, 122, 174, 190, 194, 222
probability distribution, 70
probe, 170
problem behavior, 170
problem behaviors, 170
problem solving, 172
problem-solving, 166
professionals, 170, 203, 206, 207, 208, 212, 213,
    235, 239
profit, 4, 29, 30, 34, 45, 69, 244, 245, 246, 248, 249
profitability, 37
progressive tax, 245
project, 65, 67, 75, 151, 166, 172, 212
propagation, 77
prophylaxis, 75
prosperity, x
protection, 131, 185, 246, 247, 248, 249, 257

proteins, 106, 108, 111
proteinuria, 145
prototype, 167, 276
psychiatric disorders, 160, 161
psychiatrist, 166
psychiatry, 165, 177
psychologist, 173
psychopathology, 169
psychotherapy, 157, 163, 165, 166, 174
PTSD, 165
public assistance, 20
public education, 188
public goods, 25
public health, 3, 23, 155, 177, 197, 221, 227, 231
public interest, 257
public life, 170
public service, 25, 26
public support, 25
pulmonary edema, 145
pulmonary embolism, 150, 189, 190, 194
pumps, 100, 105
purchasing power, 252

Q

qualifications, 257
quality improvement, 45, 73, 181
quality of life, 73, 107, 118, 141, 157, 161, 171, 172, 174, 175
questioning, 191
questionnaire, 123, 194, 198

R

race, 38, 138
radiation, 247
radiography, 264
rape, 246
rating agencies, 121
reactions, 163
real income, 245
real time, 23
reality, 45, 159, 164, 171, 186, 211, 235, 236
reasoning, 207
recession, 83, 92, 210
recognition, 46, 74, 121, 151
recombinant DNA, 252
recommendations, 64, 71, 74, 130
recovery, 17, 46, 80, 97, 98, 107, 108, 110, 119, 121, 122, 123, 131, 163, 213, 216, 244
recruiting, 22
recurrence, 169

red blood cells, 114, 150
reform(s), x, 7, 8, 27, 83, 125, 252, 277
regionalization, 19
Registry, 73
regression, 103, 133, 134
regression model, 103, 133, 134
regulations, ix, 4, 6, 8, 20, 83, 238, 248, 275, 279
rehabilitation, 13, 14, 19, 34, 35, 38, 45, 48, 51, 53, 62, 65, 71, 72, 73, 124, 172, 228
rejection, 118
relapses, 177
relevance, 123
reliability, 75
relief, 162
religion, 2, 7
Rembrandt, 2
remediation, 181
remission, 163, 164, 166
renaissance, 276
renal failure, 127, 128
renal replacement therapy, 138
replication, 147, 180
reproduction, 152
reputation, 245
requirements, 45, 62, 78, 97, 148, 206, 247, 257, 258
research facilities, 185
researchers, 54, 174
resentment, 6, 237
reserve currency, x
resilience, 163
resistance, 62, 220, 225, 227
resolution, 279
resource allocation, 46, 164
resource utilization, 179
resources, ix, 7, 12, 19, 24, 26, 34, 37, 41, 42, 43, 44, 47, 54, 62, 63, 64, 70, 72, 76, 80, 85, 87, 90, 92, 143, 147, 163, 165, 169, 185, 196, 202, 206, 207, 208, 211, 213, 225, 227, 235, 236, 244, 257, 260, 261, 264, 266, 275, 277, 278, 279, 280
respiration, 114
respiratory disorders, 141
respiratory distress syndrome, 144
response, 21, 23, 24, 67, 122, 137, 163, 169, 177, 192, 193, 256
restrictions, 238, 251
restructuring, 175
retardation, 226
retirement, 215, 256
retribution, 208
revenue, 17, 18, 20, 52, 66, 67, 68, 69, 188, 235, 237, 248
rights, 8, 249, 277

risk, 7, 8, 35, 44, 48, 63, 76, 80, 85, 86, 89, 90, 92,
    95, 96, 97, 98, 107, 108, 110, 115, 131, 143, 144,
    145, 146, 147, 150, 151, 152, 153, 154, 155, 159,
    160, 161, 165, 169, 170, 176, 177, 179, 184, 188,
    201, 206, 207, 222, 245, 257, 266
risk assessment, 35
risk factors, 35, 44, 48, 76, 98, 160, 165, 170, 176,
    177, 206
risk profile, 207
risks, 38, 63, 151, 175, 212
Romania, 219
rotations, 281
routes, 148
rules, 4, 128, 131, 247, 248
rural areas, 13, 63, 68, 75, 254
rural population, 63, 74
Russia, 113, 219, 282

S

safety, 49, 75, 107, 108, 109, 119, 121, 125, 136,
    148, 151, 170, 171, 177, 184, 235, 238, 271
sample survey, 137
savings, 7, 38, 46, 64, 65, 87, 95, 97, 98, 107, 108,
    166, 170, 172, 192, 194, 198, 257
savings account, 257
scarce resources, 23
schema, 209, 210
school, 8, 207, 254, 257, 275
schooling, 171
science, 125, 136, 171, 257
scientific progress, ix
scoliosis, 267, 268, 272
scope, 150
security, 184, 189, 192, 214
sedative, 173
sedentary lifestyle, 159
seizure, 7
self-consciousness, 175
self-management behaviors, 162
self-monitoring, 175, 176
Senate, 26, 27, 46
senescence, 169
sensitivity, 52, 56, 62, 68, 70, 192, 215, 216
sepsis, 147
serum, 143, 145
service industries, 245
service provider, 220, 221
SES, 161
sex, 133, 206, 214, 215
short supply, 257
shortage, 22, 71, 117, 119, 124, 135, 187, 251, 252,
    253, 254, 255, 256, 257, 258
shortfall, 7, 119
shortness of breath, 168
showing, 121, 164, 187, 188
side effects, 159
signals, 257
signs, 114, 118, 152, 168, 172, 190
silver, 49
simulation, 52, 67, 69
Singapore, 110, 139, 188, 203
skimming, 248
skin, 222, 223
sleep apnea, 96, 141
smoking, 63, 141, 159
social care, 169
social coping, 34
social justice, 277
social security, 186, 261
social services, 163, 164
social stigmatization, 141
social structure, x, 276
social support, 163
social workers, 165
socialism, 247
socialization, 176
societal cost, 64, 161
society, 7, 8, 45, 70, 83, 166, 207, 210, 275
socioeconomic status, 161
software, 14, 70, 173
solidarity, 207
solution, 46, 71, 238, 241, 251
South Africa, 204
Southeast Asia, 11
Soviet Union, 9
Spain, 56, 58, 59, 194, 195, 205, 215, 218
specialisation, 189
specialists, 18, 22, 23, 164, 199, 237, 239
species, ix, 122
speech, 62
spending, 3, 83, 119, 138, 152, 158, 253
sphincter, 145
spinal cord, 100
spinal fusion, 111, 261, 267, 268
spinal stenosis, 267, 268, 270, 272
spine, 85, 88, 89, 90, 91, 92, 93, 95, 96, 97, 98, 100,
    107, 110, 111, 113, 114, 115, 259, 260, 261, 263,
    264, 265, 266, 267, 268, 269, 272, 281
spondylolisthesis, 270, 271, 272, 273
sputum, 223
stability, 4
stabilization, 21, 100, 267
staff members, 235
staffing, 20, 62, 122, 124, 137, 183, 185, 186, 189,
    191, 193, 202

stakeholders, 4, 13, 25, 26, 123
standard deviation, 65, 67, 103
standardization, 218, 260
state, ix, 13, 14, 15, 17, 18, 19, 24, 25, 38, 39, 44, 45, 46, 47, 50, 76, 87, 107, 114, 118, 121, 128, 143, 144, 167, 231, 234, 248, 250, 252, 255, 257
state intrusion, x
state of emergency, 76
states, 4, 13, 21, 23, 24, 30, 38, 47, 48, 107, 141, 152, 153, 155, 168, 212, 235
statistics, 9, 47, 48, 70, 155, 193, 202, 243
statutes, 238
stenosis, 268, 269, 270
stethoscope, 191
stockholders, 248
strategic planning, 237
stratification, 179
stress, 125, 136, 144, 162, 169, 171, 173, 212, 237, 245
stressors, 168
striatum, 178
stroke, 25, 29, 30, 34, 35, 37, 38, 39, 40, 41, 43, 44, 45, 46, 47, 48, 49, 51, 52, 53, 54, 55, 56, 57, 58, 59, 61, 62, 63, 64, 65, 67, 68, 70, 71, 72, 73, 74, 75, 76, 77, 78, 80, 81, 82, 141, 158, 188, 191
stroke symptoms, 45, 46, 63
structure, ix, 4, 14, 25, 46, 62, 84, 175, 239, 276
style, 177, 239
subacute, 73
subcategorization, 266
subsidy, 254
substance use, 178
substitutes, 254
suicidal ideation, 164, 178
supervision, 76, 171, 220
supervisor, 207
suppliers, 76, 251, 252
supply curve, 254, 255, 256
support staff, 234, 236
surgical intervention, 89, 90, 92, 114, 214, 267
surgical technique, 148
surplus, 17, 21, 236
surveillance, 35, 48, 143, 151, 155, 222
survival, 11, 12, 23, 52, 64, 70, 71, 81, 118, 151, 266
survival rate, 151, 266
survivors, 151
susceptibility, 223
sustainability, 26, 70
Sweden, 14, 56, 57, 58, 59, 183, 188, 189, 191, 194, 202, 269
swelling, 146
Switzerland, 280
sympathetic nervous system, 77

symptoms, 63, 114, 162, 163, 164, 167, 168, 171, 172, 175, 176, 184, 185, 188, 189, 221, 248
syndrome, 145, 151, 154, 164, 167
Syria, 282

T

takeover, 7
tangles, 168
Tanzania, 222, 230
target, 163, 169, 177, 207
target population, 207
tax increase, 245
taxation, 6, 237
taxes, 5, 186
taxpayers, 245
teachers, 275
team members, 130, 164
teams, 12, 53, 85, 95, 98, 129, 162, 164, 186, 239
techniques, 63, 151, 174, 175, 268
technological advances, 97
technological change, 119
technological developments, 97
technologies, ix, 45, 51, 109, 218, 234, 235, 260
technology, 4, 45, 49, 52, 64, 67, 119, 124, 230, 235, 245, 249, 252, 265
telephone, 75, 76, 147, 163, 169
tendon, 192
tension, 29, 30, 162, 234, 269
tensions, 235, 240
testing, 45, 143, 144, 152, 174, 179, 181, 191, 198, 204, 222, 223
textbook, 252
theatre, 126
therapeutic approaches, 180
therapeutic interventions, 84
therapeutic process, 174
therapist, 62
therapy, 30, 39, 48, 56, 63, 70, 73, 75, 80, 118, 123, 127, 128, 145, 166, 172, 174, 175, 184, 186, 187, 188, 191, 194, 198, 220, 221, 228, 230
threats, 163
thrombolytic therapy, 45, 52, 61, 65, 70, 71, 74, 76
thrombosis, 87, 120, 150, 155, 192
tissue, 45, 49, 53, 63, 71, 75, 76, 114, 192
tissue plasminogen activator, 45, 53, 71, 76
titanium, 268
tobacco, 3
Tort Law limitations, x
total costs, 18, 45, 132, 134, 201, 217, 221
total revenue, 67
tourism, 9
toys, 253

TPA, 48
tracks, 252
trade, 8
trainees, 255, 257
training, 3, 8, 11, 14, 25, 62, 97, 124, 129, 171, 173, 174, 175, 178, 179, 180, 182, 188, 252, 253, 254, 255, 256, 257, 258, 281
training programs, 11, 254, 255, 256
trajectory, 83
transformation, 63, 74, 83, 176
transfusion, 144, 155
transient ischemic attack, 29, 30, 75
translation, 210
transmission, 184
transparency, 119, 257
transplant, 117, 119, 120, 125, 126, 127, 129, 130, 131, 134, 137
transplantation, 118, 126, 127, 128, 129, 133, 134, 137, 138
transport, 12, 13, 23, 24, 25, 64, 118, 121, 184, 205, 210, 215, 221, 222
transport costs, 118, 215, 222
transportation, 45, 46, 214
trauma, 11, 12, 13, 14, 15, 16, 17, 18, 19, 20, 21, 22, 23, 24, 25, 26, 27, 37, 38, 39, 41, 42, 43, 44, 46, 47, 48, 49, 65, 76, 114, 191, 192, 203, 255, 260, 264
Trauma Care Systems Planning and Development Act, 38
traumatic brain injury, 38, 39, 171
trial, 2, 49, 63, 65, 72, 110, 172, 178, 181, 182, 203, 267, 268, 269, 271
tuberculosis, 219, 220, 221, 222, 224, 226, 227, 229, 230, 231
tumor, 255
turnover, 123, 126, 185, 202
type 2 diabetes, 141, 143, 145, 153

U

U.S. Bureau of Labor Statistics, 119, 138
UK, 56
Ukraine, 219
ulcer, 120, 132, 133
ultrasonography, 203
ultrasound, 144, 191, 192, 202
ultrastructure, 111
UN, 243
uncontaminated water, ix
underwriting, 246
undeveloped countries, ix
unhappiness, 250
uniform, 53, 62, 70, 206, 211

uninsured, 13, 16, 17, 18, 20, 21, 22, 24
United, ix, x, 3, 26, 27, 29, 37, 38, 47, 48, 49, 52, 57, 58, 59, 63, 64, 65, 67, 68, 71, 83, 84, 90, 106, 108, 141, 142, 143, 151, 158, 160, 165, 166, 175, 180, 226, 227, 233, 235, 243, 266, 267, 278, 281
United Kingdom, 57, 58, 59, 278
United States, ix, x, 3, 26, 27, 29, 37, 38, 47, 48, 49, 52, 58, 63, 64, 65, 67, 68, 71, 83, 84, 90, 106, 108, 141, 142, 143, 151, 158, 160, 165, 166, 175, 180, 226, 227, 233, 235, 243, 266, 267, 281
university education, 186
updating, 173, 178
urban, 26, 44, 64, 74, 155, 164, 183
urban population, 155
urbanization, 35, 183
urinalysis, 209
urinary tract, 120
urinary tract infection, 120
urine, 223
USA, 1, 11, 29, 37, 38, 51, 70, 77, 83, 89, 95, 97, 99, 113, 117, 141, 157, 221, 223, 233, 243, 251, 259, 261, 267, 275
uterine cancer, 142
uterine fibroids, 154
uterus, 248

V

vaccination rates, ix
vaccinations, 208
vaccine, 253
vacuum, 146
validation, 93, 169, 266
variable costs, 52, 67, 68, 69, 70
variables, 39, 70, 89, 100, 129, 131, 133, 171, 175, 206, 211, 212, 260, 264, 265
variations, 34, 99, 101, 105, 212, 268, 270
varus, 226
vehicles, 39, 41, 42
vein, 87, 120, 150, 155, 192
ventilation, 122
Vice President, 136
victims, 12, 13, 19, 24, 46, 47, 70
Vietnam, 11
vision, 152, 162, 168, 240
visualization, 148
volunteerism, 235
vulnerability, 175

W

wage level, 255

wages, 34, 38, 186, 245, 247, 255, 256, 257
war, 54, 57, 189, 193, 203, 276
Washington, 9, 26, 88, 99, 138, 182, 240
waste, 87, 175, 248
water, ix, 209
weakness, 114, 202, 212
wear, 1, 125, 185
web, 173, 255
web sites, 255
weight gain, 145, 153
welfare, 234, 275
well-being, 144, 168, 233, 240
wellness, 163
WHO, 229, 231
windows, 63
work environment, 53, 125, 126
workers, 4, 155, 210, 224, 236, 245, 247
workflow, 191
workforce, 6, 137, 155, 171, 251, 252, 254, 258

working hours, 191, 193
working memory, 170, 174
workload, 186, 193
workplace, 204
World Bank, 228
World Health Organization (WHO), 215, 219, 243, 250
World War I, 276
worldwide, ix, x, 9, 52, 65, 68, 70, 142, 146
wound infection, 86, 87, 122, 138, 146, 148

Y

Y-axis, 143
yes/no, 133
yield, 29, 30, 46, 108, 129, 134, 212
young people, 19